Hospital Management

Volume 1

- Hospital Management: An Introduction
- Introduction to Healthcare
- Continuous Quality Improvement in Hospitals
- Hospital Planning
- Overview on Hospital Operations Management
- Accountancy for Hospital Managers
- Information Technology in Healthcare

Other Volumes in the Series

Hospital Management — Volumes 2 and 3

1. Introduction to Materials Management in Hospitals — Dr Feroz Ikbal
2. Optimization of Hospital Services through OR Techniques — Mrs Girija
3. Introduction to Strategic Management in Hospitals — Dr Manisha Saxena
4. Introduction to Hospital Information Systems — Mr Murtuza Hussain Bakshi
5. Communication Skills For Healthcare Professionals — Ms Syeda Amtul Yafe
6. Legal Issues in Hospital Management — Dr Shazan M Khan
7. Management of Job Stress and Coping Mechanisms of Healthcare Professionals — Prof Suryanarayana
8. Corporate Social Responsibility in Hospitals — Dr Surekha
9. Introduction to Activity Based Costing in Hospital Services — Dr Parthasarthy
10. Management of Technology in Healthcare — Dr GVK Acharyulu
11. Entrepreneurship and Consultancy Management in Healthcare — Dr Sandhya Maliye
12. Introduction to Hospital Financial Management — Ms Rafath Mubeen
13. Introduction to Health Insurance — Dr Shazan M Khan
14. Management Support System in Hospitals — Mr Murtuza Hussabin Bakshi
15. Structure, Process, Outcome of Select Departments in a Hospital — Ms Syeda Amtul Yafe
16. Issues of Quality Management in Support Services in Hospitals — Mrs Sujatha
17. Marketing of Hospital Services for Rural Areas — Mr Girish Babu
18. Introduction to Health Economics — Dr Subodh Kandamuthan
19. Introduction to Marketing for Hospitals — Dr Chetan Srivastav
20. Accreditation for Hospitals — Dr Feroz Ikbal
21. Introduction to Cost Accounting for Hospitals — Mrs Ghousia
22. Introduction to Statistics for Hospital Management — Mrs Girija
23. Research Methods in Hospital Management — Dr Manisha Saxena
24. Legal Aspects Relating to Organ Transplantation — Mrs Lalitha Raghuram

Human Resource Management for Hospitals

1. Introduction to Hospital HR — Manisha Saxena
2. Human Resource Policy
3. Planning and Designing of Hospital HR
4. Acquisition of Hospital HR
5. Training and Development of Hospital HR
6. Motivating Hospital HR
7. Compensation Plan for Hospital HR
8. Internal Mobility of Hospital HR
9. Human Resource Information System (HRIS) for Hospitals
10. Counseling services for Hospital HR
11. Disputes and Grievance Settlement for Hospital HR
12. Dynamics of Human Relations in Hospital HR
13. Safety and Welfare Services for Hospital HR
14. Quality Circles in Hospitals
15. Hospital HR Audit
16. Hospital HR in Mergers and Acquisitions
17. Ethical Issues in Hospital HR
18. Challenges of Hospital HR
19. Competency Mapping
20. Performance Appraisal for Hospital HR
21. Case Studies

Hospital Management

Volume 1

EDITOR

MANISHA SAXENA MA, MBA, PhD
Professor and Principal
Department of Hospital Management
Deccan School of Management
Hyderabad

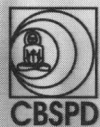

CBS Publishers & Distributors Pvt Ltd
New Delhi • Bengaluru • Chennai • Kochi • Kolkata • Lucknow • Mumbai
Hyderabad • Jharkhand • Nagpur • Patna • Pune • Uttarakhand

Disclaimer

Science and technology are constantly changing fields. New research and experience broaden the scope of information and knowledge. The editor and the contributors have tried their best in giving information available to them while preparing the material for this book. Although, all efforts have been made to ensure optimum accuracy of the material, yet it is quite possible some errors might have been left uncorrected. The contributors, the editor, the publisher, or the printer will not be held responsible for any inadvertent errors, omissions or inaccuracies.

Hospital Management
Volume 1

ISBN: 978-81-239-2301-7

Copyright © Editor and Publisher

First Edition: 2013
 Reprint: 2015, 2019, 2022, 2024

All rights reserved. No part of this book may be reproduced or transmitted in any form or by any means, electronic or mechanical, including photocopying, recording, or any information storage and retrieval system without permission, in writing, from the author and the publisher.

Published by Satish Kumar Jain and Produced by Varun Jain for
CBS Publishers & Distributors Pvt Ltd
4819/XI Prahlad Street, 24 Ansari Road, Daryaganj, New Delhi 110 002, India
Ph: 011-23289259, 23266861 Website: www.cbspd.com
e-mail: delhi@cbspd.com

Corporate Office: 204 FIE, Industrial Area, Patparganj, Delhi 110 092
Ph: 011-4934 4934 Fax: 011-4934 4935 e-mail: publishing@cbspd.com; publicity@cbspd.com

Branches

- **Bengaluru:** Seema House 2975, 17th Cross, K.R. Road, Banasankari 2nd Stage, Bengaluru 560 070, Karnataka, India
  Ph: +91-80-26771678/79 Fax: +91-80-26771680 e-mail: bangalore@cbspd.com
- **Chennai:** 7, Subbaraya Street, Shenoy Nagar, Chennai 600 030, Tamil Nadu, India
  Ph: +91-44-26680620, 26681266 Fax: +91-44-42032115 e-mail: chennai@cbspd.com
- **Kochi:** 42/1325, 1326, Power House Road, Opp KSEB, Power House, Ernakulam 682 018, Kerala, India
  Ph: +91-484-4059061-65 Fax: +91-484-4059065 e-mail: kochi@cbspd.com
- **Kolkata:** 147, Hind Ceramics Compound, 1st Floor, Nilgunj Road, Belghoria, Kolkata-700056, West Bengal, India
  Ph: 033-25633055, 033-25633056 e-mail: kolkata@cbspd.com
- **Lucknow:** Basement, Khushnuma Complex, 7-Meerabai Marg (Behind Jawahar Bhawan), Lucknow 226001, India
  Ph: 0522-4000032 e-mail: tiwari.lucknow@cbspd.com
- **Mumbai:** PWD Shed. Gala no. 25/26, Ramchandra Bhatt Marg, Next to JJ Hospital Gate no. 2, Opp. Union Bank of India Noorbaug Mumbai-400009, Maharashtra, India
  Ph: 022-66661880/89 e-mail: mumbai@cbspd.com

Representatives

- **Hyderabad** 0-9885175004
- **Patna** 0-9334159340
- **Jharkhand** 0-9811541605
- **Pune** 0-9664372571
- **Nagpur** 0-8692091830
- **Uttarakhand** 0-9716462459

Printed at Mudrak, Noida, UP, India

to

my mother

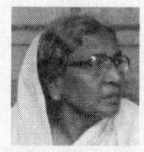

Smt. Vasundhara Saxena
whose blessings, love and affection
always inspire me in all my assignments

Contributors

Manisha Saxena
is Principal, Department of Hospital Management, Deccan School of Management, Hyderabad, which is affiliated to Osmania University. She obtained her BSW from PG College of Social Work, Hyderabad, and MA, MPhil and PhD from School of Social Sciences, University of Hyderabad. She is a postgraduate in management (MBA) and an accredited management teacher of AIMA. She has worked with the Regional Training Centre of Family Planning Association of India and Sivananda Rehabilitation Home for destitute leprosy patients. She has been associated with Department of Hospital Management, Deccan School of Management, since 1999.

Pavan Kumar
is Assistant Professor, Community Medicine, Department of Social and Preventive Medicine, Deccan College of Medical Sciences, Hyderabad. He obtained his MBBS from Al-Ameen Medical College, Bijapur, and MD from BJ Medical College, Pune, and Postgraduate Diploma in Hospital and Healthcare Management from Symbiosis, Pune.

Feroz Ikbal
is Associate Professor, Department of Hospital Management, Deccan School of Management. He took his MHA from Mahatma Gandhi University, Kottayam, Kerala, and PhD from Faculty of Management, Osmania University. He has been associated with Department of Hospital Management since 2001.

Syeda Amtul Yafe
is Associate Professor and Head, Department of Hospital Management, Deccan School of Management, Hyderabad. She holds BPharm from Jawaharlal Nehru Technological University, Hyderabad, and MHM from Osmania University. She completed her MPhil and is pursuing PhD in the area of human resource management from Osmania University.

V.R. Girija
is Assistant Professor, Department of Hospital Management, Deccan School of Management. She holds an MPhil in hospital and health systems management from BITS-Pilani and completed her Master's in Hospital Management from Deccan School of Management. She is enrolled with Osmania University for her PhD program in the area of Operations Management. She has been working with DSHM since 2007.

Ghousia
is a faculty member at Millennium Institute of Management, Aurangabad. She had earlier worked as Associate Professor and Head at DSHM. She has to her credit MBA from Osmania University, MPhil from SV University, Tirupathi, and is currently doing PhD in management.

GVRK Acharynlu
is course co-ordinator for MBA (hospital and healthcare management) at School of Management Studies, University of Hyderabad, with which he has been associated since 2007. He holds a PhD in supply chain management from Osmania University. He obtained his MBA from Osmania University and MTech from REC, Warangal. He taught at Apollo Institute of Hospital Administration and has 10 years of industrial experience.

Foreword

Hospitals have become complex organizations having adopted various managerial practices, be it the process of planning or infrastructure management or day-to-day operations. Hospital management has thus become a full-fledged academic discipline attracting students from varied backgrounds.

Hospital management as an academic discipline has grown as an offshoot of general management and contextualizes it from the perspective of the hospital. Though hospital as an organization is quite unique from that of the other services, it necessitates a different school of thought in its management. The very unique nature of its customers, both internal and external, makes the academic discipline of hospital management challenging for the academicians and students.

The academic programme of hospital management has been offered in the Indian universities since the late eighties, but there are very few textbooks from the Indian perspective which focus only on basic hospital planning and medical administration.

Hospital management has evolved as a specialization management rather than that of medicine as was envisaged earlier. Hospitals are increasingly applying modern management concepts like balanced score card to that of economic value addition.

This book, edited by Dr Manisha Saxena, will be a very useful reference book for academicians, practising managers and students of hospital management as it fills the caveat for a holistic book on hospital management covering the various perspectives like hospital planning, operations, IT, and quality, besides the basic introduction to hospital management. I am sure that all the stakeholders in the healthcare and hospital management sector will immensely benefit from the book.

I congratulate the author for her painstaking effort to compile and edit the articles in a lucid manner and hope that some more emerging issues would be covered from time to time.

Prof. V Venkata Ramana MBA, PhD
Dean
School of Management Studies
Prof. CR Rao Road, Gachibowli, Hyderabad 500 046
AP, India
Off : +91-40-2313 5000 ; Telefax: +91-40-2301 1091
E-mail: deanms@ernet.in
www.uohyd.ernet.in

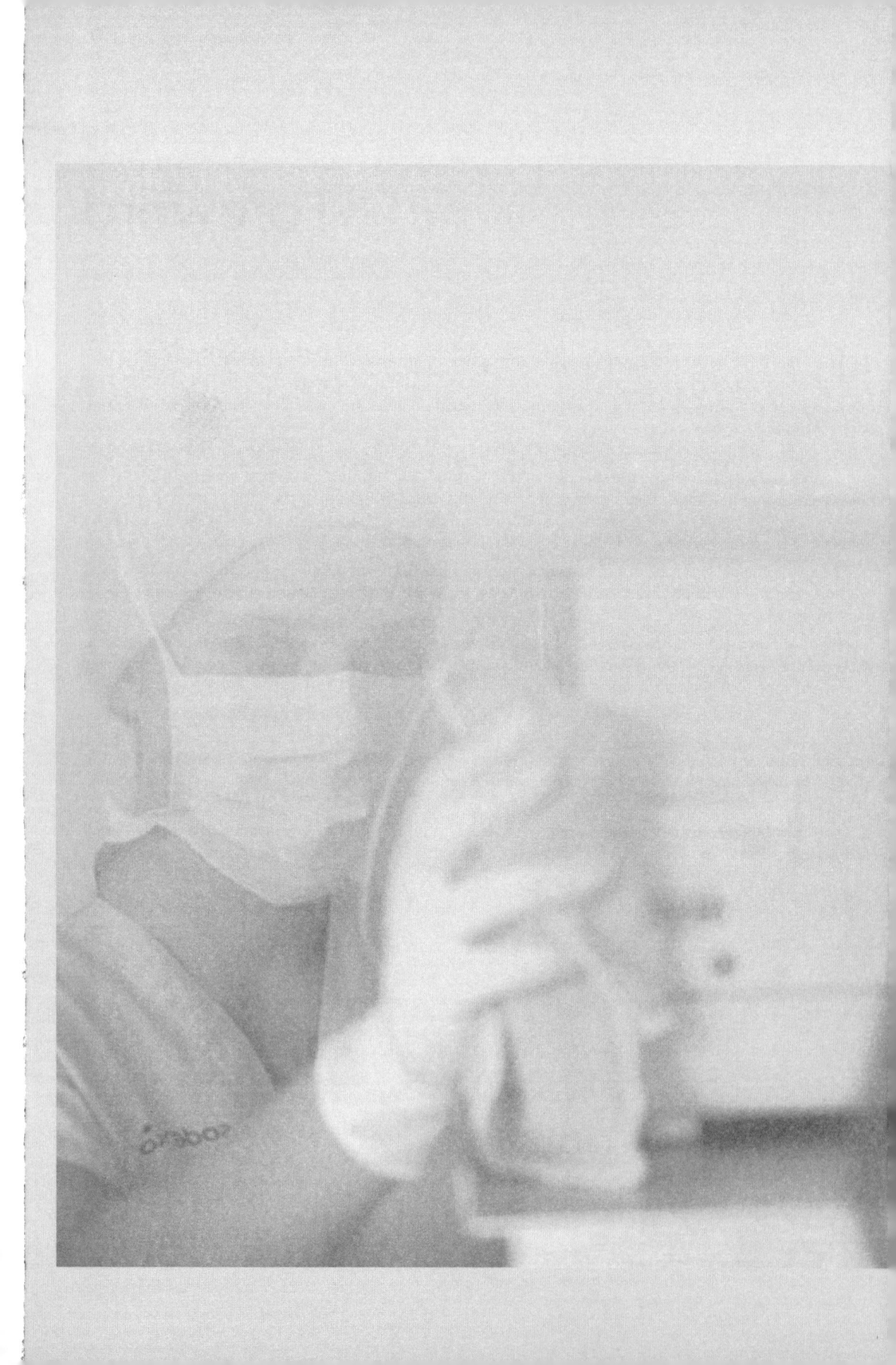

Preface

Last few years have seen the rise of hospital management as a distinct field of management in India. This is particularly due to arrival of new generation corporate hospitals. On the other side, governments both at the centre and the states is increasingly investing in hospitals from primary healthcare centers to teaching hospitals. Many hospitals in the voluntary sector are restructuring themselves to meet the realms of competition.

Hospital Management as a career is becoming highly lucrative. Earlier, the managerial positions were virtually the monopoly of medical professionals. But today, hospital management graduates are increasingly taking top managerial positions. Hospital management as a branch of management science is quite different from the management of other services and manufacturing organizations. There have been a very few textbooks pertaining to the core issues of hospital management. Many a times students of hospital management rely on conventional management books.

This book is intended to look into the select dimensions of hospital management with a holistic perspective. The authors are academicians with long standing experience in teaching and research at postgraduate level.

I hope this book will be of use to students of hospital management, healthcare management, nursing graduates, owners of nursing homes, practising hospital managers, and all those who are interested in the working of hospitals.

Authors do not claim that this book is completely original. Materials have been incorporated from various sources such as books, journals, monographs, etc. In the process there may have been some unintentional mistakes. I take full responsibility for them.

Manisha Saxena

Acknowledgements

I am deeply grateful to Darussalam Educational Trust (DET) for the resources and facilities provided to Department of Hospital Management (DHM), Deccan School of Management. Janab Assaduddin Owaisi, MP, Chairman, DET, has always encouraged the academic pursuits of our college.

I express my sincere thanks to Janab Akberuddin Owaisi, MLA and Managing Director, Deccan College of Medical Sciences and Allied Institutions, for the dynamic leadership provided by him to all the endeavors of DHM.

I am thankful to all the contributors for having spared their precious time and effort for the respective chapters.

I am thankful to the publishers, CBS Publishers & Distributors, for the meticulous work they have done.

Manisha Saxena

Contents

Contributors vi
Foreword by Prof. V Venkata Ramana vii
Preface ix

1. **HOSPITAL MANAGEMENT**
   An Introduction 1
   Definitions of Management 1
   Hospital Management 2
   Hospital as an Organization 4
   Scientific Management 5
   Management by Objectives 10
   Management Functions 12
   Ethical Issues in Hospital Management 33

2. **INTRODUCTION TO HEALTHCARE** 38
   Evidence-based Care 42
   Management Functions in Managed Care 43
   Negotiating 46
   Managing Doctors 51
   Managing Care in Hospitals 56

3. **CONTINUOUS QUALITY IMPROVEMENT IN HOSPITALS** 64
   Introduction 64
   Dimensions of Quality 64
   Concept of Quality in Healthcare 65
   Core Concepts of TQM 66
   Cost of Quality 66
   Seven Basic Tools of Quality Control 67
   Pareto Chart 69
   Control Charts 70
   Business Process Re-engineering 72
   Benchmarking 74

4. **HOSPITAL PLANNING** 77
   Major Functions of a Hospital 77
   The Changing Role of Hospitals 77
   The Changing Scene in the Hospital Field 77
   Concept of Green Building 78
   Hospital Utilisation Indices 80
   Indices Relating to the Hospital 80
   Hospital Planning Team 81
   Assessment of the Extent of Need for the Hospital Services 82
   Choosing a Site 84
   Master Plan in its Totality 84
   Distances, Compactness, Parking, Landscaping and Visual Impact 86
   Zonal Distribution and Interrelationships of Department 87
   Gross Space Requirements 88
   Climatic Consideration in Design 88
   Preparation of the Functional Brief or Architectural Brief 89
   Equipping a Hospital 92
   Construction and Commissioning 93
   General Considerations for Planning and Designing Hospital 94
   Outpatient Services 96
   Nursing Unit or Inpatient Unit 98
   Specifications 99
   Labor and Delivery Suites 101
   Accident and Emergency Department 102
   Operating Unit/Operation Theater 105
   Design Parameters 106
   Zoning 108
   Supply Air 109
   Intensive Care Unit 111
   Day Care Services 113
   Laboratory Services 114
   Blood Bank 116
   Cafeteria Unit 118
   Housekeeping and Waste Management 119

Linen and Laundry Services 122
Medical Imaging Services 124
X-ray Room 125
CT Scanning (Computerised Tomography) 127
MRI (Magnetic Resonance Imaging) 127
Angiography 128
Pet Room 128
Cyclotron 129
Central Sterile Supply Department 129
Heating Ventilation and Air Conditioning 131
Cardiac Catheterization Laboratory 135
Medical Gases 136
Space Requirements 141
Space Requirements 142
Mortuary Services 142
Space Requirements 144

5. OVERVIEW ON HOSPITAL OPERATIONS MANAGEMENT 148

Systems Concept in Operations Management 148
Brief History of Operations Management 148
Application of Computer and Advanced Operations Technology 150
Operations Strategy 152
Generic Corporate Strategy 153
Productivity and Work Measurement 161
The Power of Productivity Standards 163
Learning Curves 166
Safety and Health 166
Scope and Types of Incentive Schemes 167
Ergonomics 168
Work Study 175
Method Study 176
Chronological Sequence Analysis 176
Work Measurement 178
Value Engineering 180
Value Engineering Process 181

6. ACCOUNTANCY FOR HOSPITAL MANAGERS 148

An Introduction to Accountancy 183

7. INFORMATION TECHNOLOGY IN HEALTHCARE 210

Introduction 210
Healthcare Information Technology (HIT) 212
Components of HIT 213
Use of HIT 214
Electronic Health Record (EHR) 214
Technology in Healthcare 216
Quality and Health Information Technology 218
Telemedicine 219
Hospital Information System (HIS) 220
Organization and Information 222
Need for Hospital Information System (HIS) 225
Functional Model of a Hospital Information System 225
Applicability of Computers in Different Areas of Hospital 228
Benefits of Hospital Information Systems 228
Application of HIS 230
Radio Frequency Identification (RFID) 231
E-health 234
Latest Trends in Healthcare IT 236
The Legal Aspect of Health Informatics 236
The Future Health Information Systems 236

Bibliography 237

Index 239

Hospital Management
An Introduction

Manisha Saxena

The word 'manage' is derived from Italian word 'maneggiare' meaning to handle. This in turn was derived from Latin word 'manus' which means hand. The French word 'mesngement' helped in the development of English word 'management' during the 17th and 18th centuries.

Management is one of the most important activities of all human beings. It consists of deciding what, when, and how to do things, how to mobilize human and other resources.

DEFINITIONS OF MANAGEMENT

Management has been defined in many ways by many authorities, but the original definition by Henri Fayol is considered being the father of modern management, over seventy years ago still holds good. Fayol, in his famous book, *Administration Industrielle et Generale*, which was published in 1916, stated that:

"To manage is to forecast and plan, to organize, to command, to coordinate and to control".

Management is the accomplishment of results through the efforts of other people.
–Lawrence A. Appley

Management is the art of getting things done through and with the people in formally organized groups. –Koontz H.

Management is a process of planning organizing, actuating and controlling to determine and accomplish the objectives by the use of people and resources.
–Terry G.

Management is the process by which managers create, direct, maintain and operate purposive organizations through systematic, coordinated, cooperative human effort.
–McFarland

It is the coordination of all resources through the process of planning, organizing, directing and controlling in order to attain stated objectives. –Sisk

Management has also been defined as a decision-making, rule-making and rule-enforcing body. According to Professor Moore, management means decision-making. Appley called it personnel administration. For the sake of simplicity and convenience, we can broadly define the term thus: management is concerned with resources, tasks and goals. It is the process of planning, organizing, staffing, directing and controlling to accomplish organizational objectives through the coordinated use of human and material resources.

Scope of Management

The scope of management is quite broad and far-reaching. Management functions and principles are universal. They apply to all areas of human activities, though the techniques and procedures of their application may differ. It is important for hospital organizations as well as other service organizations dealing with education, social services, sport and crisis management. So good and professional management is essential for all the fields of human activity, such as industrial organization or government department, and hospitals are no exception. They also need good management for effective performance.

Administration vs Management

The two words have been often used synonymously. To many, administration is a higher and broader function than management. Management is considered as an art and science of development of knowledge, attitudes, skills and practices. There are three different approaches:
1. Administration is above management
2. Administration is a part of management
3. Administration and management are the same.

HOSPITAL MANAGEMENT

Hospital management has developed and grown in leaps and bounds from a nearly insignificant topic to one of the integral ones of our economy. Hospital management has evolved into a powerful and innovative force on which our healthcare organizations depends for all-round support.

"The hospital is an integrated part of a medical and social organization, the function of which is to provide for the population complete healthcare, both curative and preventive, and whose outpatient services reach out to the family and its home environment, the hospital is also a center for the training of health workers and bio-social research." (WHO, 1957).

"Medical care is a programme of services that should make available to the individual, and thereby to the community all facilities of medical and allied services necessary to promote and maintain health of mind and body. This programme should take into account the physical, social and family environment, with a view to the prevention of disease, the restoration of health and the alleviation of disability." (WHO 1959)

Patient care: The services rendered by members of the health profession and non-professionals under their supervision for the benefit of the patient. (From Dorland, 28th ed., p. 269). Nursing care is only one type of patient care. Patient care aims at patient-satisfaction and aspires for patient-delight.

Growing Significance of Management in Organizations

"Companies fail when they become complacent and imagine that they will always be successful. So we are always challenging ourselves. Even the most successful companies must constantly reinvent themselves."
–Bill Gates

Factors Contributing to Increased Significance of Management in Hospitals

1. *It helps in achieving hospital goals:* It organizes the resources, integrates the resources in effective manner to achieve organizational goals. It directs group efforts towards achievement of predetermined goals. By defining objective of organization clearly there would be no wastage of time, money and effort. Management converts disorganized resources of men, machines, money, etc. into useful enterprise. These resources are coordinated, directed and controlled in such a manner that enterprise work towards attainment of goals. The goals of a hospital can be increased bed-occupancy, increase in revenue, adding existing bed capacity, adding new technology such as PET scan, Robotic surgery, etc.

2. *Optimum utilization of hospital resources:* Management utilizes all the physical and human resources productively. This leads to efficacy in management. Management provides maximum utilization of scarce resources by selecting its best possible alternate. It makes use of experts, professionals and these services lead to use of their skills, knowledge, and proper utilization and avoids wastage. Hospitals have resources in the form of manpower, materials, machine, money and minute (time). Human resource is a scarce commodity in hospitals. Most of the hospitals find severe

shortage of nurses and doctors. Scheduling the duty of nurses, getting the prime time of consultants is an important issue in the utilization of human resources. Most of the hospitals have infrastructure like OT, ICUs, Cath-Lab, which are highly capital-intensive resources. Professional management will help in the effective utilization.

3. *Reduces costs:* It gets maximum results through minimum input by proper planning and by using minimum input and getting maximum output. Management uses physical, human and financial resources in such a manner which results in best combination. This helps in cost reduction. Cost reduction in hospitals can be done by reducing the average length of stay, better negotiation with the supplier, multiskilling and multitasking.

4. *Establishes sound organization:* There is no overlapping of efforts. To establish sound organizational structure is one of the objectives of management which is in tune with objective of organization and for fulfillment of this, it establishes effective authority and responsibility relationship, i.e. who is accountable to whom, who can give instructions to whom, who are superiors and who are subordinates. Management fills up various positions with right persons, having right skills, training and qualification. All jobs should be cleared to everyone. Most of the hospitals have matrix structure, which makes several employees to report to two supervisors.

5. *Establishes equilibrium:* It enables the organization to survive in changing environment. It keeps in touch with the changing environment. If the change is external environment, the initial coordination of organization must be changed. So it adapts organization to changing demand of market/changing needs of societies. It is responsible for growth and survival of organization. Today hospital as an industry, as well service is fast changing. There is an increase in awareness regarding quality in hospital services. Many of the hospitals are going for accreditation programs like JCI and NABH.

6. *Essentials for prosperity of society:* Efficient management leads to better economical production which helps in turn to increase the welfare of people. Good management makes a difficult task easier by avoiding wastage of scarce resource. It improves standard of living. It increases the profit which is beneficial to business and society will get maximum output at minimum cost by creating employment opportunities which generate income in hands. Organization comes with new products and researches beneficial for society. The major objective of hospital is to restore the members of the society. "Health is wealth" — only the society where the members are healthy, economic growth and prosperity will occur.

Unique Features of Hospital Management

1. Hospital management covers a large number of activities and fulfils different functions.
2. The service of the hospital is focused on the individual, rendered by professionals from the medical, nursing and other specialized backgrounds. Thus hospital management requires a great deal of tact and ingenuity.
3. Hospital service is unique as no two situations are similar.
4. The dual control by way of professional authority and the executive authority in the hospital leads to conflict, which every hospital administrator has to face.
5. Hospital has to be highly responsive to the health needs and expectations of the community.
6. There is a great concern for clarity and responsibility. The cost of making mistake inpatient care is likely to be very high with serious life and legal consequences.
7. Hospital service requires extensive coordination of efforts, resources and demands.

8. The hospital does not have single line of authority unlike other formal organizations. Thus many employees are subject to more than one line of authority.
9. The hospital generates many types of waste and disposing it is a challenging task.
10. Hospital's work being urgent in nature and cannot be postponed or interrupted, work goes on for 24 × 7 × 30 × 365 – days.

Characteristics of a Modern Hospital

1. Modern hospitals have rapidly grown in response to the increasing population.
2. Modern hospitals are more specialized hospitals rather than general hospitals.
3. Modern hospitals are dominated by consumers rather than providers.
4. Today the hospitals are placing more emphasis on quality aspects and are racing for various kinds of accreditations such as JCI, NABH, etc.
5. Because of rapid advances in science and technology modern hospitals have latest equipment and superior diagnostic and therapeutic tools. Technology is given more importance than human values.
6. Modern hospitals are managed by trained and qualified hospital managers.
7. Modern hospitals are capital intensive.
8. As modern hospitals have world class facilities and services, necessary accreditations and approvals, they attract overseas patients.
9. Due to increasing population there is tremendous growth in number of hospitals. Thus the competitiveness is growing in healthcare industry.
10. Modern hospitals are catering to patients who pay out of pocket, insurance patients and credit patients, etc.

HOSPITAL AS AN ORGANIZATION

The word 'organization' is derived from Greek word *'organon'* meaning tool.

A hospital organization is a social arrangement in which a number of people pursue collective goal of health for all by way of division of labor and function through a hierarchy, which controls its own performance to ensure health and well being.

A hospital organization is a **group of people** working together in a **structured situation** to accomplish a medical or health-related goals. Hospital organizations can range in size. There are many types of hospital organizations: teaching hospitals, corporate hospitals, public hospitals, etc.

Table 1.1: Evolution of management thought

Period	Regions	Management approach
3000–2400 BC	Sumerians	Development of written records; one of the oldest written law by Akkadian rule, Ur-Nammu
3000–1000 BC	Egyptians	Pioneered in national government, full civilization, buildings and roads and other infrastructure: Full planning involved
2700–500 BC	Babylonian	Oldest and complete set of rules by Hammurabi, an Amorite ruler
1000–200 BC	Greeks	Functional local government, democracy and government
800 BC–500 AD	Roman	Roman Republic with Senate and councils
1500 BC–1300 AD	Chinese	Good government, cultural empowerment, flourishing science and arts
450–1500 AD	Venetians	Laws related to commerce, highly dominant commerce through area

Hospital organizations have major subsystems, such as departments, programs, divisions, or teams. Each of these subsystems has a way of doing things, along with other subsystems; achieve the overall goals of the organization.

Evolution of management thought: Management has evolved through experience and research for a long time. Different regions on the globe evolved different approaches to handle situations (Table 1.1).

This evolution of management thought can be studied in the following broad stages:

A. The classical theory of management (classical approach): It includes the following three streams of thought:
  i. Bureaucracy
  ii. Scientific management
  iii. Administrative management
B. The neoclassical theory of management: It includes the following two streams:
  i. Human relations approach
  ii. Behavioral sciences approach
C. The modern theory of management: It includes the following three streams of thought:
  i. Quantitative approach to management (Operations research)
  ii. Systems approach to management and
  iii. Contingency approach to management

It is rather difficult to state the exact period of each stage in the evolution of management thought. Experts, in general, agree with the following period for each thought/school.
a. Classical school/thought: 1900 to 1930
b. Neoclassical school/thought: 1930 to 1960
c. Modern school/thought: 1960 onwards

SCIENTIFIC MANAGEMENT

Frederick Winslow Taylor (1856–1915) is the father of scientific management. He exerted great influence on the development of management thought through his experiments and writings. During a career spanning over 26 years, he arranged a series of experiments in three companies: Midvale Steel, Simonds Rolling Machine and Bethlehem Steel.

- *Time and motion study:* Since Taylor had been an operator himself; he knew how piecework workers used to hold back production to one-third its level. The workers feared that their employers would cut their piece rate as soon as there was a rise in production. The real trouble, Taylor thought, was that no one knew how much work was reasonable for a man to do. Therefore, he established the time and motion study, where every job motion was supposed to be timed by using a stopwatch and shorter and fewer motions. Thus, the best way of keeping an account of work performance was found. This had replaced the old rule-of-thumb-knowledge of the worker.

- *Differential payment:* Taylor had founded the differential piecework system and the related incentives with production. Under this plan, a worker received a low piece rate if he produced the standard number of pieces and a high rate if he surpassed the standard. Taylor also comprehended that the attraction of a new high piece rate would encourage the workers to increase production.

- *Drastic reorganization of supervision:* Taylor developed two new concepts: i. Division of planning and doing and ii. Functional foremanship. In those days, it was customary for each worker to plan his own work. The worker himself used to select his tools and decide the sequence of performance of operations. The foreman essentially told the worker what jobs were to be performed, not how they were to be performed. Taylor suggested that the work should be designed by a foreman and not by the worker. He stated that there were distinctive functions involved in doing any kind of job and that each of the foremen should give orders to the worker in his specialized field.

- *Scientific recruitment and training:* Taylor also gave importance to the scientific selection and development of the worker. He said that the management should develop and train every worker in order to bring out his best output and to enable him to perform a superior, more interesting and profitable class of work than he has done in the past.
- *Intimate and friendly cooperation between the management and workers:* Taylor said that, "a complete mental revolution" on the part of management and labor was necessary to make the organization successful. Rather than argue over profits, they should both try to increase production. Consequently, profits will also increase manifold, which will leave no room for further disagreements. Taylor realized that both the management and labor had a common interest in maximizing production.

Henry Fayol: While Taylor is considered the father of scientific management, Henri Fayol (1841–1925) is considered as the father of the administrative management theory, with a focus on the development of broad administrative principles applicable to general and higher managerial levels. Fayol was a French mining engineer-turned-leading industrialist and successful manager. In 1916, he authored a book in French titled General and Industrialist Administration.

Fayol opined that all actions of business enterprises could be divided into six groups: technical, commercial, financial, accounting, security and administrative or managerial.

Fayol's primary focus was on this last managerial activity because he felt that managerial skills had been the most neglected aspect of business operations. He explained management in terms of five functions: planning, organizing, commanding, coordinating and controlling.

Fayol's 14 principles of management are as under:

1. *Division of work:* Division of work aims at producing more and better work with the same effort. It is accomplished through reduction in the number of tasks to which attention and effort must be directed.
2. *Authority and responsibility:* Authority means the right to give orders. Responsibility is associated with authority. Whenever authority is exercised, responsibility arises simultaneously.
3. *Discipline:* Discipline means following rules, obedience and respect for the agreements between the first and its employees. Discipline also involves sanctions judiciously applied in the organization.
4. *Unity of command:* Employee should receive orders from one superior only.
5. *Unity of direction:* Each group of activities should have one objective and should be unified by having one plan and one head.
6. *Subordination of individual interest to general interest:* The interest of one employee or group of employees should not take precedence over that of the company or broader organization.
7. *Remuneration:* To maintain the loyalty and support of workers, all employees must receive a fair wage for services rendered in the organizations.
8. *Scalar chain:* The scalar chain is the chain from top management ranging from the ultimate authority to the lowest ranks. Communication follows this chain (Fig. 1.1).

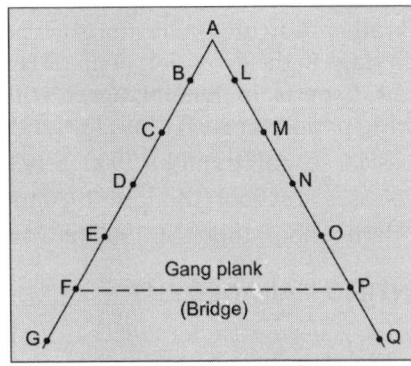

Fig. 1.1: Scalar chain

9. *Order:* Everything should be in right place at right time.

10. *Stability of tenure of personnel:* High turnover increases inefficiency. A manager who stays for long is always preferred.
11. *Centralization:* Centralization is the degree to which subordinates are involved in the decision-making. It belongs to the natural order of things. Proper proportion of centralization is needed for each situation.
12. *Equity:* It is the kindness and fairness to subordinates.
13. *Initiative:* This means allowing originating and carrying out plans to ensure its success.
14. *Espirit de corps:* This means team spirit, harmony and unity within the organization.

Concept of Bureaucracy

The concept of bureaucracy was put forwarded by German Sociologist Max Weber.

Bureaucracy is an administrative system characterized by continuous organization of official functions bound by rules, hierarchy, formalization and competent personnel.

Features of Bureaucracy

- They are selected on the basis of merit.
- Their tenure of service is determined by the rules and regulations of the organization.
- Bureaucrats have interest in the organization to the extent of their careers.
- Usually more than merit, seniority is considered for promotion.
- Compensation is given in the form of salary, which is not measured in terms of work.

Characteristics of Bureaucracy

- Administrative hierarchy
- Division of work
- Impersonal relationship
- Official rules and records
- Formal organization

Many government hospitals have bureaucratic form of functioning.

Human Relations Approach to Management

The Hawthorne plant of Western Electric in Cicero, Illinois, US was studied in 1924. Issues related to physical illumination and worker efficiency were the focus. Elton Mayo from Harvard University analyzed and reviewed the observation. Behavioral science and human relation thinking started the new management movement. Psychological factors and human needs were considered as the issues that determined why people worked. The issues related to social factors and informal group were given due importance in management.

Some Results

1. Whenever changes in working conditions were made, both good and bad, output increased.
2. In every department, the supervisor played a different role.
3. A number of employees expressed a dislike for close, coordinated supervision.

Features of Human Relations Approach

1. A business organization is not merely a technoeconomic system but also a social system and involves human element.
2. An individual employee is motivated not merely by economic incentives but also by noneconomic incentives, psychological and social interests, needs and aspirations.
3. The informal groups in the organization are more important than individuals and play an important role in raising productivity.
4. In place of task-centered leadership, the employee-centered, humanistic, democratic and participative style of leadership should be introduced as it is more effective/productive.
5. Employees are not necessarily inefficient or negative in their approach. They are capable of self-direction and control.

6. Employees performance can be raised by meeting their social and psychological needs. Cordial atmosphere at workplace is also useful for raising productivity.
7. Management needs social skills along with technical skills in order to create a feeling (among the employees) that they are a part and parcel of the organization and not outsiders.
8. Employees need respect and positive feeling from the management. For this, employees should be encouraged to participate and communicate freely their views and suggestions in the concerned areas of decision making.
9. The management has to secure willing cooperation of employees. The objective before the management should be to secure cooperative effort of its employees. For this, employees should be made happy and satisfied.

Human relations approach is a progressive development as compared to classical approach. Here, productivity is not treated merely as an engineering problem. Cooperation of employees, team spirit and their satisfaction are treated as factors useful for raising productivity. The human relations approach has put special stress on social needs and the role of management in meeting such needs.

Limitations of Human Relations Approach

1. Too much importance to employees, and social needs.
2. Employee-oriented approach to a limited extent.
3. Faulty assumption in the theory: The human relations approach is based on a wrong assumption that satisfied workers are more productive.
4. Limited importance to economic incentives.

Behavioral Approach towards Management

Behavioral approach considered understanding of human behavior vital in the professional management. The major contributions are in the areas of motivation, leadership, communication, organizational conflict, organizational change and development, group dynamics, etc. Among the prominent contributors were Maslow, Herzberg, McGregor, Blake and Mouton Bake. The major conclusions of behavioral approach are as follows:

- Job itself is a source of motivation and satisfaction to the employees.
- Most people can exercise a great deal of self-direction, self control, and creativity in their current job.
- The managers' basic job is to use the untapped human potential in the service of organization.
- The organization should provide healthy, safe, comfortable and convenient place to work.
- Employee participation.
- Job satisfaction may improve as by-product of subordinates making full use of potential.

Systems Theory of Organization

The systems approach helps in obtaining an integrated approach to management problems.

Some important contributors of the systems approach are Chester Barnard, George Homans, Philip Selznick and Herbert Simon. The following are the key concepts of this approach:

A system is a set of interdependent parts, which together form a unitary whole that performs some function. An organization is also a system composed of four interdependent parts, namely task, structure, people and technology. A system can be either open or closed. A system is considered open, if it interacts with its environment. All biological, human and social systems are open systems because they constantly intermingle with their environments. A system is considered closed if it does not interact with the environment. Physical and mechanical systems are closed systems because they are insulated from their external environment. Traditional organization theorists regarded organizations as closed systems while, according to the modern view, organizations are open systems, constantly interacting with their environments.

Each system, including an organization, has its own boundaries, which separate it from other systems in the environment. The boundaries for open systems are however, 'permeable' or 'penetrable', unlike those of the closed systems. They are quite flexible and adjustable, depending upon their activities. The confines for closed systems are rigid. The function of management is to act as a boundary-linking pin among the various subsystems within the organizational system, on the one hand and between the organization and the external environmental system, on the other. In the context of a hospital organization, it has many boundary contacts or 'interfaces' with many external systems like patients, suppliers, creditors, regulatory bodies, government agencies, etc.

Every system has flows of information, material and energy. These enter the system from the environment as inputs and exit the system as outputs. The inputs of a service organization are raw human effort, equipment, technology and information. The organization converts these inputs into outputs of services and satisfactions. This process of change is known as 'throughput'. It should be remembered that the output of a system is always more than the combined output of its parts. This is called 'synergy'. In organizational terms, synergy refers to the increase in productivity when separate departments within an organization co-operate, coexist and interact as compared to the productivity when they acted in isolation. In other words, as separate departments within a hospital organization cooperate and interact, they become more viable and productive than if they had acted in isolation. For example, it is obviously more efficient for each department in a hospital to manage one diagnostics department than for each department to have a separate diagnostics department of its own.

Contingency Theory of Organization

The contingency management approach is similar to known leadership theory called situational leadership theory. The contingency approach is applicable to leadership as well as to business management. This situational management approach is relatively a new approach to management and is an extension of systems approach. The basic theme of contingency approach is that organizations have to deal with different situations in different ways. There is no single best way of managing applicable to all situations. In order to be effective, the internal functioning of the organization must be consistent with the needs and demands of the external environment. In other words, internal organization should have the capacity to face any type of external situation with confidence.

Features of the Contingency / Situational Approach

1. Management is entirely situational. The management has to use the measures/techniques as per the situation from time to time.
2. Management should match its approach as per the requirements of the situation. The policies and practices used should be suitable to environmental changes.
3. The success of management depends on its ability to cope up with its environment. Naturally, it has to make special efforts to anticipate and comprehend the possible environmental changes. Managers should realize that there is no one best way to manage. They have to use management techniques as per the situation which they face.

According to contingency approach, management principles and concepts of different schools have no universal applicability under all situations. This means these schools have not suggested one best method of doing things under all situations and at all times. The contingency approach has provided a solution to this situation.

As per the contingency approach, the task of managers is to try to identify which technique or method will be most suitable for achieving the management objectives under the available situation. Managers have to develop a sort of situational sensitivity and practical selectivity in order to deal with their managerial problems as they develop from time to time.

Contingency approach views are applicable in designing organizational structure and in deciding the degree of decentralization in establishing communication and control systems and also in deciding motivational and leadership approaches. In brief, the contingency approach is applicable to different areas of organization and management. It is an attempt to integrate various viewpoints and to synthesize various fragmented approaches to management.

The contingency approach is the outcome of the research studies conducted by Tom Burns and G. W. Stalker, James Thompson and others.

Merits of Contingency Approach

1. Contingency approach is pragmatic and open minded. It discounts preconceived notions, and universal validity of principles.
2. Theory relieves managers from dogmas and set principles. It provides freedom/choice to manage, to judge the external environment and to use the most suitable management techniques. Here, importance is given to the judgment of the situation and not the use of specific principles.
3. The contingency approach has a wide-ranging applicability and practical utility in organization and management. It advocates comparative analysis of organizations to bring suitable adjustment between organization structure and situational peculiarities.
4. The contingency approach focuses attention on situational factors that affect the management strategy. The theory combines the mechanistic and humanistic approaches to fit particular/specific situation. It is superior to systems theory as it not only examines the relationships between sub-systems of an organization but also the relationship between the organization and its external environment.

Limitations of Contingency Approach

1. It is argued that the contingency approach lacks a theoretical base.
2. Under contingency approach, a manager is supposed to think through all possible alternatives as he has no tried principles to act upon. This brings the need of more qualities and skills on the part of managers. The responsibility of a manager increases as he has to analyze the situation, examine the validity of different principles and techniques to the situation at hand, make right choice by matching the technique to the situation and finally execute his choice. The areas of operation of a manager are quite extensive under this theory.

The contingency approach falls somewhere in between the classical theory and systems theory. It provides a synthesis that brings together the best of all segments of what Koontz has termed "management theory jungle". Contingency approach is practical, progressive and action oriented. It considers each organization as unique and gives special attention to situation around it. Finally, it integrates theory with practice in a systems framework.

MANAGEMENT BY OBJECTIVES

Management by objectives was introduced by Peter Drucker in the 1950s and written about in his 1954 book, *The Practice of Management*. It gained a great deal of attention and was widely adopted until the 1990s when it seemed to fade into obscurity.

Partly, the idea may have become a victim of its own success. It became so much a part of the way business is conducted that it no longer may have seemed remarkable, or even worthy of comment. And partly it evolved into the idea of the balanced scorecard, which provided a more sophisticated framework for doing essentially the same thing.

Using Management by Objectives

Peter Drucker outlined the five-step process for MBO as shown in Fig. 1.2. Each stage has particular challenges that need to be addressed for the whole system to work effectively.

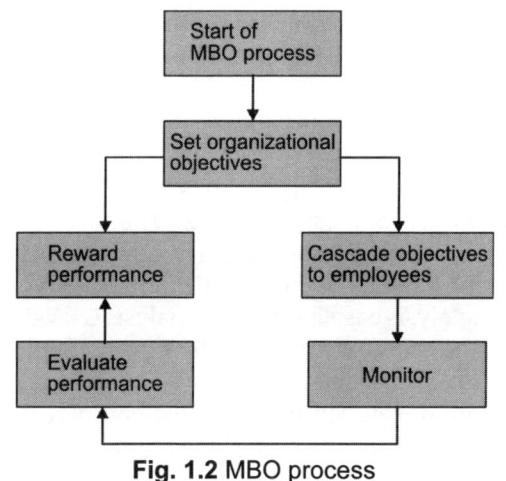

Fig. 1.2 MBO process

These steps are explained below.

1. *Set or review organizational objectives:* MBO starts with clearly defined strategic organizational objectives. If the organization isn't clear where it's going, no one working there will be clear.
2. *Cascading objectives down to employees:* To support the mission, the organization needs to set clear goals and objectives, which then need to cascade down from one organizational level to the next until they reach everyone.

To make MBO goal and objective setting more effective, Drucker used the SMART acronym to set goals that were attainable and to which people felt accountable. He said that goals and objectives must be:
- Specific
- Measurable
- Agreed (relating to the participative management principle)
- Realistic
- Time related

3. *Encourage participation in goal setting:* Everyone needs to understand how their personal goals fit with the objectives of the organization. This is best done when goals and objectives at each level are shared and discussed, so that everyone understands "why" things are being done, and then sets their own goals to align with these.
4. *Monitor progress:* Because the goals and objectives are SMART, they are measurable. They don't measure themselves though, so you have to create a monitoring system that signals when things are off track. This monitoring system has to be timely enough so that issues can be dealt with before they threaten goal achievement. With the cascade effect, no goal is set in isolation, so not meeting targets in one area will affect targets everywhere.
5. *Evaluate and reward performance:* MBO is designed to improve performance at all levels of the organization. To ensure this happens, you need to put a comprehensive evaluation system in place.

When you reward goal achievers you send a clear message to everyone that goal attainment is valued and that the MBO process is not just an exercise but an essential aspect of performance appraisal. The importance of fair and accurate assessment of performance highlights why setting measurable goals and clear performance indicators are essential to the MBO system.

MANAGEMENT FUNCTIONS

Management is the process of achieving organizational goals through planning, organizing, leading, and controlling the human, physical, financial, and information resources of the organization in an effective and efficient manner (Fig. 1.3).

The successful manager must actively perform basic managerial functions. One of the earliest classifications of managerial functions was made by Fayol, who suggested that planning, organizing, coordinating, commanding, and controlling were the primary functions. Some others theorists identified additional management functions, such as staffing, communication, or decision making. But now generally, there is agreement that the basic managerial functions are: planning, organizing, leading, and controlling (Fig. 1.3).

Planning

A plan is a predetermined course of action which provides purpose and direction.

Planning is foreseeing future circumstances and requirements, then, setting objectives, making long and short term plans and determining the policies to be followed with standards to be set.

It involves making a systematic process for achieving the organization's goals.

- In planning, managers receive and store information, monitor and disseminate the information.
- A manager makes decisions on strategy and allocation of resources and initiate planned changes.
- Strategic planning is the process of developing and analyzing the organization's mission, overall goals.

General Strategies and Allocating Resources

A strategy is a course of action created to achieve a long-term goal.

- Goals are the things that the organization strives to achieve.
- Strategic planning requires a lot of information gathering, exploring alternatives and emphasizing future implications of its current decisions.

Steps in Planning

1. *Define the organization's mission and vision:* A mission is the purpose of the organization. It explains why the organization exists. Vision is the future goal or achievement of an organization. It guides the mission of the organization by defining measurable strategic and financial objectives.
2. *SWOT analysis:* Analyze the strength, weaknesses and identify opportunities and threats of the organization, i.e. SWOT analysis baseline. SWOT analysis is used as the basis for future improvements, setting goals and objectives. Goals and objectives are developed to bridge the gap between current capability and the mission.

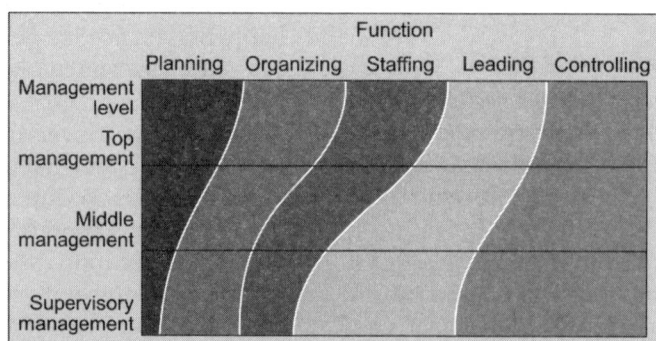

Fig. 1.3: Relative amount of emphasis placed on each function of management

3. Objectives are statements describing results and the way in which they will be achieved. They are more specific and narrower than goals.
4. Develop a strategy information collected from the environmental scan is used to match strengths with opportunities and address weaknesses while trying to minimize threats to its existence make superior profits by getting a competitive advantage over competitors.
5. *Implementation of strategy:* Strategy is implemented by developing programs, budgets and procedures. It involves organizing the firm's resources and motivating staff to achieve the firm's objectives.
6. *Evaluating/monitoring and control:* Evaluation and control consists of defining parameters to be measured. Defining the target values of those parameters and performance measurement. Then the results are compared to pre-defined standards and necessary changes are thereby made.

Organizing

Organizing is the managerial function of making sure there are available resources to carry out a plan. "Organizing involves the assignment of tasks, the grouping of tasks into departments, and the allocation of resources to departments" (Richard Daft). Managers must bring together individuals and tasks to make effective use of people and resources. Three elements are essential to organizing:
- Developing the structure of the organization.
- Acquiring and training human resources.
- Establishing communication patterns and networks.

People are an organization's most important resource, because people either create or undermine an organization's reputation for quality in both products and service.

In addition, an organization must respond to change effectively in order to remain competitive. The right staff can carry an organization through a period of change and ensure its future success. Because of the importance of hiring and maintaining a

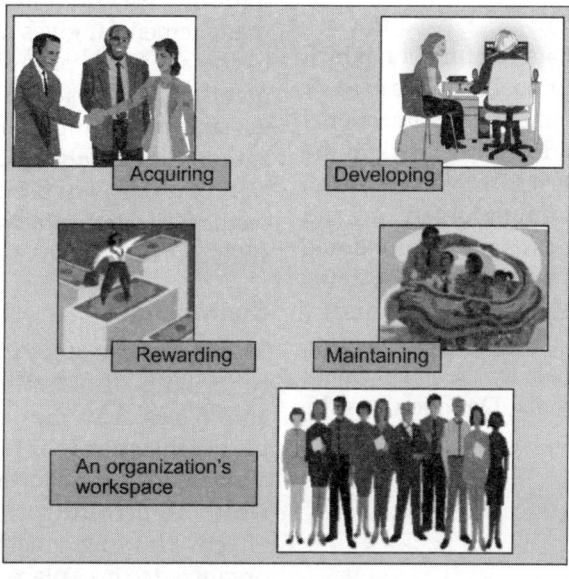

Fig. 1.4: Staffing

committed and competent staff, effective human resource management is crucial to the success of all organizations.

Staffing is the management function devoted to acquiring, training, appraising, and compensating employees. In effect, all managers are human resource managers, although human resource specialists may perform some of these activities in large organizations. Solid HRM practices can mold a hospital's workforce into a motivated and committed team capable of managing change effectively and achieving the organizational objectives (Fig. 1.4).

Understanding the fundamentals of HRM can help any manager lead more effectively. Every manager should understand the following three principles:
- All managers are human resource managers.
- Employees are much more important assets than buildings or equipment; good employees give a hospital the competitive edge.
- Human resource management is a matching process; it must match the needs of the organization with the needs of the employee.

Directing

1. It is that part of managerial function which actuates the organizational methods to work efficiently for achievement of organizational purposes. It is considered life-spark of the enterprise which sets it in motion the action of people because planning, organizing and staffing are the mere preparations for doing the work. Direction is that inert-personnel aspect of management which deals directly with influencing, guiding, supervising, motivating subordinate for the achievement of organizational goals. Direction has the following elements:
    - Supervision
    - Motivation
    - Leadership
    - Communication

Supervision: Implies overseeing the work of subordinates by their superiors. It is the act of watching and directing work and workers.

Motivation: Means inspiring, stimulating or encouraging the sub-ordinates with zeal to work. Positive, negative, monetary, non-monetary incentives may be used for this purpose.

Leadership: May be defined as a process by which manager guides and influences the work of subordinates in desired direction.

Communications: It is the process of passing information, experience, opinion, etc. from one person to another. It is a bridge of understanding.

Coordinating

Effective coordination and also integration of activities of different departments are essential for orderly working of an Hospital Organization. This suggests the importance of coordinating as management function. A hospital manager must coordinate the work for which he is accountable. Coordination is rightly treated as the essence of management. It may be treated as an independent function or as a part of organisations function. Coordination is essential at all levels of hospital management. It gives one clear-cut direction to the activities of individuals and departments. It also avoids misdirection and wastages and brings unity of action in the organization. Coordination will not come automatically or on its own special efforts are necessary on the part of hospital managers for achieving such coordination.

Controlling

The final phase of the management process is controlling. "Controlling means monitoring employees' activities, determining whether the organization is on target towards its goals, and making correction as necessary" (Richard Daft). Controlling ensures that, through effective leading, what has been planned and organized to take place has in fact taken place.

Three basic components constitute the control function:

Elements of a Control System
- Evaluating and rewarding employee performance.
- Controlling financial, informational, and physical resources.

Controlling is an ongoing process. An effective control function determines whether the organization is on target toward its goals and makes corrections as necessary.

All these managerial functions are necessary and are related and interrelated to each other and are applicable to healthcare organizations.

The **Planning** function is applicable in healthcare organizations in the following ways:
1. Purpose or mission oriented plans identify the functions of the organization, usually mission is expressed in the mission statement of the organization.

   Example: The mission of Owaisi Hospital is:
   - To provide effective and advance healthcare of the high equality to all segments of our society, irrespective of their economic status.
   - To create a platform for training all healthcare professionals by modern method of healthcare.
   - To perform research and investigate on various liver diseases. To evolve with effective treatment strategies and to make necessary procedures for transplantation.
   - To treat every individual with respect and humanity.
   - To make available, necessary services for treatment of all ailments under one roof.
2. Objectives and goals of the organization have to be planned. Once the board has approved vision and mission statements, development and prioritization of goals become the next challenge. A goal identifies an end to which the organization aspires, what is hoped to be achieved. For purposes of clarification, this is distinguished from an objective, which is an activity necessary to reach the goal.

   For instance, the objective may be to reduce the incidence of nosocomial infections. The goal may be to bring it down by 5%.
3. *Strategic planning:* A hospital/health system should plan for its future to:
   - Improve the hospital's performance
   - Determine the hospital's future direction
   - Provide high quality healthcare services
   - Optimize resource allocation
   - Meet accreditation and regulatory requirements
   - Meet the hospital's vision and mission statement
   - Maximize its chances for success
   - Policy planning
   - Procedures planning
   - Rule planning
   - Programme planning
   - Budget planning
4. *Facilities planning:* More commonly known as bricks-and-mortar planning, facility planning is heavily oriented towards design and construction of physical facilities. The major emphasis during this stage is on the replacement or expansion of physical facilities. The focus on expansion of physical facilities is dictated by the growth of hospitals in every direction coupled with capacity shortages, technological and medical advances. Architects and engineers are the major players in facilities planning.
5. *Operational planning:* The purpose of the operational plan is to provide organization personnel with a clear picture of their tasks and responsibilities in line with the goals and objectives contained within the strategic plan (Fig. 1.5).

On the other hand, the operational plan does present highly detailed information specifically to direct people to perform the day-to-day tasks required in the running of the organization. Organization management and staff should frequently refer to the operational plan in carrying out their everyday work. The operational plan provides the what, who, when and how much:

- **What** — the strategies and tasks that must be undertaken
- **Who** — the persons who have responsibility of each of the strategies/tasks
- **When** — the timeliness in which strategies/tasks must be completed
- **How much** — the amount of financial resources provided to complete each strategy/task

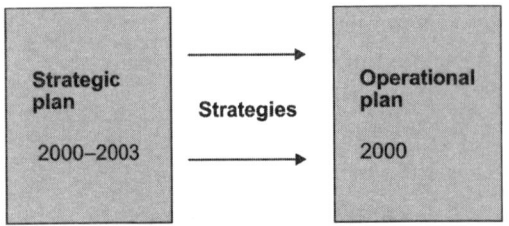

Strategies are the end point of the strategic plan but the start point of the operational plan

Fig. 1.5: Strategic and operational planning

6. *Budget planning:* Making a hospital budget is only the second to medical delivery systems in a hospital. In fact, if a budget is not properly written, the hospital may be unable to deliver medical services at all. So many expenses and sources of revenue must be taken into consideration, hence the budget process takes an expert to get through it successfully.

Similarly organizing, staffing, directing, coordinating and controlling are also very much practically applicable in healthcare organizations.

Organization Concepts and Processes

Samson (2005) described organizing as "the management function concerned with assigning tasks, grouping tasks into departments, and allocating resources to departments" (p. 25).

Organization is a rational combination of the activities of a number of people for the achievement of a common purpose or goal, by division of labor and function, and through a hierarchy of authority and responsibility.

Hospital organization involves systematizing of all clinical, administrative, and supportive services and personnel to achieve patient satisfaction and employee satisfaction.

- Organizational structure refers to levels of management within a hospital. The structure helps one understand the hospital's chain of command. Organizational structure varies from hospital to hospital. Large hospitals have complex organizational structures. Smaller hospitals tend to have much simpler organizational structures. Hospital departments are grouped in order to promote efficiency of facility. Grouping is generally done according to similarity of duties. Common categorical groupings are
  - Administrative Services
  - Informational Services
  - Therapeutic Services
  - Diagnostic Services
  - Support Services

Modern hospitals in India have been organized along British lines having stringent hierarchical structure. In the past decades, the organization of hospitals in India has been severely criticized. Increasing specialization is leading to fragmentation. As modern hospitals have to perform more complex functions, engage skilled human resources and provide superior facilities, their organizations have grown increasingly complex and their operations more costly.

How Hospital is Different from any Other Organization

1. In a hospital there are a number of heads, such as medical head, administrative head, departmental head, etc.

2. There is an absence of single line of authority and presence of two chains of command.
3. The hospital organization is characterized by high interdependence of individuals and departments.
4. The inflow and outflow of the patients is more by chance than planned.
5. Hospital organization is both authoritative and permissive, highly formalized yet loose.

Organizational Chart

It is an abstract illustration of the structure. It is the depiction of specific positions in an organization, their states within the organization and the reporting relationship between a subordinate and his superior.

Structure and Context Factors

Organizational context is defined as the social and economic setting in which organization chooses to operate. While studying about organizational structure, four aspects needs to be mentioned. They are:

External environment: It includes economic, political and legal conditions, demographic and cultural factors, multi-institutional arrangements (mergers, corporate influence structures, health insurance arrangements), and changes in the medical technology.

Organizational assessment: It deals with the mission of the hospital and reconsiders it in relation to its future environment. It also deals with the goals and specific strategies developed by the organization on one hand and the quality, quantity and types of service to be provided on the other hand. In this case problems are related to the current structure and internal process of hospital may be identified, e.g. communication barriers, delay in making decisions, etc.

Human resources: It involves evaluating the capabilities and potential of key persons in the organization.

Political process: It involves a systematic assessment of the informal internal dynamics of the hospital. The informal groups and leaders who influence the programmes in the hospital needs to be identified.

The structural dimension of an organization purposes:
- To channelize information to the appropriate managers, so that their level of uncertainty is reduced when they make decisions.
- To effectively distribute the authority to make decisions.
- Is a managerial tool that aids in guiding the organization towards its goals.

Organizational structure defines and governs the relationship among the various work units, ensuring that all work is assigned and completed in an orderly fashion, which in turn, contributes to effective overall organizational performance.

Constituent Elements of Organizational Structure

- *Formalization:* It represents the extent to which jobs are governed by rules and specific guidelines.
- *Centralization:* It is a measure of distribution of power within the organization.
- *Specialization:* It refers to the extent to which an organization favors division of labor. In hospitals there is a high level of specialization at all levels.
- *Complexity:* It refers to the extent of knowledge and skills required for occupational roles and their diversity.
- *Configuration:* Organization structure occurs in a limited number of configurations.

Mintzberg (1983) proposed a rational approach to the formation of structure, which is composed of five elements.
- Strategic apex
- Operating core
- Middle line
- Techno structure
- Support staff

Organizational Designs

- *Functional design:* This arrangement is prevalent in hospitals with less than 200 beds, where the workers are divided into specific functional departments, such as Finance, Nursing, Pharmacy, Housekeeping, etc. This design facilitates decision making in a centralized or hierarchical manner, and the role of the manager is clearly demarcated. This design is appropriate for hospitals offering single specialty, or few specialties.
- *Divisional design:* This is found in large teaching hospitals and sometimes in a few private hospitals. It is most appropriate where clear divisions can be made within the organizations, and semiautonomous units can be created. Each division will have its own internal management structure.
- *Design based on products:* This is usually seen in manufacturing industry, but now introduced in hospitals, e.g. University hospital of Cleveland, where the hospital is divided into six management centers—pediatrics, medical and surgical departments, psychiatry, obstetrics and gynecology, integrated health systems, and hospital services —each under a general manager.
- *Corporate design:* This is increasingly found in hospitals. In this design there will be a governing body and the top management.
- *Matrix design:* It was developed initially for aerospace industry, which is characterized by dual authority system where individuals have two or more bosses.
    - Matrix design is useful in specialized technological area. It helps in multidisciplinary team approach. Disadvantages are: 1. Two bosses for employees, who create conflicting expectations and ambiguity and 2. It can be expensive (Fig. 1.6).
    - The other organizational designs include design based on geographical location; by type of customers, and parallel design, which are seldom used in hospitals.

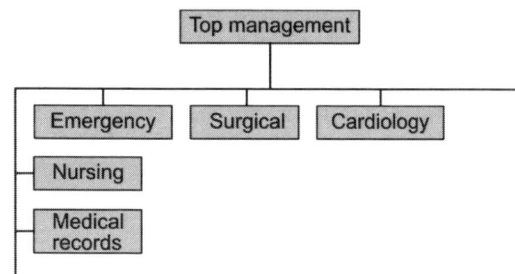

Fig: 1.6: Matrix design

Formal and Informal Organizations

Formal organization means the intentional structure of roles in a formally organized enterprise (Koontz, 1998), however, it does not imply inflexibility or rigidity.

According to Chester Barnard, informal organization is any joint personal activity without conscious joint purpose, even though contributing to joint results.

Line and Staff Relationships

Line functions are those that have direct impact on the accomplishment of the objectives of the organization and staff functions are those which help the line personnel work more effectively in accomplishing the objectives.

In hospital, the line function is performed by doctors and nurses, whereas staff includes the supportive and managerial functionaries. However, it is very difficult to clearly draw a line between line and staff functions.

Line and staff is an issue of authority relationships, the activities do not characterize a department as line or staff. Line organization is the backbone of the hierarchy. Staff and functional organization merely supplements the line.

Decision Making

Decision making can be regarded as the mental processes (cognitive process) resulting in the selection of a course of action among several alternative scenarios. Every decision making process produces a final choice. The output can be an action or an opinion of choice.

Decision making is the key to all managerial and administrative functions. It is the duty of the hospital administrator to take the necessary decisions as and when they arise in the hospitals (Fig. 1.7).

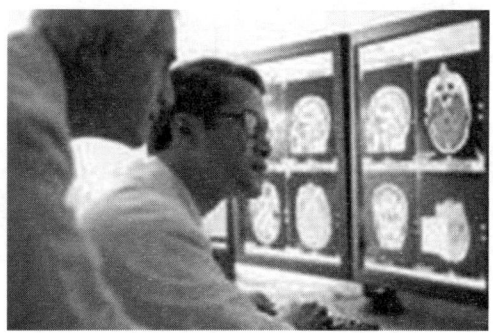

Fig. 1.7: Two doctors examining an X-ray

Decision making is defined as **the selection of a course of action from alternatives**. There are 3 phases in decision-making process, based on the timeframe. They are:

- *The past:* In which problems developed, information accumulated, and the need for a decision was perceived.
- *The present*: In which alternatives are found and the choice is made.
- *The future:* In which decisions will be carried out and developed.

Herbert Simon, described the activities associated with decision making in three major stages (Fig. 1.8):

- Intelligence
- Design
- Choice activities

Types of Management Decisions

1. *Personal and organization decisions*: According to Bernard " personal decisions cannot ordinarily be delegated to others, whereas organization decisions can often, if not always be delegated, e.g. of personal decision—decision to resign, take leave, e.g. of organizational decision: regarding recruitment, promotion, etc.

2. *Basic and routine decisions*: Basic decisions are those which are unique, decisions involving long-term commitments of relative performance or delegation or those involving large instruments, e.g. location of hospital, organizational structure, usually all top management decisions are basic divisions.

3. *Routine decisions*: These are everyday highly repetitive management decisions by which they themselves have a little impact on overall organization. However, taken together routine decisions play important role in the success of organizations, e.g. scheduling of elective surgeries, purchase of material, drugs.

4. *Programmed and non-programmed decisions*: According to Simon programmed decision are typically handled through structured techniques (standard operating process). Non-programmed decisions must be made by managers using available information and their own judgment.

Gresham's Law

An important principle of organization design that relates to managerial decision making is Gresham's Law of planning. This law states that there is a general tendency for programmed activities to overshadow non-programmed activities. Hence, if a series of decisions are to be made, those that are more routine and repetitive will tend to be made before the ones that are unique and require considerable thought. This happens presumably because you attempt to clear the desk so that you can get down to the really serious decisions. Unfortunately, the desks very often never get cleared.

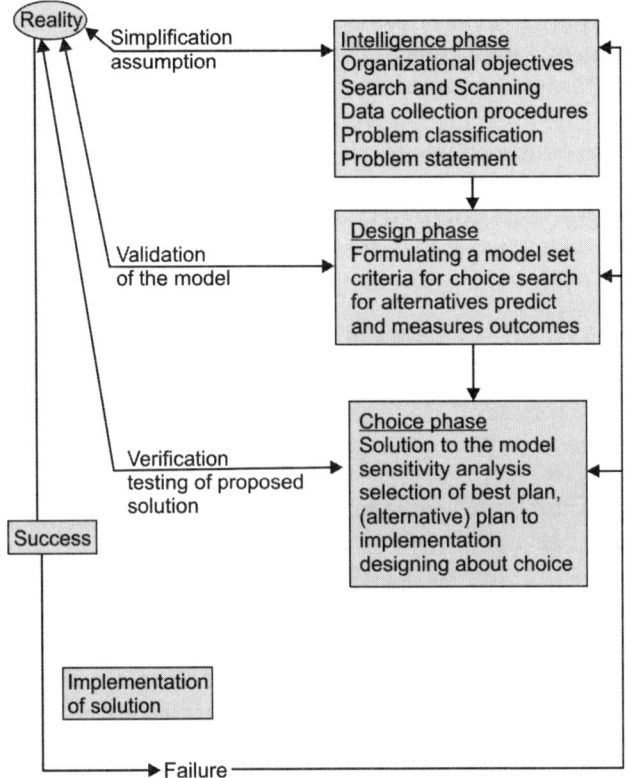

Fig. 1.8: Decision-making process

- *Mechanistic decisions:* It is one that is routine and repetitive. Most of mechanistic decisions, problems are solved by habitual responses, standard operating procedures or clerical routines, e.g. scheduling surgeries, preparing patients for surgeries, etc.
- *Analytical decisions:* It involves problems with a large number of decisions variables. Operations research techniques are usually used for taking analytical decisions, e.g. waiting problems in OPD, diagnostics.
- *Judgment decisions:* It involves a problem with a limited number of decision variables, but the outcomes of decision alternatives are unknown, e.g. marketing and investment decisions (Table 1.2).
- *Adaptive decisions:* It involves problems with a large number of decisions variables, where outcomes are not predictable, e.g. large-scale expansion, research and development.

Decision Making Under Different Stages of Nature

The three stages of nature for decision making are:
- Decision under certainty
- Decision under risk
- Decision under uncertainty

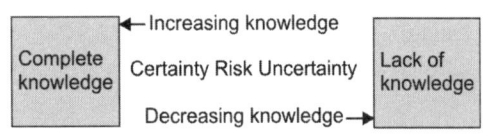

Decision under certainty: When manager knows the precise outcome associated with each

Table 1.2: Judgmental and adaptive decisions

	Judgmental Decisions	Adaptive Decisions
Uncertainty High	(For example, marketing, investment, and personnel problems)	(For example, research and development and long-term corporate planning)
	Mechanistic decisions	Analytical decisions
Outcome Low	(For example, daily routines and scheduled activities)	(For example, complex production and engineering problems)
	Low Problem	Complexity High

alternative course of action. Exact results are known in advance with 100% certainty, e.g. investment in CT scan machine by a viable hospital.

Decision under risk: A decision is made under conditions of risk when a single action may result in more than one potential outcome, but the relative probability of each outcome is known, e.g. most of the decisions pertaining to clinical care.

Decision under uncertainty: A decision is made under conditions of uncertainty when a single action may result in more than one potential outcome, but the relative probability of each outcome is unknown, e.g. decision to undergo angiogram by patient.

Decision-making Techniques and Processes

Identification of alternatives: There are three methods for generating alternatives. These are:

1. *Brain storming:* Developed by F. Alex. It involves the use of a group whose member is presented with a problem and is asked to develop as many potential solutions as possible. Members of the group may be all the employees of the same firm or outside experts in the same. Brain storming is based on the premise that when people interact in a free and uninhabited atmosphere they will generate creative ideas. Brain storming is governed by important rules such as:
   - Criticism is prohibited.
   - Quantity is wanted: The greater the number of ideas, the greater the likelihood of outstanding solutions.
   - Combination and improvement are sought.
   - The wider the idea the better

   Brain storming usually involves 6–8 participants and run from 30 minutes to one hour. It is usually effective when a problem is simple and specific. It produces a specific solution usually which can be solved by selecting group members who are familiar with the problem.

2. *Synectics*: Developed by William J.J. Gordon, it is a formalized creative technique for the generation of alternative solution. The term synectics is derived from a Greek word meaning "the fitting together of diverse elements". Members of a synectics group are typically selected to represent a variety of background and training.

   An experienced group leader plays a vital role in this approach. The leader states the problem for the group to consider. The group reacts by stating the problem as they understand it. Only after the nature of the problem is thoroughly reviewed and analyzed does the group proceed. To offer potential solution leader should ensure that the group members deviate from their traditional way of thinking. With this role, other thought provoking exercises are also conducted.

It stimulates creative alternatives. It is from this complex set of instructions that a final solution hopefully emerges. A technical expert is present to assist the group in evaluating the feasibility of ideas. Thus in constant to the brain storming where the judgment of ideas is withheld until all ideas have been generated. Judicial evaluation of member's suggestion does take place from time to time. Synectics is appropriate for complex and technical problems and is seldom used when compared with brain storming.

3. Nominal grouping developed by Anderbellberg and Andrew Vandiven. Nominal grouping differs from both brain storming and synectics in two important ways. It does not rely on free association of ideas and purposeful attempts to reduce verbal interactions. From this it received its name; it is a group "in name only".

Five Stages in Nominal Grouping

- *Stage-I*: 7–10 individuals with different backgrounds and training are brought together and familiarized with the selected problem.
- *Stage-II*: Each group member is asked to prepare a list of ideas in response to the identified problem. Working silently and alone.
- *Stage-III*: After a period of 10–25 minutes group member share the ideas at a time in a round-robin manner. A group records the ideas on a blackboard/flip for all to see. Round-robin continues until all ideas are presented and recorded.
- *Stage-IV*: A period of structural interaction follows in which group member openly discuss and evaluates each recorded idea. At this point ideas may be rewarded combined, deleted or added.
- *Stage-V*: Each group members voted by on priority ideas, i.e. ranking the presented ideas in order of their perceived importance. Following a brief discussion of the vote, a final secret ballot is conducted, the group preference in the mathematical outcome of individual voter. Nominal grouping is effective in situations requiring a high degree of innovation and idea generation.

Quantitative Techniques for Decision Making

- *Operation research (OR)*: The quantitative study of an organization in action carried out in order to find ways in which its functions can be improved is called OR.
- *Decision tree*: Involves a series of steps, the second step depending on the outcome of the first, and soon and often uncertainty surrounds each step. It is a graphical method for identifying alternative action, estimating probabilities and indicating the resulting expected payoff. Decision maker falls uncertainty.
- *Linear programming*: It is used in optimum allocation of resources in the organization.
- *Game theory*: It is helpful in making decisions under competitive situation. It provides an answer to the question, what may be considered a rational course of action for an individual confronted with a situation whose outcome depends not only on his own action but also on the action of others who in turn are faced with similar problem of choosing rational course of action.
- *Queuing or waiting line theory*: It involves mathematical study of queues or waiting line. "A group of items waiting to receive service". It is either due to much demand for facilities.

- *Creative thinking*: For creative thinking managers have to use creative and analytical thinking, conscious and subconscious mind and seek group as well as individual involvement in decision making evaluation of alternatives may be performed by a single manager or by a group.

Advantages and Disadvantages of Group Decision Making

There are two phenomenon associated with group decision making. They are:
1. **Risk shift phenomenon**: Which says that groups make riskier decisions than individuals.
2. **Group think**: Discussed by James refers to a model of thinking in a group in which the seeking of concurrence among members become so dominant that it overrides any realistic appraisal of alternative course of action (Table 1.3).

Degree of Participation

- No participation
- Benevolent dictatorship (opinions taken but not considered)
- Occasional involvement
- Participation in minor and major decisions
- Complete involvement

Barriers to Effective Decision Making

- Elbing (1978) has identified several road blocks to effective decision-making.
- The tendency to evaluate before investigation.
- The tendency to equate new and old experience.
- The tendency to use available solution rather than consider new or innovative ones.
- The tendency to deal with problems at face value, rather than ask questions that might illuminate reasons behind the more obvious aspects of the problems.
- Tendency to direct decision towards single goal, but most problems involve multiple goals.
- Tendency to confuse symptoms and problems.
- Tendency to overlook unsolvable problem, *Strategies to overcome the barriers.*
- Group leaders can encourage each member to evaluate critically of the various proposals.
- When groups are given a problem to solve leaders retain from stating their own position and instead encourage open enquiry and impartial probing of a wider range of alternatives.

Table 1.3: Advantages and disadvantages of group decision making

Advantages	Disadvantages
Group can accumulate more knowledge and facts.	Group often works more slowly than individual.
Group have broader perspective and consider alternative solutions.	Group decision involves considerable compromise which may lead to less than optimal decision.
Individuals who participate in group decisions are more satisfied with decision and more likely to support it.	Groups often determined by individual, or thereby negating the virtues or group procedures.
Group decision process serves an important communication function as well as political function.	Overreliance on group decision making inhibits managements ability to act quickly and decisively when neccessary.

- The organization can give the same problem to the two different groups and compare the results.
- Outside experts can be brought in.
- At every group meeting one member could be appointed as devil's advocate to challenge the majority positions.

Various committee in a hospital
- Purchase committee
- Infection control committee
- Medical Audit committee

Managers are poor decision makers due to psychological phenomenon:

Cognitive Bias
- Prior hypothesis bias
- Escalating commitments
- Representativeness
- Illusion of control
- Reasoning by analogy

Group Think

Without a proper question and assumption, a group makes an initiative or takes a course of action, e.g. cabinet members.

Leadership

The key function of a leader is to serve in enabling others by helping them discover, develop, and effectively use their God-given gifts (Fig. 1.9).

A simple **definition of leadership** is that leadership is the art of motivating a group of people to act towards achieving a common goal.

"Management is doing things right, leadership is doing the right things."
(Warren Bennis and Peter Drucker)

- Autocratic:
  - Leader makes decisions without reference to anyone else.
  - High degree of dependency on the leader.
  - Can create de-motivation and alienation of staff.
  - May be valuable in some types of business where decisions need to be made quickly and decisively.
- Democratic:
- Encourages decision making from different perspectives — leadership may be emphasised throughout the organisation
  - Consultative: Process of consultation before decisions are taken.
  - Persuasive: Leader takes decision and seeks to persuade others that the decisions are correct.
- Democratic:
  - May help motivation and involvement.

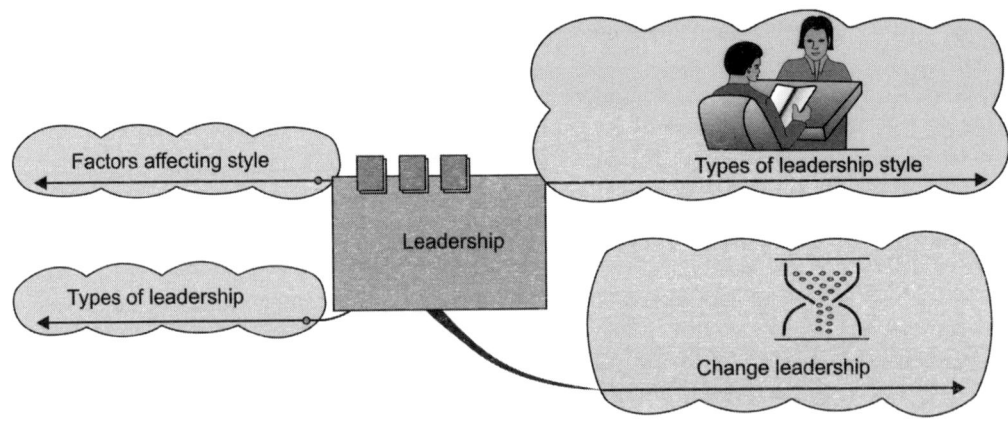

Fig. 1.9: Leadership

- Workers feel ownership of the firm and its ideas.
- Improves the sharing of ideas and experiences within the business.
- Can delay decision making
• Laissez-faire:
  - 'Let it be' — the leadership responsibilities are shared by all.
  - Can be very useful in businesses where creative ideas are important.
  - Can be highly motivational, as people have control over their working life.
  - Can make coordination and decision making time-consuming and lacking in overall direction.
  - Relies on good team work.
  - Relies on good interpersonal relations.
• Paternalistic:
  - Leader acts as a 'father figure'.
  - Paternalistic leader makes decision but may consult.
  - Believes in the need to support staff (Fig. 1.10).

Change Leadership

- The most challenging aspect of business is leading and managing change (Fig. 1.11).
- The business environment is subject to fast-paced economic and social changes.
- Modern business must adapt and be flexible to survive.
- Problems in leading change stem mainly from human resource management.
- Leaders need to be aware of how change impacts on workers.
- Series of self-esteem states identified by Adams et al. and cited by Garrett.

Theories of Leadership

The trait model of leadership is based on the characteristics of many leaders—both successful and unsuccessful and is used to predict leadership effectiveness. The resulting lists of traits are then compared to those of potential leaders to assess their likelihood of success or failure. Scholars taking the trait approach attempted to identify physiological (appearance, height, and weight), demographic (age, education and socio-economic background), personality, self-confidence, and aggressiveness), intellective (intelligence, decisiveness, judgment, and knowledge), task-related (achievement drive, initiative, and persistence), and social characteristics (sociability and co-operativeness) with leader emergence and leader effectiveness. Successful leaders definitely have interests, abilities, and personality traits that are different from those of the less effective leaders. Through many researches conducted

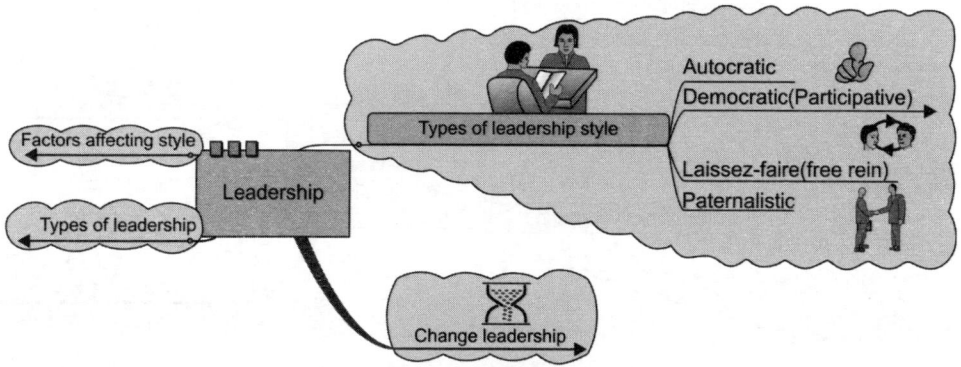

Fig. 1.10: Types of Leadership Styles

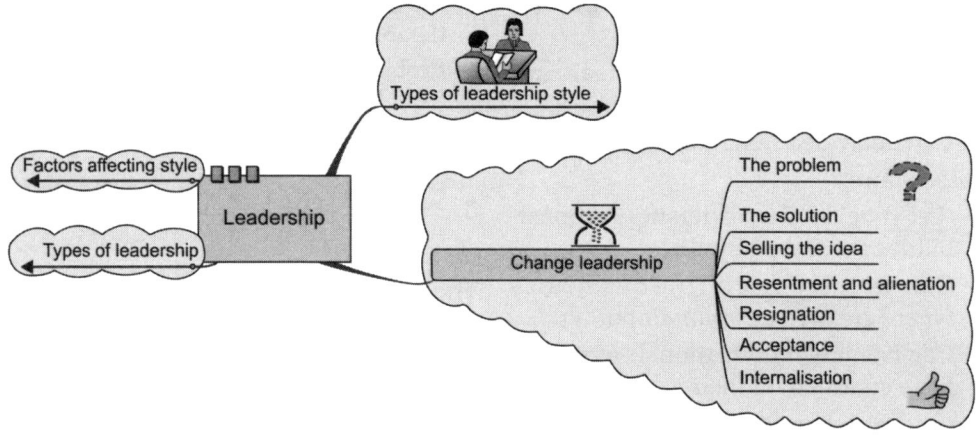

Fig. 1.11: Change Leadership

in the last three decades of the 20th century, a set of core traits of successful leaders have been identified (Fig. 1.12).

Among the core traits identified are

- Achievement drive: High level of effort, high levels of ambition, energy and initiative.
- Leadership motivation: An intense desire to lead others to reach shared goals.
- Honesty and integrity: Trustworthy, reliable, and open.
- Self-confidence: Belief in one's self, ideas, and ability.
- Cognitive ability: Capable of exercising good judgment, strong analytical abilities, and conceptually skilled.
- Knowledge of business: Knowledge of industry and other technical matters.

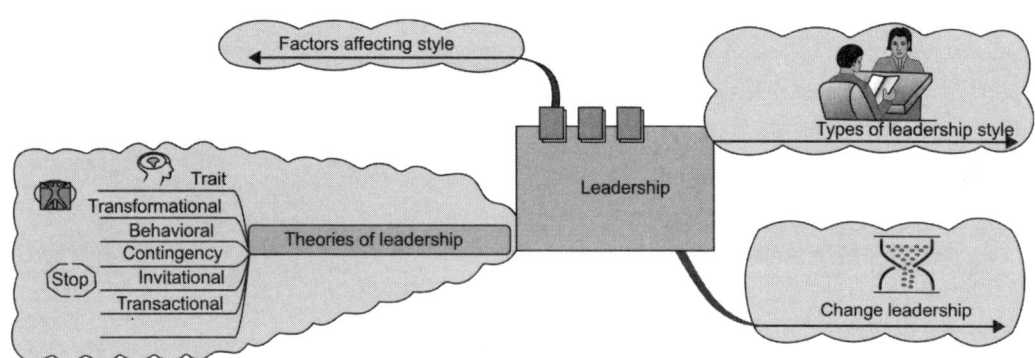

Fig. 1.12: Theories of Leadership

- Emotional maturity: Well adjusted, does not suffer from severe psychological disorders.
- Others: Charisma, creativity and flexibility.

Strengths/Advantages of Trait Theory

- It is naturally pleasing theory.
- It is valid as lot of research has validated the foundation and basis of the theory.
- It serves as a yardstick against which the leadership traits of an individual can be assessed.
- It gives a detailed knowledge and understanding of the leader element in the leadership process.

Limitations of the Trait Theory

- There is bound to be some subjective judgment in determining who is regarded as a 'good' or 'successful' leader.
- The list of possible traits tends to be very long. More than 100 different traits of successful leaders in various leadership positions have been identified. These descriptions are simply generalities.
- There is also a disagreement over which traits are the most important for an effective leader.
- The model attempts to relate physical traits such as, height and weight, to effective leadership. Most of these factors relate to situational factors. For example, a minimum weight and height might be necessary to perform the tasks efficiently in a military leadership position. In business organizations, these are not the requirements to be an effective leader.
- The theory is very complex.

Behavioral theory: It implies that leaders can be trained too on the way of doing things:

- Structure based behavioral theories: Focus on the leader instituting structures—task orientated.
- Relationship based behavioral theories: Focus on the development and maintenance of relationships—process orientated.

Contingency theories

- Leadership as being more flexible: different leadership styles used at different times depending on the circumstance.
- Suggest leadership is not a fixed series of characteristics that can be transposed into different contexts.

Managerial Grid Theory was developed by Robert Blake and Jane Mouton (1978). This model uses two variables of leadership orientation. Concern for people and Concern for production. A managerial grid is formed by the axes of concern of people and concern of production. By plotting various locations on the grid formed by the variables, there are five leadership styles.

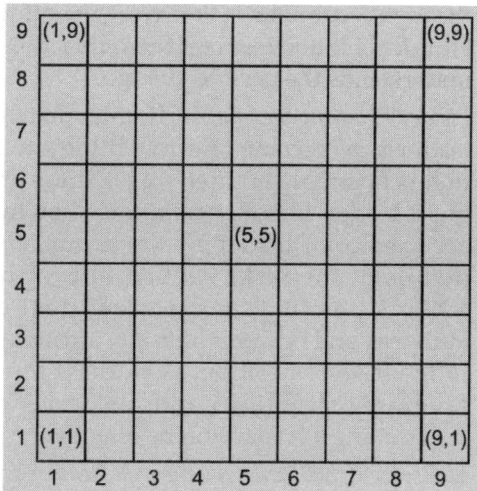

- *1, 1 – Impoverished management leader:* It is neither concerned with production nor people. They avoid taking sides, and stay out of conflicts.
- *1, 9 – Country club management leader:* It is primarily concerned for people and has a little concern for production. The leaders major responsibility is to establish

harmonious relationship among subordinates and to provide a secure and pleasant work atmosphere.

- *9, 1 – Task management leader:* Managers in this position have a great concern for production and a little concern for people. They desire tight control in order to get tasks done efficiently. They consider creativity and human relations unnecessary.
- *5, 5 – Middle of the road management leader:* Leaders in this position have medium concern for people and pro-duction. They attempt to balance their concern for both people and production, but are not committed to either.
- *9, 9 – Team management leader:* This type of leadership is considered to be the ideal. Such managers have concern for both people and tasks. He is concerned to see that the work accomplishment is from committed people, interdependence through a 'common stake' in organization. He is flexible and responsive to change and understands the need to change.
- *Fielder's contingency theory:* It states that the leader may become effective if the situation is favorable in three ways. These are good leader–member relations showing acceptance of leader by the group, the details of the tasks spelled out to the leaders position, and a great deal of authority and power is formally attributed to the leaders position. With these three favorable situations and his styles of functioning a leader will be effective.
- *House–Mitchell path goal theory of leadership:* This theory states that the leadership smoothes out the path towards goals and provide rewards for achieving them. Robert House called this theory as path goal because he believed that "The motivational function of the leader consists of increasing personal payoffs to subordinates for work-goal attainment and making the path to these payoffs easier to travel by clarifying it, reducing road-blocks and pitfalls and increasing opportunities for personal satisfaction en route.

This theory relies on the results of the Ohio State University and University of Michigan. The path goal theory sees the leader as having three motivational functions. The leader can increase the **valences** associated with work. Goal attainment, **instrumentalities** of work goal attainment and the **expectancy** that effort will result in work goal attainment.

House and Mitchell identified the role leadership plays by noting that followers are motivated by leader behavior to the extent this behavior influences expectancies.

Path goal theory is a situational theory because its basic premise is that the effect of leader behavior on follower performance and satisfaction depends on situation, specifically including follower, subordinate characteristics and task characteristics. According to House and Mitchell there are four categories of leader behavior each is best suited to particular situations:

- *Directive leadership:* It describes the behavior of leader who tells followers what they must do, tells them how to do it, requires that they follow the rules and procedures, etc.
- *Supportive leadership:* It describes the behavior of the leader who is friendly, approachable and exhibits consideration for the status, well being and needs of followers.
- *Participative leadership:* It describes the behavior of leaders who consult with the followers, ask for the opinions and suggestions and considers them.
- *Achievement-oriented leadership*: It describes the behavior of leader who establishes challenging goals for followers, accepts excellent performance and exhibits confidence that followers will meet expectations.

Turnaround leadership

It is a concept developed by Rosabeth Moss Kanter of Harvard Business School. When organizations are in crisis, they need leaders more than managers. Down beat companies needs re-engineering and strategies, but what need even more is a CEO who can restore confidence in employees. She has studied the turnaround of several corporates like BBC, Gillette, etc. Organizations decline usually start with a decline in company's fortune. Then people begin pointing fingers and deriding colleagues

The resulting tensions lead to a downward spiral in confidence and attitudes. Organizational pathologies—secrecy, blame, isolation, avoidance, passivity and feeling of helplessness arise during a difficult time, re-enforcing one another in a way that the company enters a death spiral. Even companies that were once successful suddenly seem to fall into a losing streak, to the external halo effect. This is the aura that surrounds a successful person or organization. When the going is good it hides its weakness. When the going is bad, it hides its strengths. But it needs great leaders to allow organizations to discover their hidden strengths.

The first task of turnaround leaders is to open the channels of communication. He or she should not find out scapegoats for previous mistakes. Turnaround leaders must move people towards respect.

Functions of Leadership in Hospital and Healthcare Organizations

- Developing an internal consensus on organizational priorities.
- Enlisting internal and external support for organizational purposes.
- Selecting an optimal service and patient mix.
- Locating responsibility for the organizations direction and performance.
- Developing effective planning strategies.
- Selecting competitive strategies to pursue.
- Managing conflicts between economic and professional interests.
- Negotiating reimbursement with TPA's and insurance companies.
- Managing change.
- Developing strategy to overcome competition.
- Rising to the aspirations of changing patient needs.
- Retaining talent in the organization.

Behavioral Concepts and Theories

The **behavioral management theory** is often called the human relations movement because it addresses the human dimension of work. Behavioral theorists believed that a better understanding of human behavior at work, such as motivation, conflict, expectations, and group dynamics, improves productivity.

The theorists who contributed to this school viewed employees as individuals, resources, and assets to be developed and worked with—not as machines, as in the past. Several individuals and experiments contributed to this theory.

Abraham Maslow, a practicing psychologist, developed one of the most widely recognized **need theories,** a theory of motivation based upon a consideration of human needs. His theory of human needs had three assumptions:

- Human needs are never completely satisfied.
- Human behavior is purposeful and is motivated by the need for satisfaction.
- Needs can be classified according to a hierarchical structure of importance, from the lowest to the highest.

Maslow broke down the needs hierarchy into five specific areas:

- *Physiological needs:* Maslow grouped all physical needs necessary for maintaining basic human well-being, such as food and drink, into this category. After the need is satisfied, however, it is no longer is a motivator.

- *Safety needs:* These needs include the need for basic security, stability, protection, and freedom from fear. A normal state exists for an individual to have all these needs generally satisfied. Otherwise, they become primary motivators.
- *Belonging and love needs:* After the physical and safety needs are satisfied and are no longer motivators, the need for belonging and love emerges as a primary motivator. The individual strives to establish meaningful relationships with significant others.
- *Esteem needs:* An individual must develop self-confidence and wants to achieve status, reputation, fame, and glory.
- *Self-actualization needs:* Assuming that all the previous needs in the hierarchy are satisfied, an individual feels a need to find himself.

Maslow's hierarchy of needs theory helped managers visualize employee motivation.

Douglas Mc Gregor was heavily influenced by both the Hawthorne studies and Maslow. He believed that two basic kinds of managers exist. One type, the Theory X manager, has a negative view of employees and assumes that they are lazy, untrustworthy, and incapable of assuming responsibility. On the other hand, the theory Y manager assumes that employees are not only trustworthy and capable of assuming responsibility, but also have high levels of motivation.

An important aspect of McGregor's idea was his belief that managers who hold either set of assumptions can create **self-fulfilling prophecies**—that through their behavior, these managers create situations where subordinates act in ways that confirm the manager's original expectations.

> **"Don't waste your time on jealousy. Sometimes you're ahead, sometimes you're behind. The race is long and, in the end, it's only with yourself."**
> Mary Schmich, "Chicago Tribune", 1 June 1997 in a piece now known as "the Sunscreen Speech" which has been made into a record by the film director Baz Luhrmann.

As a group, these theorists discovered that people worked for inner satisfaction and not materialistic rewards, shifting the focus to the role of individuals in an organization's performance.

Herzberg's two factor theory is a "content theory" of motivation." Herzberg analyzed the job attitudes of 200 accountants and engineers who were asked to recall when they had felt positive or negative at work and the reasons why.

From this research, Herzberg suggested a two-step approach to understanding employee motivation and satisfaction:

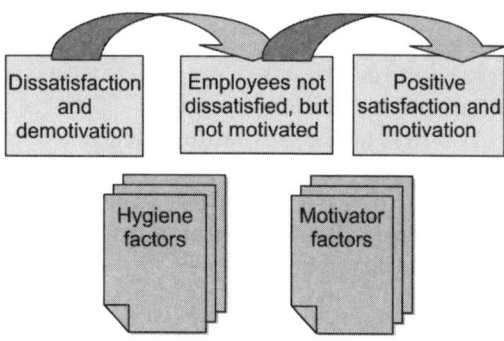

Hygiene Factors

Hygiene factors are based on the need for a business to avoid unpleasantness at work. If these factors are considered inadequate by employees, then they can cause dissatisfaction with work. Hygiene factors include:
- Company policy and administration
- Wages, salaries and other financial remuneration

- Quality of supervision
- Quality of interpersonal relations
- Working conditions
- Feelings of job security

Motivator Factors

Motivator factors are based on an individual's need for personal growth. When they exist, motivator factors actively create job satisfaction. If they are effective, then they can motivate an individual to achieve above-average performance and effort. Motivator factors include:
- Status
- Opportunity for advancement
- Gaining recognition
- Responsibility
- Challenging/stimulating work
- Sense of personal achievement and personal growth in a job.

There is some similarity between Herzberg's and Maslow's models. They both suggest that needs have to be satisfied for the employee to be motivated. However, Herzberg argues that only the higher levels of the Maslow Hierarchy (e.g. self-actualisation, esteem needs) act as a motivator. The remaining needs can only cause dissatisfaction, if not addressed.

Applying Herzberg's Model to Demotivated Workers

What might the evidence of demotivated employees be in a business?
- Low productivity
- Poor production or service quality
- Strikes/industrial disputes/breakdown in employee communication and relationships
- Complaints about pay and working conditions.

According to Herzberg, management should focus on rearranging work so that motivator factors can take effect. He suggested three ways in which this could be done:
- Job enlargement
- Job rotation
- Job enrichment

Motivating Medical and Paramedical Personnel
The strength of your team depends on how much effort you place in training and development. Obtain positive results for your organization by developing a policy to strengthen your medical office staff.

Be sure your policy includes a continuing education program to make sure all employees are kept up-to-date on office policies, compliance and job specific requirements.

One area that promises positive results in your strengthening efforts is cross-training staff. Cross-training is the most valuable training tool that an employer can offer for the benefit of the entire organization.

Continuity of service is an example of one of the benefits cross-training your staff can offer. The quality of care your patients receive should not be less than excellent due to 1 or 2 absent employees.

Cross-training also improves morale. Employees feel they are a valuable asset to the organization when they are given the opportunity to expand their skills or knowledge.

Another way to strengthen the medical office staff is by reassigning or removing unproductive employees. The team is only as strong as it's weakest link. Unproductive employees can compromise quality of care and lower employee morale.

This does not necessarily mean the employee needs to be terminated. Evaluate your unproductive employees to find out their strengths and weaknesses. Sometimes employees are placed in a mismatched position or haven't been properly trained.

With proper training and development, your medical office staff can reach their maximum.

Social Responsibilities of Management

A hospital administrator encounters many ethical problems. The issues of medical ethics involve life and death. Serious ethical issues pertain to a few issues like, patient rights, informed consent, negligence, etc. Ethics focuses on what is right choice, in the given circumstances, at a given time in a given culture. Ethics are based on values.

Medical ethics is derived from values in healthcare. It is concerned with the obligations of the doctors and the hospital to the patient, other health professionals and the society. (Francis, CM and De Souza, 2004) Properly embedded, socially responsible behavior across the hospital's value chain ensures that the role of private hospitals as legitimate healthcare providers will be accepted by both government and electorates alike. It will:

- Preserve access to patients and their demand for services provided because patients will not feel 'scalped'.
- Guarantee the supply of willing and motivated staff because employees will feel the hospital is doing what is 'right' to patients and staff.
- Keep government 'on side' as they will not have political repercussions to fear.
- As a result, provide access to quality partners and investors from around the world, happy to be associated with organizations that respect the environment, the laws and conventions of the countries in which they operate and provide good care for both patients and staff, thus ensuring a benign political environment.

Social objectives and responsibilities of management with special reference to hospitals

- A hospital, unlike other organizations, deals with the immediate life of the people has to be highly responsive to the societal needs.
- Social responsibility embraces multitude of internal and external relationships of the firm. Organizations conscious of their social responsibility, would seek to comply with the laws concerned with employment of women, non-discrimination in employment, ecological effect of production/service, consumers, and employee welfare and in general would think of the impact of their action on society.
- Running the enterprise in a "socially responsible" manner implies that the activities of the organization are in tune with what is generally perceived as in the public interest. It also implies that the firms respond positively to emerging societal priorities and balances the interest of various stakeholders. Hospitals purpose of existence is to provide healthcare to the community. In discharging its duties, hospitals should see that it follows the ethical standards, and it provides its service to all sections of society to a larger extent.
- If the organizations ignore the changing priorities and expectations of society, the results could be greater public criticism and more onerous regulation by governments, e.g. regulation of scan centers through PNDT act, proposal to regulate hospitals through clinical establishment regulatory act.

Corporate social responsibility is seriously considering the impact of the organisation's action on society.

- Social responsiveness: It means ability of an organisation to relate its operations and policies to the social environment in ways that are mutually beneficial to the organisation and to the society. The main difference between social responsibility and social responsiveness is that the latter implies actions and how enterprise responses.
- Concern for social responsibility has led to the development of formal procedures to monitor corporate compliance with changing social demand.
- Bauer and Fen define social audit as a commitment to systematic assessment of and reporting of some definable domain of

an organisation's activities that have a social impact. In India TISCO was the first company to conduct some sort of social audit.
- Social audit is more or less a formal device for judging how a corporate entity has implemented its social policy and programme. It is in the interest of organized business to undertake social audit for it would help the management to determine areas where the firm will be vulnerable to public criticism.

Culture and Management

Culture of the country or the region affects the management philosophy. The countries which were able to incorporate their cultural ethos into their management philosophy, are found to be successful, e.g. Japan.

American Culture and Management Philosophy
- High divorce rate
- Poor job security
- Nuclear family
- There is an insecure feeling in the minds of Americans, which makes them hard-working.' Hire and Fire' is the labor management style followed in the U.S., which can be referred to as **contractual style**. The greatest positive feature of American culture is the importance they give to 'Merit', and the opportunities it gives to people irrespective of religion, race, caste, and location. There is no room for complacency and incompetency.

Management Ethics

How can organizations maintain high standards of Ethical conduct?

The word 'Ethics' is derived from greek word 'Ethos', which means character and sentiments of society. According to concise Oxford dictionary, ethics is relating to morals, treating moral questions and being morally correct and honourable.

Ethics is
- Rightness or wrongness
- Goodness and badness of human conduct
- About standards and ideals
- About norms and values of certain seriousness
- A standard of behavior and ideals
- Principle of conduct governing an individual or profession
- Where a significant number of people do not look disdainfully
- Keeping promises
- Respecting sentiments of others
- Distribution of benefits and burdens in a fair and equitable way.
- A diagnostic tool that establishes and makes:
  – Moral standards
  – Norms of behavior
  – Judgments on moral behavior
  – Opinions and attitudes about human conduct.

Matters of hospital management do not figure prominently on the medical ethics agenda. However, management decisions that have to be taken in the area of hospital care are in fact riddled with ethical questions and do have significant impact on patients, staff members, and the community being served.

ETHICAL ISSUES IN HOSPITAL MANAGEMENT

The specific social setting of the hospital abounds in ethical problems and conflicts that neither involve, nor are caused directly by, the hospital management. Rude behavior towards patients during rounds, sloppy informed consent procedures before the inclusion of patients into clinical trials, or tensions within medical teams frequently do not even reach the management level. Nevertheless, hospital managers carry an exceptional responsibility for all activities in hospitals, because of their position in the institutional hierarchy and their decisive influence on the concrete framework within which the delivery of healthcare is taking place. Although it is less probable that decisions of the management will directly harm individual patients than a mistake by the medical staff, responsible decision making on the part of the hospital management is surely an important pre-condition if it is to be possible for hospital staff to integrate ethics into their daily work. The hospital manager bears responsibility to at least three parties: the patients who are being treated in the hospital; the staff; and the community that provides the funding for the institution. The long standing guidelines on ethical conduct and relationships for healthcare institutions of the American Hospital Association, (AHA) (first version issued in 1973), describe three corresponding areas of ethical concern: the responsibility of healthcare institutions for their patients; organizational issues within the hospital; and the community role of healthcare providers. These areas mirror the relevant interests which come together in the hospital. The interest of society to have effective healthcare institutions; the interest of patients to be treated adequately in the hospital; and the interest of hospital staff to work in an institution with appropriate ethical and social standards. What do these three areas mean in the context of everyday decisions that have to be taken by hospital managers? As far as the first area is concerned, healthcare institutions have a special accountability to their patients, due to the particular nature of the relationship between patients and healthcare providers in the hospital setting, which is usually highly asymmetrical, in terms of knowledge and authority. To protect the patients' personal rights, the AHA's code of conduct mentions several instruments, including: informed consent for diagnosis and therapy; the use of advance directives; confidentiality regarding patients' private data; and respect for social, spiritual, and cultural needs and beliefs. In addition, hospital managements have to ensure continuity of healthcare for all patients; and at the same time they should enable doctors to offer patients possible treatment alternatives and engage in the improvement of the quality of care and therapy.

As for the second area, organizational and staff issues, the hospital management has to make sure the institutional mission statements and policies do not conflict with the professional ethical codes of—for example—doctors and nurses. Beyond this requirement, hospital managements should aim to encourage and promote initiatives from medical staff to implement ethical guidelines in their daily work. Anyone familiar with the impact of rationing in medicine knows, however, that the scarcity of resources for healthcare produces ethical problems—either of resource allocation, or of a lack of working hours, which may limit staff engagement in activities that are ethically important. Hospital management can use its influence to reduce such problems and to maintain ethical standards. As in any other enterprise, employees and medical staff deserve fair compensation, fair benefits, and the opportunity to take part in continuing education in order to steadily improve the quality of healthcare.

As far as the third area is concerned, the community role of healthcare providers requires hospitals to structure their healthcare provision so as to adequately meet the needs of the society in a specific local setting, in order to fulfill their public functions. Given that there are no clear upper limits to the demand and supply of medical goods as illustrated—for example, by the much discussed definition of health offered by the World Health Organization (WHO)—it is necessary to use some rational criteria for resource allocation. Healthcare institutions must also give special consideration to the needs and medical problems of vulnerable groups, whether their vulnerability results from a specific lack of autonomy (as in the case of the very young, the elderly, or psychiatric patients), or from social marginalization, as in the case of poor or inadequately insured people.

Finally, healthcare institutions are financed by the fees of the insured or by other kinds of public funding and have therefore special duties to make "fair and effective use of available healthcare delivery resources". Hospital management is responsible to the public, at least in cases when it is the public which makes possible the existence and running of hospitals. In sum, hospital managers can exercise influence aimed at promoting ethical healthcare over a wide range of organizational features. Although medical ethics mainly deals with conflicts between the patients and their healthcare providers. It is clear to us that the features which frame the institutional setting, such as the hospital, in which such conflicts take place, are of considerable importance as well for finding appropriate solutions. The emergence and formulation of common and consensual codes of conduct in many hospitals today can be interpreted as a sign of a growing consciousness of such a wider perception of factors shaping moral conflicts in medicine.

Corporate Social Responsibility in Hospitals

Being responsible means finding the right balance between what patients want and what government can afford, and that staff are willing to provide the care needed. Doing this affects the entire hospital value chain.

"A business that does not show a profit at least equal to its cost of capital is irresponsible; it wastes society's resources. Economic profit performance is the base without which business cannot discharge any other responsibilities, cannot be a good employer, a good citizen, a good neighbor. But economic performance is not the only responsibility of a business. Every organization must assume responsibility for its impact on employees, the environment, customers, and whomever and whatever it touches. That is social responsibility."
— Peter Drucker

At the heart of delivering good private healthcare lies an apparent contradiction. Hospitals for profit are expected to make money, arguably capitalizing on patients' misfortune and suffering. Some may feel that being socially responsible means providing unlimited healthcare without paying attention to profit. Yet as Peter Drucker's quotation above shows, they would be wrong because being socially responsible is first and foremost about using scarce resources well and this applies to not-for-profit hospitals just as much as it does to profit-making hospitals. The advantage of profit-making hospitals is that normally profits are a good signal that what is being provided is valued and being done efficiently. Yet in this area too, there is a problem because some treatments cannot be justified on the ground of profits (Table 1.4).

Who are the Stakeholders?

So what do we really mean by corporate social responsibility (CSR) in the hospital context? Perhaps the easiest way to answer the question is to consider who the stakeholders of healthcare are. First and foremost they are customers (patients and families) served by hospitals, employees working in hospitals and government who have a vital interest in public health of electorates that can vote them out of office if they are dissatisfied with the health service they receive. Shareholders are also primary stakeholders, but in many countries they are regarded as less important because much of society still has to come to terms with the idea of making money from people's suffering.

Customers

In business, as opposed to healthcare the focus is on creating and retaining loyal customers. Again in the words of Peter Drucker:

Hospital Management

Table 1.4: CSR and the hospital value chain

R and D	Purchasing	Production	Outpatient Care	Marketing and Sales	Management Policies
Natural Capital					
• Biopracy • Patenting traditional remedies	• Environmental damage • Waste • Pollution • GHGs	• Pollution/Spills • Emissions/GHGs • Use of water • User of energy • Bandage/parts disposal			• 3 Rs – Reduce – Reuse – Recycle
Social Capital					
• Computation • Intellectual property • Abuse of indigenous people's knowledge	• Corruption • Social inequity • Abuse of indigenous people	• Corruption • Social inequity	• Corruption • Social inequity • Ethical marketing • Generics V. brands	• Corruption • Social inequity • Ethical marketing • Generics V. brands	• No competition • Obey the law • Avoid politics • Support
Human Captial					
• Discrimination • Human Rights • Union Rights • Health and Safety	• Discrimination • Human Rights • Unicon Rights • Health and Safety	• Discrimination • Human Rights • Unicon Rights • Health and Safety	• Discrimination • Unicon Rights • Health and Safety • Working hours	• Discrimination • Human Rights • Health and Safety • Working hours	• Diversity and inclusion • Meritocracy • Respect Union Rights • Good health and safety • Good working hours • Pay for performance

"It is the customer who determines what a business is. For it is the customer, and he alone, who though willing to pay for a good or a service, converts economic resources into wealth, things into goods. What the business thinks it produces is not of the first importance—especially not to the future of the business and to its success. What the customer thinks he is buying, what he considers 'value' is decisive—it determines what a business is, what it produces and whether it will prosper.

The customer is the foundation of a business and keeps it in existence. He alone gives employment. And it is to supply the consumer that society entrusts wealth-producing resource to the business enterprise." — Drucker: the Practice of Management.

There are, however, problems when we apply this thinking to healthcare:
- Patients demand the best care regardless of economic justification and are often unable to pay for it, looking to government to meet the bill.
- Government are finding they can no longer afford to do this.
- Successful healthcare reduces the number of patient visits; it does not try to maximize loyalty or retention, unlike business. We cannot, therefore, adopt a customer focussed approach designed to maximize repeat purchase.

The first responsibility is to use scarce resources well and private hospitals have the benefit of the profit mechanism to signal they are doing this. Being responsible means finding the right balance between what patients want and government can afford, ensuring that society as a whole has good standards of public health, and that staff are willing and able to provide the care needed. It affects the entire hospital value chain. Doing this well guarantees access to patient demand and employee supply and ensures public acceptability and acceptance of private medicine, thus ensuring the long term success that shareholders demand if they are to get an adequate return on their investment.

Conclusion

Hospital as an organization is highly complex. It is an organization which continuously engages with its end customers, i.e. patients. Most of the core activities of the hospital are unplanned, but at the same time requires highest level of coordination which makes managing hospitals highly challenging.

References

American Hospital Association (AHA). AHA management advisory—ethical conduct for healthcare institutions. Chicago: AHA, 1992. http://www.hospitalconnect.com/aha/resource_center/resource/resource_ethics.html (accessed 21 Jan 2004).

Biller-Andorno N, Lie R, ter Meulen R. Evidence based medicine as an instrument for rational health policy. Health Care Anal 2002: 10:261–75.

Biller-Andorno N, Karageorgiou A. Evidence based medicine in Germany. Paper presented at the European Union EVIBASE project State of the Art and Health Care; 2001 Feb 2–3; Maastricht.

Biller—Andorno N. Evidenz-basierte Gesundheitsversorgung—kritische Nachfragen vor medizinethischem Hintergrund. Wien Med Wochenschr 2002;152:161–4.

Dickenson D, Vineis P. Evidence based medicine and quality of care. Health Care Anal 2002; 10:243–59.

Francis CM, MarioC de Souza Hospital Administration, Jaypee Brothers, Medical Publishers (P) Ltd., New Delhi, 2000.

George, MA: The Hospital Administrator, Jaypee Brothers, Medical Publishers (P) Ltd., New Delhi, 2008.

Glaeske G. Evidence based medicine aus Sicht der Krankenkassen—ein Rahmen für qualifizierte Therapiefreiheit und verbesserte Wirtschaftlichkeit? Z Arztl Fortbild Qualita

Leititis JU. Stationa̋re Leistungserbringung unter DRGs. Krankenhaus 2002; 152:161–4.

Leititis JU. Evidence for health policy: evidence based medicine/healthcare and the cost effectiveness debate. Commentary presented at the EVIBASE Workshop: Evidence based medicine as an instrument for rational health policy; 2001 Sept 28–29; Goettingen.

Llewellyn-Daview, R, Macaulay, H.M.C.: Hospital Planning and Administration, World Health Organization-Geneva, Jaypee Brothers, 1995.

Mintzberg, Henry et.al., The Strategy Process, 4th edition, Englewood Cliffs, NJ: Prentice Hall, 2002.

Sakharkar BM,: Principles of Hospital Administration and Planning, Jaypee Brothers, Medical Publishers (P) Ltd., New Delhi, 2000.

2
Introduction to Healthcare

Pavan Kumar

The Practice of Medicine

For centuries, the subject of medicine was more art than science. Doctors applied fashionable nostrums, blend their patients or starved them. In general, these remedies were ineffective, sometimes fortuitously beneficial or extremely harmful. The prestige of a doctor rested more on the status of his patients and the confidence of his assertions than on the evidence of his cures. But in the last fifty years, the application of scientific method to medical subjects has transformed their effectiveness. Medicine is now a practical subject. The experience and judgment of a good doctor is as important as the extent of his knowledge and the quality of his training.

Until recently, the evolution of clinical practice has been piecemeal and uncoordinated, driven by individual clinicians. Towards the end of the nineteenth century, groups of physicians in the Western World, notably in the USA and the UK banded together to form specialist boards and colleges that laid down codes of conduct and practice for their members. The American Boards and the Royal Colleges take on the responsibility of ensuring that only those specialists registered with them are allowed to practice. They also produce guidelines for the management of common conditions and take action against those practitioners who indulge in malpractice or have been medically negligent.

The Indian Scene

Unfortunately, in India, clinical practice is still disorganized, uncoordinated, unregulated and unchecked. Regulatory bodies exist, but only on paper and even the Medical Council of India are unable to enforce codes of practice on registered physicians. Judicial delays mean that even those patients and their relatives who are willing to take on errant practitioners are made to run from pillar to post even to obtain a hearing in court. Invariably, by the time a judgment is passed, the patient has either died or given up the frustrating task of bringing the culprits to book. Rampant malpractice and criminal negligence is the order of the day.

However, the consumer, i.e. patient, is gradually becoming more and more knowledgeable, sophisticated and aware of his/her rights. Increasing incomes have encouraged patients and their relatives further to seek redress from the higher courts. Consumer forums have sprung up in many cities willing to take on the might of the establishment. Patients are less likely to accept a medical mistake for granted without compensation. There is thus a need for some kind of regulation or monitoring of clinical personnel at the local level since neither the Government, nor the judiciary, nor are even the medical bodies willing to take charge of the situation. Those responsible for managing and funding healthcare, both in the public and private health sector, are becoming aware of the need to develop a new relationship within which clinicians and managers within hospitals can work together to guide the course of clinical practice.

The Need for Healthcare

Worldwide, the need and demand for healthcare is increasing. In India, the rate of growth of both need and demand is faster than the rate of increase in resources available for providing it. The main reasons for the increase in healthcare need and demand are:

Population ageing: This is the singlemost important factor 'increasing the need for healthcare. As the number of older people increases, so does the need for healthcare.

New technology and knowledge: Advances in medicine increase the need for healthcare. The knowledge that an effective intervention exists for a disease previously thought to be incurable leads to public and professional demand for that service to be provided. Sometimes the application of a new technology will result in lower health costs or in lower costs elsewhere in the economy. However, there is often an increase in cost in the short term.

Patient expectations: This is rising day by day, reflecting societal changes in attitude towards the provision of goods and services, a trend usually called consumerism. Patients expect:
1. Easy access to services
2. High quality services
3. Compensation in case there is failure, or a perceived failure of service professional expectations: These are influenced by patient expectations. If 90 year aged wants hip replacements, this will affect professional attitudes and expectations about the services that should be offered. There may also be a negative effect. The threat of litigation may stimulate an increase in the practice of defensive medicine, i.e. excessive, unnecessary investigations and inappropriate treatments that will push up the cost of healthcare.

Healthcare Problems

The challenges to the provision of healthcare such as population ageing, rising patient expectations and the advent of new technologies are not restricted to the developed nations alone. Healthcare in India has not *only* to address the above problems but also more pressing issues such as high infant and maternal mortality rates and prevention and management of infectious diseases. As problems associated with the delivery of healthcare increase, the solutions being sought by the government can be characterized by certain features; measures for cost control Development of systems to prevent the burden of cost falling on the individual encouragement of public to take up healthcare insurance plans. The need for purchasers of healthcare to manage the evolution and development of clinical practice in partnership with clinical professions increased public and political interest in the evidence on which decisions about the effectiveness and safety of healthcare are based.

The Indian healthcare system is undergoing a revolution today. There are an increasing number of paying patients owing to a higher standard of living. These patients are also knowledgeable and sophisticated, demanding care of the highest quality. The days are gone when patients meekly accepted the doctor's word irrespective of the effect of the treatment on them. Consumer associations and forums are growing at an exponential rate, educating people on their rights and representing them in cases of negligence or malpractice.

The burgeoning growth of the private sector with more and more people joining private firms rather than settling for government jobs has resulted in a mushrooming of employee healthcare plans and contracting of healthcare services with local established hospitals. These corporate clients and companies demand the best for their employees both in terms of healthcare and quality of ancillary services such as cleanliness of rooms, decor, food, etc.

The opening of the insurance sector to private and foreign investors has added another referral and purchaser of healthcare services in the country.

Insurance companies are actively soliciting members and entering into contracts with preferred providers who have been vetted in terms of healthcare provision. Added to this is the growing cost of healthcare that is rising at an alarming rate.

Rapidly developing expensive technology increasing ageing population with a concomitant increase in chronic ailments.

Increasing medicolegal litigations leading to the practice of defensive medicine.

This includes excessive, expensive, unnecessary investigations and extra treatments that could have been avoided.

Managed Healthcare

Clinical decisions are the product of healthcare. They are of direct and immediate importance to patients and are also of importance to those who manage and fund health services since one outcome of clinical decision-making is expenditure by health services. No service has infinite resources and the health service certainly is no exception to this rule. It has been shown that in any health system with finite resources, changes in the volume and intensity of clinical practice constitute the major factor driving the increase in healthcare costs that can be controlled (Eddy 1993). There is also an increasing public and political interest in the evidence on which decisions about the effectiveness and safety of healthcare are based. This has created a need to manage, in a standard manner, the care of patients who suffer from the same condition. This is known as managed healthcare. By itself, managed healthcare is a misnomer. Healthcare has to be managed by someone. When the patient treats himself or herself, for example, when you take paracetamol for a headache, you are practicing self-care, when the patient goes to a clinic or hospital and is treated by the doctor there, it is called formal care. In both instances the patient or the doctor is managing care.

Managed care, however, refers to an external or third party managed care where in addition to the physician and the patient, a third party, usually the insurance company of which patient is a member, is involved in the clinical decision-making process. This is particularly true in America where over 40% of the populations have medical insurance. Other countries in Europe are following suit. The whole aim is to make savings based on the provision of cost effective care. It is an undeniable fact that no matter how much managed care practitioners extol the virtues of their art on the basis of quality, patient satisfaction or value, the biggest driver for managed care is the need to control costs. This has generated heated opposition from doctors and other healthcare professionals, who wish to retain the discretion to make their own decisions on the management of a patient's condition.

Within a managed care system, standard care is delivered to a group of patients who have certain common conditions for which it is possible to define a core set of interventions and services which those suffering from that condition should receive. For example, BUPA, the largest health insurance company in the UK, laid out clinical criteria for hysterectomy in 1999 with the approval of the Royal college of Obstetricians and Gynecologists. The criteria do not differ from the college guidelines and ensure that this operative procedure is performed only for well-defined indications. Thus all gynecologists will perform a hysterectomy only for certain conditions and not as and when they wish to. The only difference between the guidelines or protocols set out by a managed care plan produced by an insurance company such as BUPA and those produced by medical bodies such as the American Boards or the Royal Colleges in the UK is that the guidelines of the insurance company have teeth. In other words, policing of the regulations will be much tighter and sanctions more common in managed care.

Origins of Managed Healthcare

Managed healthcare originated in the USA. The 20th century in the USA witnessed the transformation of medical practice from generalist to specialist, from solo to group practice, from direct payment for healthcare to group insurance and from a predominantly cottage industry to increasing emphasis on the corporate management of medical care. Managed medical care is strictly an outgrowth of the private sector, dating back over 70 years. The year 1929 witnessed the establishment of the first rural farmers' cooperative health plan in Oklahoma. In the same year, two Californian physicians in Los Angeles entered into a prepaid contract to provide comprehensive health services to about 2000 water company employees. These two plans were harbingers of managed care eventually serving about 40% of the American public in the early 1990's.

Several other prepaid group practice plans started between 1930 and 1960.

Prominent amongst these were the Group Health Association in Washington D.C. in 1937 and the Kaiser-Permanente Medical Care Program in 1942.

Managed Care in the West

Some of the main types of healthcare systems in the USA are:

Health Maintenance Organizations (HMOs)

HMOs are organized healthcare systems that are responsible for both the financing and delivery of a broad range of comprehensive health services to an enrolled population. An HMO can be viewed as a combination of a health insurer and a healthcare delivery system. Whereas traditional healthcare insurance companies are responsible for reimbursing covered individuals for the cost of their healthcare, HMOs are responsible for providing healthcare services to their covered members through affiliated providers who are then reimbursed. HMOs must therefore ensure that their members have access to covered healthcare services. In addition, HMOs generally are responsible for assuring the quality and appropriateness of the health services they provide to their members.

Preferred Provider Organizations (PPOs)

PPOs are entities through which employer health benefit plans and health insurance carriers contract to purchase healthcare services for covered beneficiaries from a selected group of participating providers. In contrast to traditional HMO coverage, individuals with PPO coverage are permitted to use non-PPO providers. Although higher levels of co-insurance or deductibles routinely apply to services provided by these non-participating providers.

PPOs, as a recent development in managed care, are often considered to be evolving HMOs. The PPO in its simplest form is a contractual arrangement between professional and/or institutional healthcare providers and employers, insurance carriers, or third party administrators to provide healthcare services, often at discounted rates. The PPO first appeared in the medical marketplace in the late 1970s. Unlike the HMO, however, the PPO reimburses the patient for covered services obtained from any provider at the discounted rate set for preferred providers; the patient then has to pay out of pocket the balance between the scheduled fee and the billed amount.

Exclusive Provider Organizations (EPOs)

EPOs is similar to PPOs in their organization and purpose. Unlike PPOs, however, EPOs limit their beneficiaries to participating providers for all healthcare services.

Individual Practice Associations (IPA)

A variant of the prepaid group practice plan appeared in 1954, when a prototype IPA (individual practice association) was established in California. A relative value fee schedule for guaranteeing payment was adopted and a sincere attempt was made to monitor the quality of care.

Both prepaid groups and IPAs was the opening wedge for a new kind of health delivery in the United States, whereby physicians shared the risk of financing healthcare for an enrolled population. These models led to widespread dissemination of managed care plans. HMOs assumed responsibility for providing a comprehensive range of health services to voluntarily enrolled populations at a fixed annual premium.

The evolution of these pioneer practice plans in the private sector was one of the most extraordinary developments in the history of medical care organization in the world. Physicians were, and are, given career choices between a fee-for-service practice and payment under corporate control.

Conclusion

There is no doubt that the major reason for promulgating managed care is to make savings on healthcare. Unlike any other service, the demand for healthcare can never be satisfied. The more the services, the more the needs and demands of the population that they serve. Unfortunately, resources for the provision of healthcare are limited, both in the public and private sectors.

Although managers understand this, the public and even the professionals do not. They seem to assume that there is a bottomless pit from which resources can be drawn at will. With increasing expenses in medical care and the use of more sophisticated and expensive instruments, a time will come when even in developing nations like India, managed care needs to be practiced if we are to provide healthcare to the majority of the community. Resources need to be spread out to provide the greatest good to the greatest majority. With the advent of private healthcare insurance companies in the country, managed care will assume prime importance in the years to come.

EVIDENCE-BASED CARE

The Need for Evidence

As consumerism increases, there is pressure on professionals, especially doctors, to show proof that the treatments they prescribe or the operations that they carry out are based on good quality research work or approved by fellow specialists in the field. Written evidence must be available that concurs with the physician's management of a particular condition. No longer it is enough for a physician to stand up in court and attribute his or her actions to clinical experience. Treatments and procedures must be backed up with research evidence from peer-reviewed journals or follow the guidelines laid down by the august bodies such as the American Board or the Royal Colleges. We are now entering an era of evidence-based practice.

Even today, many healthcare decisions are based on values and resources, this is called opinion-based decision-making. As the pressure on resources increases, decisions will have to be made publicly and explicitly; those who take decisions will need to be able to produce and describe the evidence on which each decision was based. There has to be, therefore, a transition from opinion-based decision-making to evidence-based decision making.

Definition

Evidence-based clinical practice is an approach to decision-making in which the clinician uses the best evidence available in consultation with the patient, to decide upon the option that suits the patient best.

"Evidence-based medicine is the process of systematically reviewing, appraising and using clinical research findings to aid the delivery of optimum clinical care to patients."
(Rosenberg and Donald, 1995)

The practice of evidence-based healthcare enables those managing health services to determine the mix of services and procedures that will give the greatest benefit to the population served by that health service. To ensure that a population receives the maximum health benefit at the lowest possible risk and cost from the resources available, both evidence-based healthcare and quality management are essential practices.

Evidence-based healthcare + Quality management = Maximum health benefit at lowest risk and cost.

Evidence-based Care in India

Evidence-based care is not restricted to the developed nations. There is a much greater need for such practice to be initiated and propagated in third world countries such as India. Its major role is in the field of public health. There are a number of interventions that have been shown to do more good than harm at reasonable cost but which are not yet widely adopted in countries with developing economies such as India. These include the administration of aspirin that reduces the health and economic burden resulting from stroke; and vitamin A supplementation that reduces morbidity and mortality in children.

Conversely, there are other interventions that have not yet been shown to be effective but which are in routine use—these interventions of unproven effectiveness consume resources that could be expanded on those which do more good than harm at a reasonable cost, such as routine anti-malarial chemoprophylaxis during pregnancy. Thus evidence-based decision-making has a role in the provision of healthcare in all countries, irrespective of the stage of their economic development.

The best healthcare is that
1. From which, based on the best evidence available, all ineffective interventions have been eliminated.
2. In which the interventions undertaken are of the highest possible effectiveness.
3. In which all services are delivered at the highest possible quality.

However, the health of a population is determined by four factors, only one of which is healthcare. The others are:
- Physical environment
- Social environment and lifestyle
- Genetics

Thus even the provision of the best healthcare will not necessarily ensure optimum levels of health in a population. However, by using evidence-based care, we can at least seek to improve the health of the population and reduce the horrendously high morbidity and mortality statistics. Efforts made in this direction through managed healthcare will be a start on the long road to health recovery.

MANAGEMENT FUNCTIONS IN MANAGED CARE

Planning in Hospitals

Managed healthcare elements in any hospital are intended to control the inappropriate use of healthcare services. It is generally accepted that the mission of managed healthcare is to deliver high quality health and medical care services at a competitive price. Hospital managers need to design a set of objectives for the organization. The process calls for a continuous input from physicians, hospitals and consumers in response to changes in the internal and external environment.

Strategic Planning

This is the process of setting long-term objectives for the future. Strategic planning, when carried out effectively, necessarily influences the future professional and business prospects of a managed medical care plan. Risks are involved in strategic planning, but even greater risk results from not planning strategically.

Resource Planning

This involves the acquisition and allocation of fixed capital. Equipment capital, human capital and operating capital in the healthcare arena in which the managed care process must function. Managers must give physician recruitment and retention a very high priority.

Facility Planning

Step down care is part and parcel of facility planning. By its very nature, either in a nursing home, at home or ambulatory care, it is less expensive than a hospital bed. This would ensure continued care of the patient but at a lesser cost. Consideration may be given to providing step down care facilities within the hospital itself. This would ensure continued revenue to the hospital, patient satisfaction as he or she would not have to leave the hospital before being declared fit to do so and encourage more insurance companies and other purchasers to negotiate contracts.

Financial Planning

Financial planning in managed healthcare has many facets but has to focus on the budget as its main planning tool. The opportunity for innovation in management-oriented cost accounting is not impeded by the traditional encumbrances of hospital accounting. Investment in innovation may provide exceptionally good opportunities to enhance the performance of managed healthcare in general and to improve the quality of medical care in particular. Communicating the importance of financial planning to physicians should be the main goal for managed medical care plans if they are to make low-cost and high quality healthcare accessible to patients.

Planning in Insurance Companies

The growth of managed care mirrors the growth of the insurance industry in the United States. There is a greater need for insurance companies to manage the care provided in hospitals and by consultants as this is the only means by which they retain profitability. Every health insurance company must have some elements of managed care, if not a full-fledged set up, in its organization to ensure the provision of cost effective care.

Insurance companies operate in a different way from corporate purchasers of healthcare. Instead of negotiating contracts for services to employees, there are health plans that cover those people (called members) who pay the premiums of the insurance company. Health insurance policies have coverage criteria by which the companies fine-tune the categories of services covered and seek to balance cost control with the provision of a range of services attractive to members.

It is upon these coverage criteria that guidelines, protocols and clinical policies are developed and a system of managed care created.

Coverage criteria are the means insurers use to promote evidence-based healthcare. Evidence obtained from randomized controlled trials, systematic reviews of trials and convincing non-experimental evidence is taken to be sufficient to demonstrate good quality healthcare (Eddy 1996).

There is sufficient evidence to draw conclusions about the intervention's effects on health outcomes. The evidence demonstrates that the intervention can be expected to produce the intended effects on health outcomes. The intervention is the most cost effective method available to address the medical condition. The intervention's expected beneficial effects on health outcomes outweigh the expected harmful effects. Who is managing the patient?

Shifting the responsibility for medical care from each individual practitioner to corporate control, either via the hospital or the insurance company, raises issues of an ethical nature in many physicians' minds.

One of the fears of the medical profession is that evidence-based healthcare and managed healthcare will be used as a means to remove individual professional liberty. This is an issue being hotly debated in the USA in response to the greater control exerted there, but it is also beginning to be joined in by other countries as different techniques, such as the production of "critical pathways" are introduced by those who manage or purchase healthcare.

In general, physicians see managed care as a general threat and a pain in the neck. The issue of loss of or impingement on autonomy is perhaps the most emotionally charged one.

Undoubtedly changing the mindset of consultants is a cumbersome task. Physicians are unique with their strong need for autonomy and control, potential for role conflicts and ingrained practice habits (Kongstvedt, 1995).

From being a sole decision-maker, the consultant would now have to provide clinical details to a third party to confirm eligibility for the procedure. Lipkin in 1996 aptly described this transition in the fortunes of American physicians over the years. From being free spirits and flying high, they are amongst the most tightly controlled in the world, a change described as "from pegasus to Sisyphus".

Managed care at times places the physician in an adversarial relationship with a patient. This is uncomfortable because physicians are not trained for it. It most often comes up in the guise of clearly unnecessary or medically marginal care that is demanded by the patient, dispute may also occur when something is medically necessary but not a covered benefit. Most doctors, if not all, are faced with this situation in their clinics at fairly regular intervals. The insistence on antibiotic prescription for common colds and other viral infections is the best example of an unnecessary treatment being forced by the patient.

Some physicians have a real fear that managed care can lead to a decreased quality of care. This has never been proven. On the contrary, there is data to show good quality of care along with lower utilization (Ware *et. al.*, 1987, Clancy and Hillier, 1989). Nevertheless the fear remains and coupled with this is the fear of increased malpractice liability if guidelines are not followed to the letter. This fear is again unfounded.

Healthcare companies practising managed care are well aware that no two patients are the same. It is not possible to impose strict guidelines on doctors.

There is enough flexibility in the protocols for clinical judgment that even the courts acknowledge. What managing care achieves is to ensure that there is no gross negligence or wildly inappropriate treatment, e.g. removing the gall bladder without investigating the cause for abdominal pain.

The Doctor–Manager

Organizational skills are essential for the successful operation of any medical practice and are especially important in managed healthcare plans.

Increasingly, physicians with organizational skills are being recruited to assume responsibility for top-level managerial positions, for motivating others, for assessing performance and for developing good working relationships with other health professionals. Physicians are uniquely prepared to manage specific problems arising from clinical practice, diagnostic procedures and therapeutic interventions. The role of the medical director, though vital in healthcare organizations, will remain a challenge until enough physicians are recruited or trained to function as managers as well as clinicians.

Quite often, doctors do not wish to work as managers or medical directors. However, it must be realized that medical directors by virtue of their knowledge, training and experience can resolve many of the operational problems that occur in managed care systems. The non-physician chief executive of a hospital should thus delegate full clinical authority to his/her medical director. But it should be kept in mind that the non-physician manager will be legally liable for contracting for doctors' services or for defects in the design or implementation of cost containment mechanisms.

Managing the Doctor

The directing function in managed healthcare plans requires skill in delegating authority appropriately while continuing to assume responsibility for both operating activities and clinical care. The problem of distinguishing authority from responsibility can be resolved by observing that one can delegate the authority to perform tasks but one cannot be relieved of the responsibility for them. Some say it is a truism that the manager must always retain responsibility for any task assigned to a subordinate. Although the non-physician manager can delegate the authority for delivering patient care to a physician, only a licensed physician can provide such a service.

So how should a non-clinical manager deal with a doctor?

It may become easier if we understand the different styles of management. A direct management style makes clear the rewards and punishments affecting the quality of performance.

A middle approach offers subordinates the manager's friendship, concern and approachability. The manager may at times consult with the employee on how to carry out a certain task.

At the other end of the spectrum, a positive management style assumes that an employee has the capability to perform a task and will accept the responsibility.

Many health professionals are trained to perform with a minimum of supervision and a high degree of autonomy when undertaking clinical tasks. Under these circumstances, style will not be successful.

The importance of the coordinating ability of the manager cannot be overemphasized. Ambiguity and conflict constitute core characteristics of complex organizations such as managed healthcare. The larger the hospital, the more the managers and doctors, the greater the potential for differences of opinions.

Great skill is required to minimize internal organizational conflicts.

Coordinating functions are also essential for opening and maintaining vertical and horizontal lines of communication.

NEGOTIATING

Definitions

The word 'provider' is used to describe a doctor or a clinic or hospital. In essence, it refers to anyone who is providing a healthcare service to the patient.

Purchaser identifies a company or corporate group who is purchasing healthcare in bulk for their members or employees.

Purchaser does not refer to the individual patient. The patient or person seeking healthcare is regarded as a client, consumer or customer.

Referrer is usually applied to general practitioners or insurance companies who link with specific hospitals or consultants and ensure that their members or patients obtain healthcare only from these hospitals or specialists.

In all healthcare textbooks, including this module, the above terms are used frequently. In order to provide services to the population where they are located, providers enter into contracts with purchasers and referrers to ensure a steady stream of customers (patients).

Contract-based networks are a hallmark of managed care. The provision of healthcare services from providers (doctors or hospitals) who are not under contract can be a real barrier to effective medical management if the volume of such service is high.

Advantages of Contracts with Consultants or Hospitals

- Ability to negotiate discounts through providing an agreed volume of referrals.
- Guarantee payments for authorized services for covered benefits. This eliminates uncertainty.

- Provide a regular revenue stream depending on the volume of work and the payment mechanism. This can be a powerful incentive especially in an overcrowded medical market or for a new hospital or consultant.
- Prevent competitors from gaining market share.
- Ability to guarantee quality of healthcare by contracting with selected providers.

Types of Reimbursements for Doctors

Fee-for-service

Hospitals in developed nations usually have a fee-for-service plan. There are different rates for different types of treatments and operative procedures.

These are listed in a code book produced by the hospital and are based on disease categories in the International Classification of Diseases, Tenth Revision (ICD-IO) code or Diagnosis Related Groups (ORCS). Separate codes are provided for diagnoses or disorders and a fee is fixed for each code depending on the severity of the illness.

Consider back pain as an example. Sudden (acute) back pain may be due to a simple muscle spasm (also called non-specific back pain) or due to a herniation of the intervertebral disc (disc prolapse). Non-specific acute back pain will have a certain code with a fee of, say (x) amount. Disc prolapse, on the other hand, is a much more severe condition that may require surgery. Hence the fee may be (2x). Specialists are thus paid according to the nature of the disease and the complexity of the treatment or surgical procedure.

In a system where economic reward is predicated on how much one does, particularly if procedural services pay more than cognitive ones, it is only human nature to do more, especially when it pays more. The reward is immediate and tangible. A larger bill is made out and it usually gets paid. Doing less results in getting paid less.

The other side of the coin is that fee-for-service distribution results in the distribution of payment on the basis of expenditure of resources. Thus a physician who is caring for sicker patients will be paid more, reflecting that physician's greater investment of time, energy and skills.

Problems with Fee-for-service Plans

There are two significant problems with using fee-for-service in managed healthcare. These problems can become markedly exacerbated if the hospital or insurer starts to get into financial trouble. Both can be resolved to some extent by managing the care provided by doctors.

The first problem is churning. This simply means that physicians perform more procedures than are really necessary and schedule patient revisits at frequent intervals. A few doctors consciously churn, but it does happen, even if unconsciously.

The second major problem is up coding and unbundling. Up coding refers to a slow creeping upward of impairment codes that pay more; for example, a routine office visit becomes an extended one, a cervical smear becomes a full gynecological examination or an ovarian cyst removal becomes a laparotomy. In the example of back pain given above, the doctor may treat the condition as non-specific back pain but may list the code for disc prolapse. As treatment modalities for back pain vary widely depending on the doctor concerned, it is difficult, even for another specialist in the same field, to judge the correct diagnosis based on the treatment given.

Unbundling refers to charging for services that were previously included in a single fee without lowering the original fee, e.g. a single outpatient visit is split into a charge for consultation, application of dressing, prescription charge, etc. instead of billing all under one heading. Thus even if there is a contract for a lump sum fee for outpatient services, the hospital or insurer ends up paying more.

Management of Fee-for-service Plans

All hospitals have accounts and billing departments while insurance companies have claims departments. The majority of insurers also have some personnel involved in data collection on their members' claims. Thus the claims department in coordination with the data analysis department is best placed to monitor these problems. Hospitals, however, rarely have systems in place to capture data other than the clinical audits carried out by their own doctors.

It has been said that over 80% of the costs borne by hospitals are due to physicians and the treatments they offer to their patients. If hospitals wish to be profitable, they need to look into the clinical practice and billing procedures of their professionals.

Two useful approaches are

The first is to look for trends by providers. Individuals who are trying to game the system will usually stand out. If there is one physician also has a 40% increased length of stay in hospital compared to the others in the same department, it is worth investigating.

The second approach is to automate the claims system to re-bundle unbundled claims and to separate for review any claims that appear to have a gross mismatch between services rendered and the clinical reason for the visit.

The only effective approach to churning is tight management (or switching to capitation). Some hospitals develop physician peer review committee to review utilization. The committee have the authority to sanction physicians who abuse the system. This has some slowing effect. The actions of such committee should follow a process that includes warnings and a probationary period in which expectations for improvement are clearly outlined.

An even better method is to manage the process such that a few sanctions are necessary. This means controlling referrals, controlling hospital and institutional utilization and negotiating effective discounts with providers and hospitals. It also means close monitoring utilization and billing patterns and acting when necessary. It requires the setting up of a utilization management (UM) team comprising of nurses and a medical director to oversee all aspects of patient care.

Capitation

One alternative for the problems of fee-for-service plans is to use a capitation fee. Although it is initially harder to calculate and harder to gain acceptance from doctors, this system has less likelihood of leading to over-utilization than fee-for-service.

Here the provider is paid a set amount per patient per month. If done properly, it can be valuable both to the consultant and/ or hospital and the insurer, a genuine win-win situation. If done poorly, it can be a source of perennial problems.

One must first calculate the expected volume of referrals, the average cost, ability to control utilization and relative negotiating strength. Past data is required and the services of an actuary would be useful to determine the correct capitation amount.

Capitation has the advantage of allowing one to budget for expected medical costs and to place a degree of risk and reward on the provider. The financial incentives encourage the provider to be a more active participant in contributing utilization.

Problems of inappropriate underutilization must be guarded against effective monitoring and an effective quality assurance system.

Retainer

This is the payment of a set amount to a provider every month and evaluates at periodic intervals the actual utilization. In other words, the specialist is paid a monthly salary. This ensures availability of the provider and provides for the steady income desired by the provider while still allowing payment on the basis of actual utilization.

Flat Rate

A flat rate is used for a well-defined set of procedures. It is usually done as part of a negotiation for a discount on charges, e.g. an obstetrician may be charged a flat rate for either a vaginal delivery or a caesarean section. The charge for either procedure will be the same regardless of how much or how little time and effort are spent.

Global Fee

Global fees must be carefully defined as to what they include and what may be billed outside them. For example, if an ultrasound scan is billed outside the global fee for obstetrics, one will need to monitor its use to determine whether any providers are using and billing for an abnormally high number of ultrasound scans per case.

Relative Value Scale (RVS)

In this system, each procedure or treatment, as defined by the procedure codes, has a relative value associated with it. The plan pays the physician on the basis of a monetary multiplier for the RVS value.

Relative values for different treatments are arrived at by consensus with leading specialists in the respective fields. Values are assigned depending on the complexity or duration of treatment and also take into account any special expertise required of the doctor that his or her colleagues in the same field may not possess. For example, not many surgeons are trained and skilled in extended cancer surgery of the head and neck. This is an area requiring special expertise. It is also a time-consuming operation and can be very complex.

Hence the relative value for this procedure is much higher than for a routine simple procedure such as tonsillectomy.

Relative values have a much wider acceptance amongst consultants than fee for service plans. Costing of procedures is done after much debate amongst professionals in the field and appropriate weightage is given for the type of treatment offered. The approach is much more scientific and logical than the arbitrary allocation of fees based on ICD or DRG classifications. Payment is based on the treatment provided. This appeals to the doctors, as there may be several methods of management of the same condition.

Another advantage of using RVS is in negotiations. 'U' a procedure has a value of 4 and the multiplier is ₹ 12, the payment is ₹ 48. Changes in fees involve negotiation of the multiplier, which is easier and does not undermine the value of the procedure.

A major problem with RVS is the imbalance between procedural and cognitive services. In other words, there is less payment to a physician performing a careful history and examination than for a minor surgical procedure. This has changed in the USA with the adoption of the resource-based relative value scale (RBRVS).

RBRVS has addressed to some extent the imbalance between cognitive and procedural services, i.e. lowering the value of some surgical procedures and raising the value of cognitive ones such as outpatient visits.

Hospital consultants can thus be paid in a variety of ways. It is apparent, however, that whatever system is used, there must be some means of crosschecking that the physician concerned has rendered appropriate involves the use of managed care techniques.

Types of Reimbursements for Hospitals

Corporate clients, large companies and insurance groups often negotiate contracts with hospitals in order to reduce the charges per employee or member. Corporate clients may deal directly with hospital managers or go through their insurance brokers who strike a deal for them.

Discounted Fee-for-service

This is applicable to insurance companies or brokers.

There are two variations here:
- A straight discount on charges, e.g. 15 or 20%.
- A discount based on volume or a sliding scale. For example, up to 10 cases per month there could be a 10% discount, from 10–20 cases per month this could increase to 15%. Thus the greater the volume of patients referred to the hospital, the more the discount.

Package Pricing

This refers to reimbursement for the entire procedure such as cardiac bypass surgery. The full fee covers all hospital charges, anesthetist and surgical fees and all pre and postoperative.

The advantage of package pricing is that there are no financial surprises at the end of the patient's stay in hospital. Furthermore, if the patient has a postoperative complication or needs to stay in longer in hospital, the hospital will have to absorb the cost and cannot pass on the same to the insurer or purchaser.

A major disadvantage is that even if the patient is discharged earlier, the full price agreed to must be paid. The cost of providing care is solely dependent on the number of patients treated and there is no leeway to make savings.

Straight Per Diem (day) Charges

This is a single charge for a day in the hospital regardless of any actual charges or costs incurred. The key to making *this* system work is predict ability. If you can accurately predict the number and mix of cases, you can calculate a per diem rate. The per diem is simply an estimate of the charges (or costs) for an average day in that hospital minus the amount of discount you feel is appropriate.

A disadvantage is that the per diem must be paid even if the billed charges are less than the per diem rate. For example, if the cost per day is ₹ 800 for a medical admission for five days, the total reimbursement comes to ₹ 4000 even if the hospital bills only ₹ 3300 for services rendered. This is acceptable as long as the average per diem rate represents an acceptable discount.

Sliding Scale Per Diem

Like the sliding scale discount on charges discussed earlier, this is also based on total volume. In this case, you negotiate an interim per diem that you agree to pay for each day in the hospital. Depending on the total number of bed days in the year, you will either pay a lump sum settlement at the end of the year or withhold an amount from your final payment for the year to adjust for an additional reduction in the per diem from an increase in total bed days.

Differential by Day in Hospital

Most hospitalizations are more expensive on the first day especially for surgical cases. This type of reimbursement is generally combined with a per diem approach, but the first day is paid at a higher rate. For example, the first day after surgery usually requires more intensive monitoring. The charge for the first postoperative day may be fixed at ₹ 1000. From day two of surgery the charge is reduced to ₹ 600 per day, as there is less need for close nursing supervision.

Diagnosis Related Groups (DRGs)

DRGs may be used to pay for inpatient care. Publications of ORG categories and criteria can be used to negotiate a payment mechanism.

There are disadvantages with this method:

If the intention is to reduce unnecessary utilization, this may not occur if only ORCS are being used.

If the payment is fixed on the basis of diagnosis, any reduction in days will result in a loss to the purchaser. Unless careful audits are performed regularly, code creeping may occur.

Conclusion

Opportunities for implementing research-based evidence are thus offered by managed care, in which a systematic approach to care management is taken and a greater use is made of clinical guidelines. Strategies employed by managed care ensure that:

Opportunities offered by managed care promote evidence-based clinical decision-making.

Contracting with providers ensures a reduction in charges.

Data collection and analysis by dedicated utilization management teams to identify outliers and processes created to take action against errant providers.

MANAGING DOCTORS
Introduction

The practice behavior of physicians in a managed healthcare plan is the most important element in controlling cost and quality. Selecting physicians who already practice high quality, cost effective medicine is the best way to achieve success. However, even in the best of hospitals, one cannot be assured that every physician participating in the plan will be solid gold. There will be some B players rather than all A players.

The best contractual arrangements in the world will be of no use if there are poor utilization patterns or a lack of cooperation with policies and procedures.

Some doctors will not modify practice behavior. Others will be hostile and may even try to sabotage plans. The majority, however, will cooperate and will be valued participants.

Financial incentives are a useful method of influencing behavior. Non-financial approaches are equally important and will be discussed here.

Professional Barriers

Berwick et al. (1992) described four barriers to quality improvement:

Time

The time that is most valued by clinicians and their patients is the time spent together. But the usefulness of this time will diminish unless we recognize the interdependencies in which we work. Quality improvement tackles those aspects of interdependency; emphasizing the relation between collaborative work and good care; and the need to be able to change how we work together if care is to be improved. Physicians need to spend adequate time with their patients, but at the same time realize that time, as a resource, is limited. Proper management of time is essential if they wish to provide quality service to the majority, if not all, of their patients.

Territory

The professions guard their territory jealously. Over the years, the medical profession has been notorious for its closed ranks and secretive style of functioning. This is no longer tenable. The contract that healthcare professions have with society is being questioned. Clinical professions may thus have to accede to transparency in self-regulation and to develop new partnerships with each other.

Tradition

Healthcare is as old as the human race itself. Through the ages, remedies and concoctions have passed hands from generation to generation. It is only in the last couple of centuries that efforts have been made to systematically analyze the utility of these treatments. The last century has seen an explosion in medical science with new treatments and procedures being replaced by newer ones almost as fast as they appeared. Doctors, however, are usually reluctant to embrace new advances even if there is sufficient proof of their usefulness.

The older the doctor, the more the resistance to change in practice.

Trust

The nobility of the profession and the social urge to serve humanity has elevated the doctor to the status of a demi-god. The patient has implicit trust and faith in the doctor. Although this still holds good in most parts of the world, people are beginning to question the degree of trust that they have in their doctor. Treatment failures, mismanagement of cases and gross negligence or malpractice at times have fuelled this apprehension. Nowhere is this more apparent than in the United States where litigation is at an all time high. The public are now regarding the medical profession just as another service provider and are demanding high standards in the quality of care provided.

The majority of patients are treated on the basis of good evidence. This is contrary to the widely held belief that only 15–20% of clinical practice is based on good research. Failures in clinical decision-making are due to the three factors that drive clinical practice.

$$P = \frac{M \times C}{B}$$

Where performance (P) is directly related to a professional's competence (C) and motivation (M) and inversely related to the barriers (B) that the professional has to overcome. Some clinicians may lack motivation; others lack competence in newer techniques and treatments and a large majority need to overcome innate psychological barriers to continuing medical education and advances and change their practice accordingly.

The Problem with Doctors

Autonomy

Physicians are trained to function in an autonomous manner, and to be the authority. It is difficult for them to accept a role where someone else has control over their professional activities. Managed care introduces elements of management control that clearly reduces the doctor's autonomy.

Role Conflict

Doctors are said to be the patient's advocate. The issue of advocacy arises when a doctor feels that the needs of the patient and the hospital policy are in conflict. This occurs most frequently when patient's request or demand treatments that are not really necessary or are medically marginal. Although a difficult situation, some physicians handle it better than others. Because of poor provider understanding of the insurance function, this conflict arises when the physician feels a service is medically necessary but is not covered by benefit. At times it is not clear whether the treatment is merely convenient or is actually medically necessary. No hospital or healthcare organization would deny truly needed services that would be covered under the schedule of benefits anyway; in fact, denial of such services would be unethical or even illegal.

Poor Practice Habits

Most doctors have habits and patterns in their practices that are not cost effective but are difficult to change. Keeping patients in for longer than is necessary, outdated operation techniques that have been proven to have no value, over-treatment with antibiotics and steroids to achieve a quicker result, these are some of the poor practices that should be changed.

Resolving Problems

Enlisting the doctor's help in achieving cost effective goals is possible by empowering the physician within the system. Doctors should be involved in:

Recruitment of Medical Staff

Cost Control of Patient Care

Frequent and regular communication will be of great help. Discussing cases and suggesting and soliciting alternatives for case management will yield better results than arbitrary demands for improving quality management programmes especially those concerned' with patient care. Some of the problems of role conflict arise from a poor understanding of insurance policies as mentioned earlier. All policies have certain exclusions and limitations of coverage. For example, a member may require three months of inpatient psychiatric care but the plan may cover only 30 days. Again, most insurers do not cover transplant operations even though they are deemed medically necessary. Sometimes policies may make exceptions but these are done rarely and after much thought.

In some cases it would be cost effective to do so. For example, agreeing to step down care at home for treatment of postoperative wound infections by paying for dressings and nursing care (which are not normally covered).

Helping a doctor understand insurance policies and limitations of coverage would go a long way to resolving most role conflicts. Management could also contact the patient concerned to explain the reasons for denial of benefit; this would assist in changing their impressions about the doctor who they would have perceived as being stubborn or less knowledgeable.

Insurance policies aim at cutting the fat out of the system. The doctor is charged with conserving the resources, to ensure availability to those who truly need them. It is the doctor who will be able to determine what is really needed. This will help provide more appropriate allocation of resources. All policies should thus be aimed at aiding the physician carry out this function.

Practice Guidelines

These may be diagnostic or therapeutic and are used to guide physicians in the care of patients with defined diseases or symptoms or as surveillance tools to monitor practice on a retrospective basis. The initial reaction to guidelines is negative. Doctors feel that this would lead to cookbook medicine and does not allow for clinical judgment in individual cases. There is also the fear of malpractice suits, as the guidelines will provide a template against which all clinical decisions will be judged.

Implementing practice guidelines is not easy, even when disseminated by medical and surgical bodies such as the American Medical Association or the Royal Colleges in the UK. There is frequent lack of enthusiasm on the part of physicians and the actual ability to monitor guidelines is limited. There is some evidence that even publication of guidelines may predispose physicians to consider changing their practice behavior but they will not effect rapid change.

It is difficult to confront a doctor with poor habits, as it appears to be questioning his/her judgment. It is preferable to lead doctors to the appropriate conclusion themselves. If you discuss the issue objectively, present supporting information and ask physicians to examine critically the difference in practice behavior, a number of them would arrive at the conclusion that their practice must change. Allowing doctors to make the change themselves reduces the risk of resistance.

At times, this may not work. Firmer action may then be needed with the involvement of the medical director or a senior medical colleague.

Counseling is preferable to imposition as the latter may lead to litigation if a patient has an adverse outcome due to the change in practice. Doctors still lack an understanding of economics in healthcare. Education on these issues is necessary. It is worthwhile translating cost effective care into how much more the doctor will earn due to the savings he/she brings to the organization. This will increase cooperation.

Increasing Consultant Performance

Managed care has placed increasing pressures on providers of healthcare to reduce costs and maintain or improve quality, as well as to find ways to protect their market share. In managed care, one is trying to practice cost effectiveness and yet provide high-quality care. Thus it is not enough to ensure that a doctor is carrying out his or her duties as per schedule. The aim of managed healthcare should be to improve performance year on year even for those professionals who are currently engaged in good prevue behavior.

Measuring outpatient productivity is one method of managing care. A common unit of measurement involves looking at the number of patient visits per unit time (e.g. visits per day). Other common measures are visits per hour, per session, per week, month or per year. The larger the time scale, the less the influence of minor factors. The problem with larger time scales is that they are slow to respond to changes and will be less sensitive indicators of current productivity. A reasonable combination is to look at visits per day or per week on average for a month and then have a rolling 12-month average for the year to date.

The whole point of the exercise is to have a reasonable expectation of outpatient productivity in relation to colleagues in the same department and not rely too heavily on it. Pressurizing productivity here will lead to sick patients being turned out at a rapid rate with scant attention being paid to their complaints, thus ending up with misdiagnoses and litigations. U studies of appointment availability show reasonable accessibility to care and if the medical expenses are well controlled, there is a little need to apply pressure to improve productivity.

On the other hand, if the waiting list for outpatient appointments for a particular consultant is considerably longer than his peers in the same department, this needs to be looked into, to understand whether the delay is because he/she is a popular specialist (due to experience, skill or method of dealing with patients) or whether he/she is slow to review cases and needs to revise his/her practice.

Similar measures could be applied for operative procedures, lengths of stay in hospital, the use of investigative procedures and patient satisfaction.

Communicating with Doctors

Most managed care plans are quite poor at providing appropriate feedback to physicians. Feedback is often sporadic, usually coinciding with annual functions or when bonuses are handed out. In fact, in some organizations, the doctors hear from the managers only when there is a problem, such as overutilization, and never at all when performance is good.

Senior Management Involvement

Senior management of any hospital should be involved with their medical and nursing staff. Frequent and regular contact either through scheduled meetings, personal visits or telephone calls will help create an environment for positive change.

If physicians hear from the top management only when there is a problem, they will try to avoid contact in the future and will have decreasing responsiveness to new plans, offer advice, suggestions and alternatives.

Involvement is a two-way proposition. Soliciting the active cooperation of doctors in management committee to help set medical policy and monitor quality will give the organization a remote sense of ownership.

Data Provision

Providing regular and accurate data about an individual physician's performance is vital to changing behavior. Most physicians will want to perform well, but can only do so when judged against their peers. The feedback must be regular to maintain credibility and sustain the changed behavior.

Communication of Cost Containment

Physicians regard cost containment as an unnecessary intrusion into their domain. Translating the goal of cost containment into terms that are both understandable and acceptable to them and to managers will lead to greater cooperation. Managing costs is particularly important in the public sector in order to ensure that economic resources will be available to compensate providers and to make services available to all patients.

Provider-relations

In most managed healthcare systems there are individuals who are solely responsible for maintaining communications with the doctors and their staff.

The roles of these provider-relations representatives are to elicit feedback from the doctors and staff, to update them on changes, to troubleshoot generally to keep things running smoothly.

The importance of this function cannot be overstated. Some care must be taken in selecting the individuals who will fill this role. Unless provider-relations staffs are mature and experienced, they may fall into the trap of forgetting for whom they are actually working. It is appropriate and necessary for them to represent the organization's point of view to plan management, but it is inappropriate if they find themselves siding against the health plan in the event of a dispute. The provider-relations staff must seek to prevent rifts not foster them.

Provider-relations must be proactive rather than simply reactive. They should have a well-developed early warning system for trouble-shooting. Such a system could include regular on-site visits by provider-relations staff (and occasionally by the medical director) and regular two-way communications.

Looking for Aberrant Behavior

Changes in patterns, particularly patterns in utilization and compliance with plan policy and procedure, will often be a sign that there is something wrong. Close monitoring of member services complaints can yield crucial information. Physicians will often tell patients what they think and what they intend to do long before they tell the higher ups in the organization.

Another function of managed care is determining who not to keep in the service. In any hospital, there will be physicians who simply cannot or will not work within the system and whose practice style is clearly cost ineffective or of poor quality. There must be a mechanism for identification of such practitioners using a combination of claims and utilization data and some kind of formal performance evaluation system.

If identified providers are reluctant to change, even after the medical director has worked closely with them, then serious consideration should be given to terminate their services.

There are a number of objections for removing a physician from the panel. Asking patients to change doctors is not easy or pleasant and invariably the doctor in question is in a strategic location. The decision often comes down to whether you want to subsidies that physician's poor practice behavior from the earnings of the other physicians or drive the rates up to unacceptable and uncompetitive levels. If these are the alternatives, then separation must occur.

Changing the Behavior of Doctors

Changing provider behavior generally involves a stepwise approach. The first and most common step is collegial discussion—discussing cases and utilization patterns in a non-threatening way. Colleague to colleague is generally an effective method of bringing about change.

Positive feedback is an even more effective tool for change but is often neglected. This means letting the doctor know when things are done well. Most managers get so involved in file fighting that they tend to neglect sending positive messages to those providers who are managing well. In the absence of such messages, providers have to figure out for themselves what they are doing right (they will usually only be contacted when they have done something wrong). This, obviously, is not optimal.

Rewards

Positive interactions or rewards are more effective in achieving long-term changes in behavior than negative interactions or sanctions. Imposing policies with sanctions alone will have disastrous effects. Firstly cooperation will be forced and not enthusiastic. Secondly, this will lead to widespread dissatisfaction and defection. Thirdly, there may be covert sabotage that will undermine the organization.

Rewards refer primarily to forms of positive feedback and communication about good performance. Good case management should yield economic rewards as well but positive feedback from senior management will be a reward in itself. The odds of cooperation will increase when the interactions between the physician and management are more positive than negative.

Persuasion is also commonly used. This is stronger than collegial discussion. Doctors are usually reluctant to send patients home for parenteral antibiotic therapy or dressings as it then becomes inconvenient for them to follow the case. Management needs to persuade them to discharge such patients in the interests of cost effectiveness.

Conclusion

Changing the behavior of doctors is crucial to the success of managed care.

Doctors have some unique attributes:
- Need for autonomy and control
- Scope for role conflicts
- Poor understanding of the economics of healthcare
- Poor practice habits

The most important step in facilitating change is to ensure that professionals want to change. The most effective way of encouraging professionals to change is to help them see decisions that they make as an intellectual challenge rather than as a management directive. It is much more effective to stimulate professionals to grow their own carrots than to force them to behave like donkeys, enticed by a carrot dangling in front and threatened by a stick from behind.

Managers should therefore:
- Be responsive to doctors' needs
- Be consistent in their policies
- Provide feedback at regular intervals
- Provide positive feedback
- Tackle problems with doctors early
- Solve problems in a stepwise fashion
- Communicate frequently and establish communication channels with medical staff.

MANAGING CARE IN HOSPITALS

Introduction

Managing the care given in hospitals is done by the purchasers of healthcare, i.e. the insurance companies or corporate human resource departments. It is in their interest to ensure that they are getting what they have contracted for. They are not paying for unnecessary treatments, shoddy practice behavior or for substandard care.

Utilization of hospital services usually accounts for over 40% of the total expenses in a health insurance care plan. That amount can even be greater when utilization is excessive. Control of these expenses is therefore prominent among most insurance managers' priorities.

The expense of any medical service is a product of the price of that service times the volume of services delivered. Simple reduction of bed days may be of value but can lull the inexperienced manager into a sense of complacency.

The Utilization Management Team

The managed care or care management (as it is known in the UK) team in an insurance company, or acting independently as in the case of brokers, is also known as the utilization management (UM) team. The title is self-explanatory. The team is responsible for ensuring the provision of good quality cost effective care to their clients. The UM team is made up of senior registered nurses with at least five years experience in nursing and with specialization in one or more fields of medicine such as oncology (cancer), urology, gastroenterology, ENT, etc. The number of nurses required depends on the geographic area covered by the insurance company, the number of members and the variety of medical specialties that need to be covered. The team also has a doctor who is appointed as the medical director. It is the responsibility of the medical director to recruit and oversee the activities of the UM nurses and provide support when dealing with difficult cases or providers.

The nurses use a number of methods discussed below to obtain information on the status of their clients who are admitted in hospital or undergoing outpatient treatment. Patient information may be obtained by telephone or by actually visiting the hospital where the client is admitted. This helps to ascertain whether the treatment being given at the hospital is eligible for benefit, i.e. covered by the insurance policy.

Their proactive stance also enables them to discuss the management of cases with the providers and suggest alternatives such as step down care (see below) that would be equally effective but less expensive.

Methods for Decreasing Utilization

The key categories are

Prospective review: This means review of a case before it even happens.

Concurrent review: Review occurs while the case is active.

Retrospective review: Review occurs after the case is finished.

Large Case Management (LCM)

This refers to managing cases that are expected to result in very large costs, such as chemotherapy courses for cancer, so as to provide coordination of care resulting in both proper care and savings.

Pre-certification refers to a requirement on the part of the admitting physician and hospital to notify the plan before a member is admitted for treatment.

Reasons for Pre-certification

To notify the concurrent review system that a case will be occurring. This will enable the Utilization Management (UM) team to prepare discharge planning ahead of time. The LCM team can also be warned in advance of a high cost case.

To ensure that care takes place in the most appropriate setting, the UM team can direct the member's admission to a unit where specialized facilities or clinicians with special expertise are available for a difficult or unusual condition. To capture data for financial accruals: By knowing the number and nature of hospital cases as well as potentially expensive ones, the plan may more accurately accrue for expenses rather than have to wait for claims to come in. This allows management to take action early and avoid nasty financial surprises.

1. To assign an estimated length of stay for inpatient surgical patients for elective procedures.
2. To verify eligibility of coverage for the member. In the case of an emergency or urgent admission, it is obviously not possible to obtain pre-certification. Most plans, however, require notification within 48 hours of admission. Failure to pre-certify usually results in a fee penalty being levied on the provider. 'U' the provider is not contracted with the plan or is not recognized, the member may have to foot the bill.

Pre-admission Testing and Same Day Surgery

This is one of the easiest and most common methods for cost control. A member requiring elective surgery has preoperative tests done as an outpatient and is admitted to hospital on the day of surgery.

In many health plans, arrangements are made for laboratory work to be done with a contracted laboratory at reduced rates or will have contracts with the hospital laboratory itself. Generally, hospitals will accept laboratory results from an accredited and licensed laboratory but members must check this beforehand to avoid having to undergo testing twice.

Mandatory Outpatient Surgery

Hospitals have lists of procedures that may only be performed on an outpatient or day case basis unless prior approval is obtained for inpatient stay. Although there is a consensus on many common procedures, there are always procedures migrating from inpatient to outpatient, hence the lists need to be revised at least yearly based on clinical evidence and practice.

Concurrent Review

This means managing utilization during the course of hospitalization.

Common Methods

Assignment and Tracking of Length of Stay

The plan assigns a length of stay (LOS) based on the admission diagnosis or operative procedure. Payment will only be made for the assigned LOS. For example, an admission for gall bladder surgery may be assigned three days. It is assumed that the patient will be admitted on the day of surgery and go home three days later. Any stay beyond that is not covered.

The LOS is determined by the International Classification of Diseases, Tenth Revision (ICD-10) code. Diagnosis related groups (DRGS) are similar in concept. Selecting a norm for the LOS is not easy given regional variations.

It is useful to collate data from a number of specialists in the field and arrive at an average LOS for different procedures and diagnoses. This would provide a more realistic expectation of the expertise of the specialists in the area and the type of patients that they see.

Advantages of using LOS

1. Allows coverage of a relatively large area with a few personnel. This is useful for new plans.
2. Has the power of legitimacy and does not require negotiation for each case.
3. Is relatively mechanical and requires less training of plan personnel problems with LOS.
4. It is easy to get complacent. Failure to evaluate preset values may result in a longer inpatient stay than necessary.
5. There is less incentive to evaluate the appropriateness of and alternatives to care even though the patient may be ready for discharge at an earlier date.
6. May achieve less than optimal results, as it is too mechanical. However, the alternative is intensive medical management by qualified personnel who are not always available.

Review by UM Nurses

The one individual who is crucial to the success of a managed care program is the UM nurse. It is the UM nurse who will be the eyes and ears of the medical management department, who will generally coordinate the discharge planning and who will facilitate all the activities of utilization control.

Staffing levels for UM nurses will vary depending on the size of the geographic area, the number of hospitals, the membership and the intensity with which UM will be performed. Usually there is one UM nurse for every 8500–12000 members. Plans that perform telephonic review only may staff at ratios that are twice that of members.

The scope of responsibilities of the UM nurse will vary depending on the plan and the personalities and skills of other members of the medical management team. In some plans, the role simply involves telephone information gathering. Information gathering includes admission date and diagnosis, doctor in charge, planned procedures or treatments, expected discharge date, discharge planning and other relevant information.

In other plans, there will be a more proactive role, including frequent communications with attending physicians, the medical director, hospitals and the hospitalized members and their families, discharge planning and facilitation and even taking rounds in selected hospitals. The latter plans have a much tighter utilization control. However, in both methods, experienced UM nurses have a little difficulty in identifying patients who need to stay longer in hospital and those who can safely be discharged. Discharges may be delayed by a day or more simply because the attending physician missed a round of the patients. Poor practice habits such as these can be picked up by the UM nurses and referred to the medical director for appropriate action.

Discharge Planning

Good discharge planning starts as soon as a patient is admitted into the hospital or even before. The admitting doctor should be considering discharge planning as part of the overall treatment plan from the outset. The planning includes:
- An estimate of how long the patient will be in hospital
- What the expected outcome will be
- Whether there will be any special requirements on discharge
- What should be facilitated earlier on

For example, if a patient is admitted with a fractured hip and it is known from the outset that many weeks of rehabilitation will be necessary, it is helpful to contact the facility where the rehabilitation will take place to ensure that a bed will be available at the time of transfer. If it is known that a patient will need special equipment on discharge, these should be ordered early so that the patient does not spend extra days in hospital waiting for it to arrive. An often overlooked aspect of discharge planning is informing the patient and family. If they do not know what to expect, they may be surprised when informed that they are being discharged. This is especially true following delivery where the patient and her family may not be prepared for the homecoming.

Discharge planning is an ongoing effort beginning with admission or preadmission screening. The UM nurse is in the ideal position to coordinate discharge planning.

In a loosely controlled plan there will be a fewer expectations of the consultant than in a tightly controlled one. The better the control of utilization, the more you have to deal with practice patterns and physician behavior. Medical Director's responsibilities in addition to monitoring all the elements discussed above, there are a few specific functions that the medical director should be performing. The medical director will have to become involved in the most difficult cases from a management standpoint. There are times when the medical director must deal with uncooperative individuals. He/she must take a compassionate, caring but firm stance when dealing with difficult people. The ability to empathies and sympathies with someone's point of view and to recognize what the real issues are in a dispute without giving in readily requires skill.

Communications

If the medical director is only heard from the time when there is a problem, his or her effectiveness will be diminished. 'U' the medical director discusses cases, suggesting alternatives if appropriate even when there is no pressing need to make a change, the participating physicians will be much more receptive to his/her opinions when a change is needed.

The usefulness of frequent contact cannot be underestimated. By asking relevant questions in a non-threatening manner, and by constantly stimulating thought regarding cost-effective clinical management, the medical director may slowly reinforce appropriate patterns of care. The aim should be to reach a point where doctors begin asking themselves the questions that the medical director would ask and begin improving their practice patterns on that basis.

Retrospective Review

Retrospective review occurs after the patient is discharged. There are two forms:

Claims Review

This refers to examining claims for improprieties or mistakes.

Pattern Review

Patterns of utilization are studied to determine where action must be taken.

For example, if three hospitals in the area perform coronary artery bypass surgery, the plan may look to see which one has the best clinical outcomes, the shortest length of stay and the lowest charges. The plan may then preferentially send all cases to the selected hospital. Pattern review also allows the plan to focus UM efforts primarily on those areas needing greater attention.

Another use is to provide feedback to providers. Although not as powerful as active UM, when combined with other management functions and financial incentives, feedback can be a useful management tool.

Large Case Management

LCM refers to specialized techniques for identifying and managing cases that are disproportionately high in cost. Examples are treatments for AIDS, bone marrow transplants, cancer chemotherapy courses, etc. Proactively contacting patients with potentially catastrophic illnesses not only can save the plan considerable expense but can also result in better medical care because the services are coordinated.

There are two ways by which LCM benefits both the patient and the managed care plan:

Use of Community Resources

These can help to provide the support structures whereby the patient can return home.

Payment of Extra-contractual Benefits

If there were limited coverage for home equipment, it would be in the plan's interest to increase cover to get the patient home and out of the hospital. The hallmark of LCM is longitudinal management of the case by a single UM nurse or department. This provides for active coordination of a variety of services that is generally required for such cases and thus enhances both the quality and cost effectiveness of healthcare.

Conclusion

Control of hospital utilization is one of the most important aspects of controlling overall healthcare costs. This is a function that must be attended to every day to achieve optimal results.

Provider Profiling

Another function of managed healthcare is provider profiling. This means the collection and analysis of data to develop provider-specific profiles. Provider here refers to doctors as well as hospitals. Such profiles have a variety of uses, but the most important one is in recruiting providers.

Other uses include

- Determining specialists to whom the company will send certain types of cases.
- Producing provider feedback reports to help them modify their behavior.
- Detecting fraud and abuse.
- Determining how to focus the utilization management program.

- Supporting performance based reimbursement systems
- Performing economic modeling

Many provider-profiling systems simply look at the behavior of the provider against certain norms. This is necessary but is a difficult task. The main problem is to define the norm and choose what to look at.

Most profiling activities focus solely on the actions of the provider. This may end up being counterproductive as patient mix and geographical area may have a role to play in outlying activities. It is much better to compare one provider's actions against those of his colleagues in the same department or in neighboring hospitals including assessment of clinical outcomes of care in order to arrive at a definitive conclusion.

Problems with Provider Profiling

Comparison of Like with Like

The doctor's specialty is not always clear, especially where super-specialization is concerned. If this is not clarified at the outset, comparisons of performance cannot be made.

Practice Differences

Habits

Referral and treatment patterns invariably differ from consultant to consultant even if the disease condition is the same. Assessment of clinical outcomes, patient satisfaction and reviews of treatment patterns to check whether evidence-based medicine is being practiced need to be considered before branding a physician as an outlier.

Case Mix

Practices may also have differences in the age and sex make-up of their patients. Geographic differences may also account for variations in utilizations. Providers with costly profiles may complain that they have the sickest and most complicated patients. Thus severity of illness is another factor that needs to be considered in the overall evaluation.

Referrals for Investigations

Links between doctors and private laboratory facilities may be responsible for a much higher referral rate. Either the doctor may own the laboratory or be given a cash incentive for sending patients to a specific laboratory. All the above factors must be considered before accusing the doctor of performing excessive investigations.

Feedback should be meaningful and useful to the plan and the provider. When the reports are clearly linked with performance expectations and when such reports can help a provider change behavior in a positive way, then feedback is successful. Providers will alter their behavior for a number of reasons:

- Natural competitiveness and peer pressure
- Opportunity to increase market share and revenue
- Fear of possible adverse actions by the plan
- Fear of medico-legal litigations by consumer forums and patients

Utilization reports are powerful tools for managers of health plans. Data collection should be simplified and only relevant information should be presented to providers. A number of associated factors must be taken into account before identifying a specialist or a hospital as an outlier.

Conclusion

Managed care may thus:
- Facilitate the introduction of evidence-based care
- Reduce the duration of hospital stay
- Counteract the vagaries of clinical care

However, there are problems with managed care. These are:

It is difficult to apply the guidelines to all aspects of care.

Clinicians view as it controls the decision-making of patient care by a nonclinical organization.

There is no doubt that managed healthcare plays a central role in the provision of cost-effective care. Absence of this policing would result in utter chaos, with each clinician being a law unto him or herself, as is the case in India and most other third world countries. Patients are usually in a vulnerable position, suffering from disease or infirmity and are generally thankful if they obtain some relief from their symptoms. They are in no condition to judge whether the care provided was of good quality, or cost effectiveness.

As discussed in the beginning of this module, medical councils worldwide and even bodies such as the Royal Colleges or the American Boards can only suggest changes in practice. They cannot enforce guidelines or criteria on practitioners. Generally action is only taken against a physician when there has been gross negligence or malpractice brought to light by an aggrieved patient or relative, by the time it is not too late.

Healthcare organizations such as health insurance companies and hospitals need managed care. Insurers, in particular, cannot do without managed care teams (also called UM teams). It is this team, which keeps providers on their toes. The profitability of insurance companies rests on the capabilities of their UM teams. Hospital managers, on the other hand, can use the techniques to recruit new staff and check the actions of their medical staff to ascertain whether they are providing cost effective, evidence-based care.

The role of the medical director is invaluable here. The medical director needs to have sufficient expertise to analyze data and identify outlying practices.

He/she also needs to have excellent communication skills in order to discuss the issues with the physician concerned without antagonizing the medical staff. Translating clinical decisions into cost activities would enable other doctors to view the provision of cost effective care in a more favorable light than to simply consider it as an intrusion to their clinical judgment. The message needs to be hammered repeatedly till physicians themselves begin to evaluate their clinical decisions on the basis of quality and cost.

Although these opportunities to influence the delivery of healthcare are tempting, their realization must be tempered with the knowledge that most clinical decisions cannot be governed by strict rules; guidelines have to remain guidelines. The introduction of managed care is undoubtedly changing the role of the physician and although change is necessary, it is vital that one of the most important, but undervalued and under-evaluated aspects of medical care—the bond between the clinician and the patient is not disrupted.

References

Berwick D.M. Einthoven A. Bunker. Quality management in the NHS: the doctor's role - n. BM 1992; 304: 304–8.

Clancy CM. Hillner B.B. Physicians as gatekeepers - the impact of financial incentives. Arch Intern Med. 1989; 149: 917–20.

Eddy D.M. Three battles to watch in the 1990s. AMA 1993; 270: 520–6.

Eddy D.M. Benefit language. Criteria that will improve quality while reducing cost. AMA 1996; 275: 650–7.

Essentials of Managed Healthcare. P.R. Kongstvedt (1995) Aspen Publishers Inc. Maryland, USA.

Evidence-Based Healthcare. A. Muir Gray (1997) Churchill Livingstone, New York, USA.

Lipkin M. Jr. Sisyphus or Pegasus. The physician interviewer in the era of corporatization of care. Ann Intern Med 1996; 124: 511–13.

Muir Gray I.A. In. Evidence-Based Healthcare. (1997), Churchill Livingstone, London, UK.

Rosenburg W. and Donald A. Evidence-based medicine: an approach to clinical problem solving. BM 1995; 310 (6987): 1122–26.

Reinhardt U.E. A social contract for 21st century healthcare: three tier healthcare with bounty hunting. Health Economics. 1996; 5(6): 479–99.

Sloss E.M. Keller E.B. *et al.* Effect of a health maintenance organization on physiologic health. Ann Intern Med. 1987; 106: 130–138.

Udvarhelyi IS. Jennison K. et al. Comparison of the quality of ambulatory care for fee-for-service and prepaid patients. Ann Intern Med. 1991, 115: 394–400.

Ware J. E. Rodgers W.H. Davies AR. *et al.* Comparison of health outcomes at a health maintenance organisation with those of fee-for-service care. Lancet I: 1017–22.

3
Continuous Quality Improvement in Hospitals

Feroz Ikbal

INTRODUCTION

Last few years saw an increase in awareness of quality in hospital industry. Increasing litigations, rising customer awareness, high patient expectations force the hospitals to focus on total quality management. Today hospitals are increasingly going for accreditation programmes like NABH and JCI as a tool to improve quality. This chapter intends to discuss the various facets of quality as well as the tools for continuous quality improvement. Several of the tools have been successfully initiated in manufacturing industries, but can be applied in hospital services also.

Quality can be defined as, 'totality of features and characteristics of a product or service that bear on its ability to satisfy stated or implied needs'.

Definition of Quality by Quality Gurus

Crosby	Conformance to requirements.
Juran	Fitness for use.
Deming	Reduction in variations
Figenbaum	Meeting customer requirements.

DIMENSIONS OF QUALITY

Accessibility: The product or service is easy to access or acquire. Accessibility of hospital includes both financial and physical accessibility.

Assurance: The staff are friendly, polite, considerate and knowledgeable. A patient coming to the hospital is highly stressed and staff has to provide him assurance of the care.

Communication: Customers are kept informed about the product or service provided. Hospitals need to communicate to its customers about its services as well as the availability of doctors.

Competence: Staff possesses the requisite knowledge and skills to provide the skill or service. Credentialing of the clinical staff should be done to ensure their competence.

Conformance: The product or service meets standards. Today in hospitals accreditation programs such as NABH, NABL, JCI, NABB, etc. ensure that hospitals confirm to established standards.

Courtesy: Politeness, respect and consideration towards customers. Employees of the hospitals need to understand that patient is the most important person for the hospital.

Efficiency: Characteristics that affect the customer satisfaction adversely. Using minimum resources hospitals should be able to provide best quality patient care.

Durability: The performance, result or outcome does not dissipate quickly. But unlike manufacturing industry, hospitals cannot give guarantee or warranty for their service.

Empathy: Staff demonstrates an understanding and provides individualized attention to customers.

Humanness: The product or service is provided in such a manner that it protect the dignity and self worth of customers. The privacy and dignity of the patient need to be protected.

Performance: The product or service does what it is supposed to do. Hospitals should be able to perform with acceptable performance indicators pertaining to mortality level, infection control rate, etc.

Reliability: Refers to ability to provide the service in a dependable and consistent manner, with minimum variation. Standard operating protocols and clinical practice guidelines will ensure the reliability of service.

Responsiveness: The timeliness of employees in providing products and services. Hospital services are emergent in nature that timely response is vital. The concept of "platinum minutes" and "golden hour" in emergency services is an example of responsiveness in hospital services.

Security: The product or service is provided in a safe setting and is free from risk or danger. Hospitals needs to follow stringent fire safety protocols and should have good disaster management plan. It needs to provide safety and security to patients, bye-standers and to its own employees.

Tangibles: The physical appearance of facilities, equipment and infrastructure of the hospital should be good enough.

According to marketing guru *Parasuraman,* firms need the right metrics to measure five things:

Customer perception of the firms offering.
Firms understanding of the customer.
Service quality standards.
Gap between actual and expected service quality.
Internal and external communication gap.

Definitions of TQM

Company wide quality management system involving all employees in activities at improvement of product, quality, production, process and services.

A comprehensive system of management that emphasizes a commitment to quality, focus on customer needs and continual process improvement enlisting all members of the organization.

TQM is a process designed to focus external or internal customer expectations preventing problem building, commitment to quality in the work force and promoting open decision-making.

Principles of TQM

- Delight the patient.
- Management by fact: Decisions are based upon facts.
- People based management: Everybody must be involved. The more the people feel involved, the greater will be their commitment to customer satisfaction. Employee should be empowered and motivated.
- Continuous improvement.
- TQM begins and ends with education and training.
- There is need for strategic quality management.
- Strong leadership.
- TQM is supported by quality system measurement and record.
- TQM cannot afford weak links/processes.
- Quality corporate culture.
- Teamwork.
- People-oriented technology

CONCEPT OF QUALITY IN HEALTHCARE

According to *Adeis donabedian,* the late quality guru in the U.S., quality in healthcare is encompassed of three critical attributes.

Structure: It refers to the "physical" aspects of healthcare delivery including infrastructure, equipment and human resources, e.g. equipment requirements as per services being offered and accessibility of facility.

Process: It pertains to the procedures and protocols that all healthcare personnel, clinical and non-clinical have to conform to, so as to ensure appropriate and adequate delivery of healthcare services, e.g. infection control procedures, protocols for patient care management.

Outcome: It pertains to the well-being of the patient after delivery of healthcare services, e.g. mortality rates, post-operative infection rates, etc.

Quality in Healthcare can also be Divided into Two Specific Parts

Clinical

- Clinical credentialing
- Clinical audit
- Clinical risk management
- Clinical outcome measurement
- Clinical care pathways

Non-clinical

- Infrastructure and facilities management
- Equipment management
- IT infrastructure and management
- Hospitality management
- Patient satisfaction
- Non-clinical risk management
- Accreditation

CORE CONCEPTS OF TQM

- *Customer satisfaction:* Internal customers are real.
- *All works are systematic:* Make it a good place to work, create a work culture which will lead to satisfied customers.
- *Measurement:* Measure the work and identify deviation and make corrections.
- *Teamwork:* Involvement of all employees.
- *People make quality:* Do it right first time, empower the employees, educate and train them.
- Continuous improvement cycle and prevention.

COST OF QUALITY

Description

The cost of quality is a shorthand formula for all business costs incurred in achieving quality of product or service. These include prevention costs, appraisal costs, internal failure costs, external failure costs, the cost of exceeding customer requirements, and finally the cost of lost opportunities. Taken together these costs can account to 20–30% drain of organizations revenue or turnover. Cutting the cost of quality is one of the central concepts of TQM.

The "cost of quality" isn't the price of creating a quality product or service. It's the cost of NOT creating a quality product or service.

Cost of Quality can be Broadly Divided into Three Heads

Cost of conformance
Cost of non-conformance
Cost of lost opportunities

Two Elements of Cost of Conformance

Cost of prevention: It is the cost of activities that prevent failure from occurring *or* the costs of all activities specifically designed to prevent poor quality in products or services.

Cost of appraisal: It is the cost incurred to determine conformance with quality standards *or* the costs associated with measuring, evaluating or auditing products or services to assure conformance to quality standards and performance requirements.

Three Elements of Cost of Non-conformance

Cost of internal failure: Those costs which occur within the organization before delivery to the external customer or failure costs occurring prior to delivery or shipment of the product, or the furnishing of a service, to the customer.

Cost of external failure: It occurs when the product or service is offered to the customer and found defective. These costs include returned products and rejected service and unhappy customers or failure costs occurring after delivery or shipment of the product—and during or after furnishing of a service—to the customer.

Cost of exceeding the customer requirements: It occurs when the organization gives the customer more than what is required. Often this cost takes the form of providing information or service which are unnecessary or for which there is no expressed or agreed requirement. Habit of sending copies of letters or documents to all instead of sending it only to the required persons, conduct studies, when the scope of implementation is very much limited.

Cost of Lost Opportunities

It refers to the loss in revenue due to an erosion of the customer base or due to the failure to get new customers because of the quality failure.

SEVEN BASIC TOOLS OF QUALITY CONTROL

Histogram

It is the visual representation of the spread or distribution of the data. It is also called frequency distribution. Histograms also illustrate the various measures of central tendency such as mean, median or mode. A frequency distribution shows how often each different value in a set of data occurs. A histogram is the most commonly used graph to show frequency distributions. It looks very much like a bar chart, but there are important differences between them.

When to Use

- When the data are numerical.
- When you want to see the shape of the data's distribution, especially when determining whether the output of a process is distributed approximately normally.
- When analyzing whether a process can meet the customer's requirements.
- When analyzing what the output from a supplier's process looks like.
- When seeing whether a process change has occurred from one time period to another.
- When determining whether the outputs of two or more processes are different.
- When you wish to communicate the distribution of data quickly and easily to others.

Check Sheet

Check sheet is a list of check off items that permit data to be collected quickly and easily in a simple standardized form that lends itself to quantitative analysis.

A check sheet is a structured and prepared form for collecting and analyzing data. This is a generic tool that can be adapted for a wide variety of purposes. Hospitals use surgical check list (Fig. 3.1).

When to Use

- When data can be observed and collected repeatedly by the same person or at the same location.
- When collecting data on the frequency or patterns of events, problems, defects, defect location, defect causes, etc.
- When collecting data from a production process.

Example:

The following check sheet shows the level of satisfaction with housekeeping among inpatients in hospital

Highly satisfied	⁄‖‖‖‖‖‖ ‖	– 12
Satisfied	⁄‖‖‖‖‖‖‖‖ ‖‖	–17
Average	⁄‖‖‖ ‖	–6
Poor	⁄‖‖‖‖‖‖‖‖	–10
Very poor	⁄‖‖‖	–05
Total		–50

Fig. 3.1: Check sheet

Stratification

It is the breaking down of (cost area of concern) into smaller related sub-group method of grouping data by common points and characteristics to better understand similarities and characteristics of data.

Stratification is a technique used in combination with other data analysis tools. When data from a variety of sources or categories have been lumped together, the meaning of the data can be impossible to see. This technique separates the data so that patterns can be seen.

When to Use

- Before collecting data.
- When data comes from several sources or conditions, such as shifts, days of the week, suppliers or population groups.
- When data analysis may require separating different sources or conditions.

Scatter Diagram

A scatter diagram is used to study the possible relationship between one variable and the other.

The scatter diagram graphs pairs of numerical data, with one variable on each axis, to look for a relationship between them. If the variables are correlated, the points will fall along a line or curve. The better the correlation, the tighter the points will hug the line.

When to Use

- When you have paired numerical data.
- When your dependent variable may have multiple values for each value of your independent variable.
- When trying to determine whether the two variables are related, such as when trying to identify potential root causes of problems.
- After brain storming causes and effects using a fishbone diagram, to determine objectively whether a particular cause and effect are related.
- When determining whether two effects that appear to be related and both occur with the same cause.
- When testing for autocorrelation before constructing a control chart.

Fishbone Diagram

This was developed by Prof. Ishikawa of Tokyo University in 1943. Fishbone diagram enables to understand the linkage between the various causes and the end result. The effect or problem is stated on the right side of the chart, and the major influences or causes are listed on the left.

The fishbone diagram identifies many possible causes for an effect or problem. It can be used to structure a brainstorming session. It immediately sorts ideas into useful categories.

When to Use

- When identifying possible causes for a problem.
- Assist both the individual and groups to see the problem of the department or the organization in depth.
- Serve as a recording device for ideas generated.
- Reveal the undetected relationship between the causes.
- Discover the origin of the problem.
- Investigate the expected results of the course of action.
- Call attention to important relationship. It helps to understand at a glance whether the problem has been thoroughly investigated.

Procedure

Agree on a problem statement (effect). Write it at the center right of the flipchart or whiteboard. Draw a box around it and draw a horizontal arrow running to it.

Brain storm the major categories of causes of the problem. If this is difficult, use generic headings:
- Machines
- Manpower
- Materials
- Measurement
- Methods
- Environment

Write the categories of causes as branches from the main arrow (Fig. 3.2).

Brain storm all the possible causes of the problem. Ask: "Why does this happen?" As each idea is given, the facilitator writes it as a branch from the appropriate category. Causes can be written in several places if they relate to several categories.

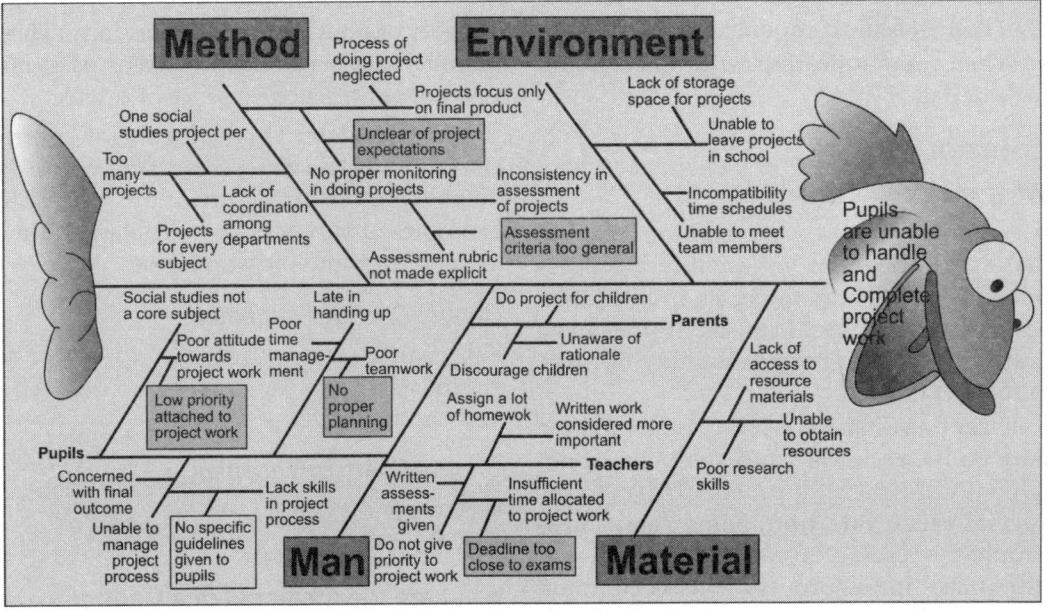

Fig. 3.2: Fishbone diagram

Again ask "Why does this happen?" about each cause. Write sub-causes branching off the causes. Continue to ask "Why?" and generate deeper levels of causes. Layers of branches indicate causal relationships.

When the group runs out of ideas, focus attention to places on the chart where ideas are a few.

PARETO CHART

Pareto analysis is fundamental in identifying the vital few, out of many problems in quality improvement studies. Pareto diagram was devised by Vilfredo Pareto, an Italian economist, who studied about the unequal distribution of wealth. He identified that 80% of the wealth is concentrated at the hands of just 20% people. He eventually identified that he had discovered a universal law — 80% of anything is attributed to 20% of the causes, e.g. 80% of absenteeism is attributed to only 20% of employees in the organization. Pareto analysis helps to identify the few causes that account for the major chunk of the problems.

A Pareto chart is a bar graph. The lengths of the bars represent frequency or cost (time or money), and are arranged with longest bars on the left and the shortest to the right. In this way the chart visually depicts which situations are more significant.

Steps in Drawing Pareto Chart

- Identify the problem
- List the causes and its frequencies in the descending order.
- Draw the bar chart.
- Construct cumulative frequency chart.

The data obtained by step 2 should be converted into percentages before going to steps 3 and 4.

When to Use

- When analyzing data about the frequency of problems or causes in a process.
- When there are many problems or causes and you want to focus on the most significant.

- When analyzing broad causes by looking at their specific components.
- When communicating with others about your data.

CONTROL CHARTS

What is a Control Chart?

A control chart is a statistical tool used to distinguish between variation in a process resulting from common causes and variation resulting from special causes. It presents a graphic display of process stability or instability over time.

Every process has variation. Some variation may be the result of causes which are not normally present in the process. This could be **special cause variation**. Some variation is simply the result of numerous, ever-present differences in the process. This is **common cause variation**.

Control charts differentiate between these two types of variations. One goal of using a control chart is to achieve and maintain **process stability**.

Process stability is defined as a state in which a process has displayed a certain degree of consistency in the past and is expected to continue to do so in the future. This consistency is characterized by a stream of data falling within **control limits** based on **plus or minus 3 standard deviations (3 sigma)** of the centerline.

Why Use Control Charts?

- Monitor process variation over time.
- Differentiate between special cause and common cause variation.
- Assess effectiveness of changes.
- Communicate process performance.

Types of Control Chart

There are two main categories of control charts, those that display *attribute data*, and those that display *variables data*.

Attribute data: This category of control chart displays data that result from counting the number of occurrences or items in a single category of similar items or occurrences. These "count" data may be expressed as pass/fail, yes/no, or presence/absence of a defect.

Variables data: This category of control chart displays values resulting from the measurement of a continuous variable. Examples of variables data are elapsed time, temperature, and radiation dose.

Control Chart for Attributes
- C chart
- Np chart
- P chart

Control Chart for Variables
- $\bar{X}$ chart
- R chart

What are the Elements of a Control Chart?

Each control chart actually consists of two graphs, an upper and a lower, which are described below under plotting areas (Fig. 3.3). A control chart is made up of eight elements.

1. *Title:* The title briefly describes the information which is displayed.
2. *Legend:* This is information on how and when the data were collected.
3. *Data collection section:* The counts or measurements are recorded in the data collection section of the control chart prior to being graphed.
4. *Plotting areas:* A control chart has two areas—an upper graph and a lower graph—where the data is plotted.
    a. The upper graph plots either the individual values, in the case of an individual X and moving range chart, or the average (mean value) of the sample or subgroup in the case of an $\bar{X}$ and R chart.
    b. The lower graph plots the moving range for individual X and moving range charts, or the range of values found in the subgroups for $\bar{X}$ and R chart.

5. *Vertical or Y-Axis:* This axis reflects the magnitude of the data collected. The Y-axis shows the scale of the measurement for variables data, or the count (frequency) or percentage of occurrence of an event for attribute data.
6. *Horizontal or X-Axis:* This axis displays the chronological order in which the data were collected.
7. *Control limits:* Control limits are set at a distance of 3 sigma above and 3 sigma below the centerline. They indicate variation from the centerline and are calculated by using the actual values plotted on the control chart graphs.
8. *Centerline:* This line is drawn at the average or mean value of all the plotted data. The upper and lower graphs have a separate centerline.

Attribute control charts are used for product or service characteristic that can be evaluated with a discrete response (pass/fail, yes/no, good/bad, etc.)

c chart
p chart
np chart

The c chart: The c chart is used to control the average number of defects in samples of fixed size taken from a process.

The formulae used are as follows:

Center line 'c': total defects/total number of samples
Upper control limit = $c + 3\sqrt{c}$
Lower control limit = $c - 3\sqrt{c}$

The p chart: The p chart is used to control the proportion of defective items samples taken from a process. The p chart allows for variable sample sizes, but to maintain constant control limits, constant sample size is required.

The formulae used are as follows:
Center line 'p' = total number of defects in all samples/total number of items inspected (sum of size of each sample)
Average sample size 'n' = sum of size of each sample/total number of samples
Upper control limit = $p + 3\sqrt{p(1-p)/n}$
Lower control limit = $p - 3\sqrt{p(1-p)/n}$

The np chart: The np chart is used to control the number of defective items in a sample of fixed size taken from a process.

The formulae used are as follows:
Center line 'np' = number of defects/number of samples
Upper control limit: $np + 3\sqrt{p(1-p)}$
Lower control limit: $np - 3\sqrt{p(1-p)}$
'p' = average defect rate per sample/common sample size

Control chart for variables: It is used when the parameter under control is some measurement of variables, such as dimension of a part, the time for work performance, etc.

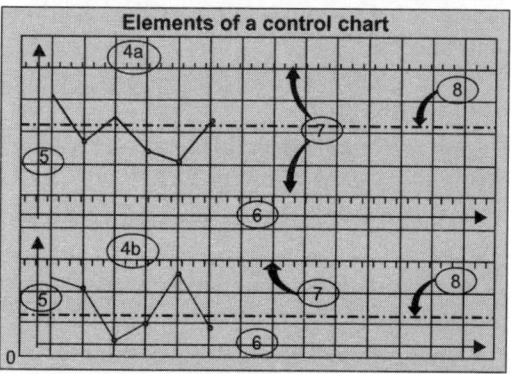

Fig. 3.3: Control chart

Table 3.1: Values for variable chart

Sample size n	X control limit A2	R chart control limits Lower D3	R chart control limits Upper D4
2	1.880	0	3.267
3	1.023	0	2.574
4	.729	0	2.282
5	.577	0	2.114
6	.483	0	2.004
7	.419	.076	1.924
8	.373	.136	1.864
9	.337	.184	1.186
10	.308	.223	1.777
11	.285	.256	1.744
12	.283	.283	1.717

Variable charts can be based on individual measurement mean values of small samples and mean values of measures of variability (Table 3.1).

$\bar{X}$ chart displays changes in the means of samples and in the variability of the sample practitioners in the field have developed short-cut methods for calculating control limits.

Center line is represented by x.

Upper control limit = $x + A2R$

Lower control limit = $x - A2R$

R chart notices and monitors the process range or dispersion, which is the display of variability of set of data.

Center line is represented by r, which is the average of all the ranges.

Upper control limit = $D4R$

Lower control limit = $D3R$

BUSINESS PROCESS RE-ENGINEERING

Business process re-engineering (BPR) is one of the buzz word in the management circle since 1990's. Michael Hammer coined the term in 1990.

"The fundamental re-thinking and re-designing of existing process tasks and operating structure to achieve dramatic improvements in process performance."

–Michael Hammer and James Charopy

The definition contains *four* key components:

1. A company or organization must fundamentally re-think the reasons for delivering products and services as it does.
2. New process must be designed.
3. As new processes are developed, full attention must be paid to the needs and values of the external customer.
4. Dramatic improvements must be the end goal of re-engineering.

Core Elements of BPR

BPR attempts radical change through organizational restructuring, work redesigning and technological retooling. These three "core elements" of re-engineering are the backbone of its success.

Core Elements

Organizational restructuring: While restructuring the organization for BPR:

Reduce or restructure organizational layers.

Realigning functions/work groups around the customer.

Driving accountability to front line.

Work re-designing: While re-designing work in organization:

Conduct "Customer value-added" process analysis of job task.

Expand job scope and ownership.

Build cross functional teams.

Technological retooling: Technological retooling requires the organization to consider:

Increasing the emphasis on process task that happen in parallel.

Gathering and communication customer related data.

Expediting access to information and data for all employees.

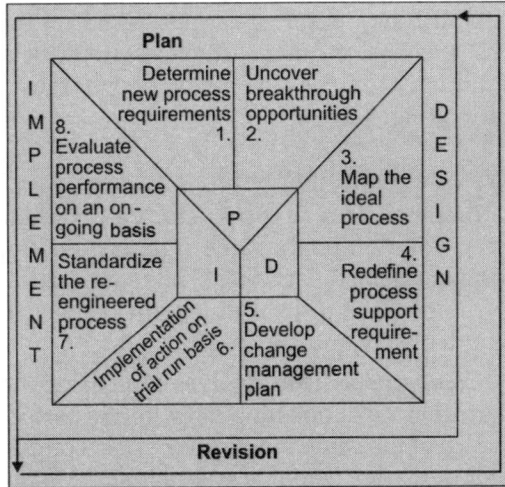

Fig. 3.4: Process re-engineering model

Selecting a process re-engineering team: The true starting point of a process re-engineering effort is putting together a team of people who will drive the effort. There are two approaches in this regard.

Core team approach: In which a small team of 3–4 members are formed.

Full team approach: In which a larger team of 8–12 or more members are involved in the process of re-engineering effort.

Phase I 1. Determine New Process Requirements

It involves uncovering what customers and the market place requires of your process, and focusing on organizations own operational requirements. The process re-engineering team should identify the internal and external customers. Who are being affected by re-engineering and how it affects them. The customer requirements includes timeliness, cost, accuracy, accessibility, etc. Customer requirements can be identified by interview/ questionnaire, etc. Organizational needs to see how their competitor is doing and in this process organization may develop new product or service. Organizations can undertake benchmarking at this juncture (Fig. 3.4).

Phase I 2. Uncover "Breakthrough" Opportunities

In this stage:

List the major process task.

Create a process flow chart, which helps to identify what happens at each step of process.

Envision the desired state — determine the new process requirements. For this undertake brain storming session with your team members as well as with the members of the corresponding department.

Identify the performance "Gaps"—compare the current process, with the ideal process. If the gap is large, prepare for re-engineering.

Phase II 3. Map the Ideal Process

Complete preliminary work, i.e. reducing the gap between the ideal and the real process.

Set new goals and establish new measures.

Create new process flow chart.

Phase II 4. Redefine Process Support Requirements

This includes:

What the organization requires from the people in the organization.

What technology/support tools the organization require.

What is the financial requirement for BPR.

Phase II 5. Develop Change Management Plan

In this:
Consider organizational impact.
Who and what will be impacted.
What are the emotional factor.
Design the change management plan.

Phase III 6. Implement on 'Trial Run Basis'

For this conduct a pilot test and assess the results and make necessary adjustments.

Phase III 7. Standardize the Re-engineered Process

Standardize means the new process become the acceptance and established process in the organization.

Phase III 8. Evaluate Performance on an On-going Basis

For evaluating hold regular meeting and celebrate progress if success is achieved.

Pitfalls in BPR

- Lack of commitment.
- Unclear rationale.
- Resistance to change.
- BPR can be used in hospitals to re-engineer various clinical and non-clinical problems.

BENCHMARKING

Definition

Xerox defines benchmarking as " the continuous process of measuring products, services, and practices against the toughest competitors or those companies known as leaders".

Robert Camp defines benchmarking as "finding and implementing best practices".

Gift and Mosel defined benchmarking as "the continual and collaborative discipline of measuring and comparing the results of key work processes with those of the best performers". It is learning how to adapt these best practices to achieve breakthrough process improvements.

All these definitions imply benchmarking
Makes systematic use of tools and knowledge.

Involves measurement, comparison and evaluation of both results and processes.

Focuses on the study and adaptation of the practices that produce the "best-in-class" results.

Strives to achieve performance improvements of breakthrough proportions.

Is best utilized on a routine basis.

Benchmarking is the search for best practices, that will lead to superior performance. Establishing operating targets based on the best possible industry practices are critical component in the success of every organization (Fig. 3.5).

Types of Benchmarking

Internal: This involves studying similar operations within the same organization, e.g. benchmarking the services of one surgical unit with another surgical unit with respect to length of stay, infections, etc.

Competitive: This involves comparing the performance of one function with the performance of the same function by direct competitor or market leader, e.g. benchmarking the diagnostic services of Owaisi Hospital with Apollo Hospital.

Functional or Generic: It involves benchmarking the similar functions/processes across different industries, e.g. benchmarking the house keeping services of a hotel with a hospital.

Collaborative: This involves conducting a benchmarking study through a voluntary network of healthcare providers in two phases —first among the members of the collaborative and then with the external benchmarking partner, e.g. 12 government hospitals jointly study the infection control procedures in their hospitals and then benchmark their infection control programme with a standard hospital which is known for infection control.

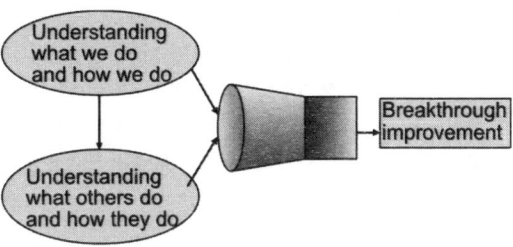

Fig. 3.5: Benchmarking model

Micro View

Organization first understands the process/product/procedure. Next the organization understands, what benchmark performers do and how they do it. Once the organization gains this knowledge, it creatively adapts the best practices found in benchmark performers into its own process, which will result in breakthrough improvements.

Benchmarking can be conducted in 11-steps, which consist of 5-phases: Planning, Analysis, Integration, Action and Maturity.

Phase I Planning: In this phase organization prepares a plan for conducting benchmarking. It first decides what to benchmark, whom to benchmark, how to collect data, etc.

1. *Identify the benchmarking subject:* Identifying the criteria to benchmark. It may be process (like discharge process), core competency (diagnostics, cardiac care, etc.), measure of performance (turnover interval, waiting time, etc.). Source may be from patient feedback, staff suggestions, etc.

2. *Identify the benchmarking partner:* Identify the immediate competitor, or the market leader. For internal benchmarking identify the department or the unit to be benchmarked.

3. *Identify data collecting method:* Generally mail survey, telephone survey and site visits are used to identify data collecting method.

Phase II Analysis: Analyzing the gap between current performance and best practice.

4. *Determine the performance gap:* Using the data collected, determine the gap between organizations performance and that of benchmarking partner's performance.

5. *Project future performance:* Based on the collected data and the anticipated customer, customer expectations, benchmarking team identify the future performance levels.

Phase III Integration: In this phase organization refines its goals and incorporates them into its planning process.

6. *Communicate results:* Communicate results to employees, shareholders and equip them for the change.

7. *Establish functional goals:* New functional goals will set to reach the new performance level.

Phase IV Action: In this phase organization implement the best practices, monitors performance and recalibrates the benchmarks.

8. *Develop action plans:* A detailed action plan will be formulated, which will contain activities to be conducted, responsibility to complete activities and their completion dates. Besides this, technical and behavioral aspects will be considered.

9. *Implement plans:* Working groups have to be formed to implement the plans.

10. *Recalibrate benchmarks:* Due to changing environment, we have to recalibrate the benchmark and modify accordingly.

Phase V Maturity: In this phase the organization will reach maturity in its benchmarking efforts.

11. *Integrate benchmarking:* Integrating benchmarking into core activities of organization, including strategic management, quality management, financial management, etc. Once benchmarking becomes integral part of organization, it has achieved a high level of sophistication in the process.

Benefits of Benchmarking

Benchmarking provides an effective approach to achieve change, which helps the organization to reach higher levels of performance.
- Benchmarking helps to set new goals and targets credibility.
- It increases customer focus.
- Benchmarking increases focus on processes that produce results and not just on results alone.
- Helps in better decision making.
- Stimulates innovation and creativity.

Pre-requisites of Benchmarking
- Commitment from leadership.
- Experience with CQI.
- A properly prepared organizational culture.
- Identification of key organizational processes.

Pitfalls
- Launching a benchmarking project without senior leadership support.
- Launching a benchmarking project without any of the pre-requisite in place.
- Conducting benchmarking for wrong reasons.
- Selecting the wrong benchmarking project.
- Selecting the wrong benchmarking partner.
- Failing to gain management approval of plans resulting from benchmark findings.

Conclusion

Hospital is a highly complex organization, whose services to a large extent are intangible. Continuous improvement in the processes will help in reducing the errors in hospitals considerably.

References

Deming, W. Edwards, "Out of the Crisis," M.I.T. Press, 1986.

Mitra, Amitava, "Fundamentals of Quality Control and Improvement," Prentice Hall, 1998.

Sridhar Bhat, Total Quality Management, Himalaya House Publications, Mumbai, 2002.

Srinivasan, N.S. and V. Narayana, Managing Quality-concepts and Tasks, New Age International, 1996.

Sundara Raju, S.M., Total Quality Management: A Primer, Tata McGraw-Hill, 1995.

4
Hospital Planning

Syeda Amtul Yafe

Hospitals are not built as monuments. It needs to be planned and constructed from the perspective of the end users, i.e. patients, doctors, nurses, bye-standers. Today most of the hospitals are built as architectural marvels, but once operations start the structure needs to be revamped.

MAJOR FUNCTIONS OF A HOSPITAL

1. Provision of medical care to the community (diagnostic, curative, preventive and promotive).
2. Education of professionals.
3. Centre for research activities.

THE CHANGING ROLE OF HOSPITALS

Earlier hospitals were merely place for the treatment of the sick. With the wide coverage of every aspect of human welfare as part of healthcare, *viz.* physical, mental and social well being, the healthcare services have undergone a steady metamorphosis, and the role of hospital has changed, with the emphasis shifting from:

 i. Acute to chronic illness.
 ii. Curative to preventive medicine.
 iii. Restorative to comprehensive medicine.
 iv. Inpatient care to outpatient and home care.
 v. Individual orientation to community orientation.
 vi. Isolated function to areawise or regional function.
 vii. Tertiary and secondary to primary healthcare.
 viii. Episodic care to total care.

Hospitals should be able to balance the "need list" of the professionals, the "want list" of the patients and the community and provide an effective, holistic, ethical, standardized, accessible, acceptable, safe and secure healthcare institute (Fig. 4.1).

THE CHANGING SCENE IN THE HOSPITAL FIELD

- Shift from providers market to consumers.
- Hospitals and healthcare institutions will become akin to industries.
- Hospitals will be catering more and more to the needs of patients which will:
  - Lead to more specialized hospitals.
  - People will shop for medical care.
  - Hospitals will require more managerial skills at all levels.
  - There will be growth of corporate hospitals.
  - Hospitals will become more capital intensive.
  - It will become more technology intensive.
  - Ascendancy of technology expectations over human values.
- Urban hospital concentration.
- Health insurance.
- Increasing role of hospitals in preventive medicine and health promotion.
- Rising mental illness, heart diseases, cancer and other chronic diseases.
- Geriatric care.
- Building new hospitals and establishing linkages.

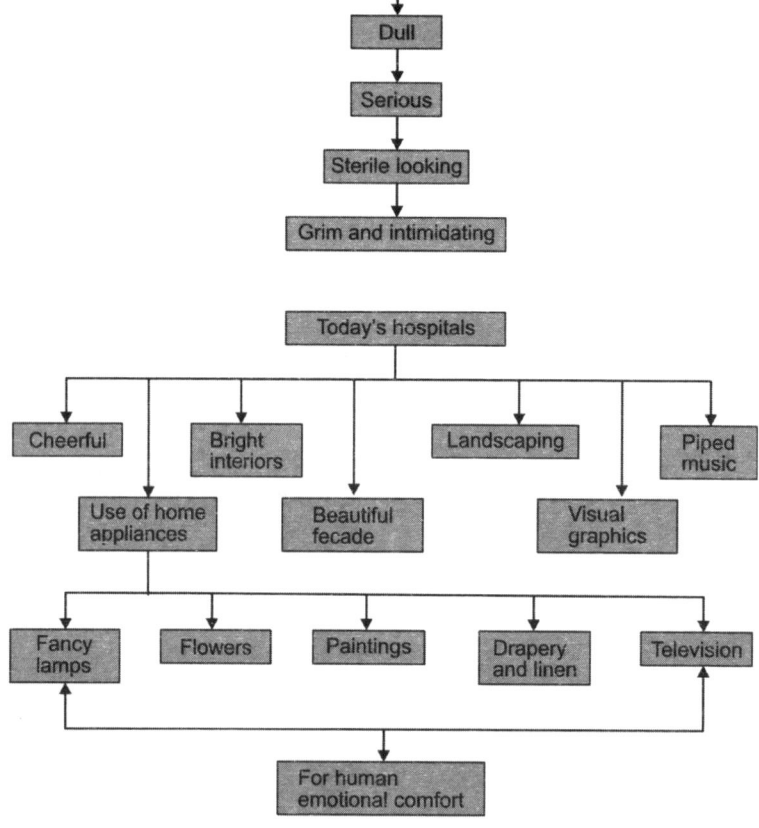

Fig. 4.1: Changing role of hospitals

- Healthcare will become non-accessible to the poorer sections of the society.
- Increasing prominence of complementary and alternate systems of medicine.
- Marketing of hospital and healthcare services.
- Consumer awareness and increased litigations against hospitals.
- Increasing costs.
- Accreditation and quality

CONCEPT OF GREEN BUILDING

It is a concept that promotes construction of building that is environment-friendly and energy-efficient. It is the practice of increasing efficiency of building and their use of energy, water and materials as well as reducing the impact of buildings on the environment and human health through better building design, construction, operation and maintenance.

Green building practices of sustainable building try to preserve and sustain the environment. They offer great benefit by way of reduction in the use of energy and water, improved air-quality and increased materials efficiency. Central to the concept of green building is the philosophy of designing building that are in harmony with the natural features and resources between a structure and built environment.

Some of the techniques associated with green building are prevention of soil erosion, rainwater harvesting, landscaping that reduces heat or helps to spread it out, reduction in the use of potable water, recycling of waste water (to be reused for non-potable purposes such as gardening, flushing toilets, etc.) and use of world-class energy efficient practices. Equally important are onsite generation of renewable energy through solar power, wind power, hydropower, etc. that can significantly reduce environmental impact of buildings. Green building emphasizes taking advantage of renewable resources such as sunlight through passive solar and active solar techniques. Site and building orientation has a major effect on building HVAC efficiency.

Green hospitals endeavor to conform to the following practices. There are 12 criteria used by the green guide for assessing green hospital candidates.

Siting: Hospital is built in a site with consideration for alternative storm water management, urban development and reducing any impact on the surrounding environment.

Water efficiency: Hospital is water efficient, taking advantage of landscaping, reduction of use of water and good use of waste water.

Energy and air pollution: Reduction in energy consumption and atmospheric pollution including chlorofluorocarbon (CFC) reductions, renewable energy, reduced energy consumption, green power and reducing ozone.

Materials and resources: Use recycled building materials and resources.

Indoor environment quality: Improve indoor air quality through increased ventilation and incorporating low-VOC (volatile organic chemical) paints, adhesives and materials to avoid off-gassing of formaldehyde and other carcinogenic com-pounds. Create comfortable temperature and enhanced day-lighting.

Healthy hospital food: Meals for patients and staff that include fresh, local and organic foods.

Green education: Hospital staff are trained in waste reduction, toxics such as mercury and PVC (which lead toxic plasticizers into fluids in IV drip bags and tubing.)

Green cleaning: Use cleaning products that do not release hazardous chemicals.

Waste reduction: Segregate medical waste and reduce, reuse and recycle general waste.

Healing gardens and green roofs: Where patients, staff and visitors can relax, reflect, drought-tolerant native plants in their healing gardens.

The following are some of the benefits of green buildings:

1. Green building practices reduce the impact of buildings on the environment.
2. They improve health of the people and hospital staff due to improved air quality and reduction in pollution.
3. They help hospitals to control or fight the menace of hospital-acquired infection. To prevent spread of infection, especially among patients with compromised immune systems, it is important to reduce exposure to germs. Green practices exactly do that.
4. There is a huge reduction in operating and maintenance cost by utilizing less energy and water. Hospital with their complex operations and medical equipment working 24 × 7 are among the greatest energy consumers. This saving will be enormous over their lifecycle.
5. They increase material efficiency.
6. It makes good business sense too. Huge economic benefit works as a good selling force for leasing or selling green buildings and properties in general.
7. Noticeable improvement in the health of community as a whole.

HOSPITAL UTILISATION INDICES

Definitions

1. *Hospital beds:* Bed which is staffed and equipped for round the clock care of patients is called hospital bed. It excludes beds in labor room, recovery room beds, beds which are not equipped and staffed for overnight use and the cots for normal, healthy, newborn babies in labor room but includes incubators and bassinets for premature babies.
2. *Bed complement:* It is the number of authorised or sanctioned beds for round the clock care of patients. It includes all adult beds, bassinets in paediatric ward, incubators and staff sick beds.
3. *Admissions:* Refer to the number per year of acceptances by a hospital of a patient who is expected to remain for one or more nights. Normal, healthy, newborn babies should not be counted as inpatient admissions, but babies requiring special care should be included among the admissions.
4. *Discharges and deaths:* The annual number of discharges includes the number of patients who have left the hospital (cured, improved, LAMA, etc.), the number who have transferred to another health or social institution, and the number who have died.
5. *Dead bed space:* Refers to beds unoccupied in a hospital due to a rigid compartmentalisation of nursing units among specialities. Such space may be up to 15 percent in large hospitals.
6. *Daily ward census (medical census):* It indicates the number of patients in the hospital on any day. It shows the number of patients in hospital at the hour of midnight because of which it is also referred to as the "midnight census" prepared by the nursing staff on night duty.
7. *Bed-days or patient-days:* It is the unit of measure denoting the service rendered to one in-patient in the hospital census between one day and the succeeding one. Sometimes the day of admission and the day of discharge are counted as one day. In other cases, a full day is counted only when admission is before midday or discharge is after midday.

In this section, the bed complement will be designated B. The annual number of admissions will be A, which can be replaced by the sum of discharges and deaths $(D + d)$; and the annual number of hospitalized patient days will be H. The daily average of beds occupied (N) will be $H/365$.

INDICES RELATING TO THE HOSPITAL

Average length of stay (L): It indicates the average period in hospital (in days) per patient admitted. Ideally it is calculated as follows: cumulative number of bed-days of all discharged patients (including those dying in hospital) during 1 year divided by the number or discharged and dead patients over a period of time. The formulae can be as follows in different countries or institutions:

a. Total number of bed-days in the year divided by the number of admissions in the same year:
$$L = H/A$$
b. Total number of bed-days in the year divided by the number of discharges and deaths in the same year:
$$L = H/(D + d)$$
c. Total number of bed-days in the year divided by half the sum of admissions and discharges (including deaths) in the same year:
$$L = H \times \frac{1}{½(A + D + d)} = 2 \times \frac{H}{A + D + d}$$

Bed-occupancy rate (O): Expresses the average percentage occupancy of hospital beds. It is calculated by dividing the daily average number of beds occupied by the bed complement and multiplying by 100:
$$O = \frac{N}{B} \times 100$$

Turnover interval (T): Expresses the average period, in days, that a bed remains empty, in other words, the average time elapsing between the discharge of one patient and the admission of the next. This figure is obtained by subtracting the actual number of hospitalization days from the potential number of hospitalization days in a year and dividing the result by the number of discharges (and deaths) in the same year:

$$T = \frac{B \times 365 - H}{D + d}$$

when the bed-occupancy rate is 100, turnover interval is zero and it becomes negative when the bed-occupancy rate is over 100.

Indices Relating to the Population at Risk

Admission rate: Also known as the hospital frequentation rate or hospital attendance rate. It is the number of hospital admissions per 1000 of the population per year.

$$Fn = \frac{A}{P} \times 1000$$

where P is the population at risk.

Hospitalization rate per person: This index expresses the volume of hospitalization in terms of number of hospitalization days per person per year.

$$Hc = \frac{H}{P}$$

where H is the total number of hospitalization days.

Bed-occupancy ratio: It is the average daily number of persons hospitalized per unit of population (usually per 1000 population). It is obtained by dividing the average daily number of beds occupied (average daily census) by the mean population in the same year and multiplying by 1000.

$$B_c = \frac{N}{P} \times 1000$$

Bed/population index: Expresses the availability of hospital beds in terms of the number of beds per 1000 of the population.

$$I_{b/P} = \frac{B}{P} \times 1000$$

where B is the bed complement.

Guiding Principles in Planning

- High quality patient care
- Effective community orientation
- Economic viability
- Orderly planning
- Early employment of the architect
- Operational plan and functional plan must precede architectural plans
- A sound architectural plan

HOSPITAL PLANNING TEAM

The first step in planning a hospital project is to assemble a planning team. The nucleus of the team consist of a hospital consultant, a person who is professionally trained in hospital administration with at least 10–15 years of experience and one or two medical and lay administrators, a nursing administrator, and hospital architect. An architect can be of value only if he has experience of hospital architecture and construction. In the early stages a core group could be formed with hospital consultant and a medical administrator. As the project progresses the core group can be expanded.

Hospital Project: Planning to Commissioning

In general, a hospital project undergoes the following phases.

- Inception
- Feasibility studies
- Outline proposal
- Scheme design
- Detail design
- Tender action
- Construction
- Commissioning
- Shake-down.

These phases can be grouped in the following six stages from A to F:

Stage A
Functional content : Project team
Outline brief : Assessment of functional content
: Submission to owners (Government, private organization, etc.) for approval
: Site appraisals, gross floor areas
: Building space. Draft master plan
: Estimation of cost and phasing
: Appraisal of work by owners

Stage B
Operational policies : Operational policies
Development plan : Departmental and interrelated activities
: Departmental and hospital policies
: Development control plan
: Budget cost
: Continuous informal discussion with owner through stage B.

Stage C
Schedules of accommodation, : Schedules of accommodation
Sketches, final cost estimate : Sketch drawing
: Equipment schedules component estimates
: Cost, revenue and staffing estimates
: Final cost approval

Stage D
Detail design working : Working drawings
drawings, tender action : Engineering detail
: Bills of quantities
: Calling tenders

Stage E
Contract and construction : Assessments of tenders
: Award of contract
: Construction
: Engineering commissioning

Stage F
Commissioning : Staff assembly and training
: Equipment and supplies assembly
: Testing of installations
: Opening

ASSESSMENT OF THE EXTENT OF NEED FOR THE HOSPITAL SERVICES

One of the first task of the planning team is collection of data to assess the extent of need for the particular hospital and the range of services required. There are two methods of assessing the extent of functional need for a hospital. They are: 1. the empirical method which applies the norms of the past and rules of thumb to the problem, with appropriate modifications to suit local conditions, and 2. analytical method which makes a more fundamental, systematic approach to the problem.

Elements requiring consideration and analysis: *Morbidity Statistics*

Prevalence of	: Communicable diseases
	: Degenerative diseases: Accident rate
	: Specific diseases/disorders
Measurement of	: Death rate
	: Birth rate
	: Maternal mortality rate
	: Infant mortality rate
Demographic	: Age and sex profile
	: Population density
	: Occupational characteristics
	: Extent of urbanization
	: Extent of migratory population
	: Economic development of the area
Socio-economic statistics	: Economic status of the community
	: Literacy and educational standard
	: Social habits and socio-cultural grouping
	: Housing conditions
	: Styles of living
	: Industrialization
Hospital statistics	: Type of existing services
	: Admission rates
	: Disease-specific admission rates
	: Hospital beds in the region
	: Utilisation of existing health and hospital services
	: Extent and effectiveness of general practitioner service

Factors Influencing Hospital Utilisation

1. Hospital bed availability
2. Population coverage and bed distribution
3. Age profile of population
4. Availability of medical services other than hospitals
5. Customs and attitudes of medical profession
6. Method of payment for hospital services
7. Availability of qualified medical manpower
8. Housing
9. Morbidity pattern
10. Hospital bottlenecks
11. Internal organisation
12. Public attitudes

Geographical, Environmental and Miscellaneous Factors

1. Meteorological information
   - Temperature
   - Rainfall
   - Humidity
2. Geographical information
   - Exiting road and rail communications
   - Terrain: mountainous, riverine, plain
   - Surrounding district bodies
   - Ecology-atmospheric pollutants from adjoin industries and other sources, proximity of sources of noise such as air-fields or rail tracks.
   - Building height restrictions due to proximity of airports
3. Miscellaneous availability of
   - Trained manpower
   - Water
   - Electricity
   - Sewage disposal.

Feasibility Report

It should bring out:

1. The potential of the planned institution.
2. Medical facilities that are lacking and need to be made available.
3. The migration pattern of patients.
4. Competition from the existing hospitals and new entrants.
5. Identify the need and demand of the healthcare services.

CHOOSING A SITE

General consideration: The second task of planning team will be to choose the site for the hospital. Site should be large enough to enable future expansion and growth. In dense urban areas, a large site near the periphery of the present town is also suitable, as it will be difficult to find a viable site in the central location of the city. Close collaboration with local town authorities will be useful in the identification of the site. Accessibility should be another factor, which should be given due consideration, while choosing a site. The site should be free from noise, smoke, vapors, and other annoyances. A site acquired cheaply or received as gift may ultimately turn out to be far more expensive than a highly priced plot.

Land requirements: In rural and semi-urban areas, plentiful land may be available permitting the hospital to grow horizontally. However, in urban areas there will always be great premium on land and the only available avenue will be a vertical growth.

Site cover on a plot of land is expressed as percentage as under

Site cover percentage =

$$\frac{\text{Total ground floor area of all buildings}}{\text{Total area of site available}} \times 100$$

The degree of crowding on a site is considered in terms of floor area ratio (FAR). It is the ratio of the total covered area on all floors of a building to the total area of the site.

Soil structure: A preliminary soil survey to determine sub-soil water level and the "bearing" quality of the soil will help determine the type of foundation, possibility of constructing basement and effectiveness of sewage plant if required.

Public utilities: The other important considerations in site selection are availability of water supply, sewage disposal system and electric power.

Water: For planning purpose the overall requirement of water in hospital is estimated at about 300–400 litres per bed excluding requirement for A/C, fire fighting, gardening and steam. ISI suggests 455 litres of water per consumer day (LPCD) for hospital up to 100 beds and 340 LPCD for hospitals of more than 100 beds. Storage capacity for 3 days must be built at the site.

Sewage disposal: Solid waste from hospitals is approximately 1 kg per bed per day. Liquid effluents will be about the same as the hospital requirements are between 300 and 400 L per bed per day. If a public sewage system does not exist in that area, hospital will have to build and operate its own sewage disposal plant.

Power: Requirement of electric power is approximately 2–5 kW on a per bed per day basis. This includes needs for all departments like X-ray, operation theatres, laboratories, C.S.S.D, laundry and kitchen. Besides this, stand-by generator is also a necessity.

Electrical substation: A hospital will have its own transformer and electrical substation for distribution of power to various areas. The total substation area depending on the transformers capacity is given in Tables 4.1 and 4.2.

MASTER PLAN IN ITS TOTALITY

In the next step, the hospital planning team will prepare the draft master plan document. The approximate volume of the buildings will be calculated. Master plan takes into consideration the future development of the hospital. Master plan will show whether hospital is a concentration of the multi-storeyed building or a loose conglomeration of spread-out structures over larger areas on the ground employing low buildings. With these the master plan should take into account the circulation routes, areas to be allotted for each department, relative dispositions of departments into functional zones, also considering light, wind, hospital engineering and hygiene aspects.

Circulation routes — the utility and success of a hospital plan depend to a larger extent on

Table 4.1: Area for electrical substation

Transformer capacity	Area for transformer	Total substation area
1 × 500 kVA	24 sq m	80 sq m
2 × 500 kVA	36 sq m	130 sq m
2 × 800 kVA	40 sq m	135 sq m
2 × 1000 kVA	40 sq m	150 sq m

Table 4.2: Electric load estimates for a 200-bed state-of-the-art

HVAC	1200 kW
General lighting (i/c external)	320 kW
General lights and power plugs	350 kW
MRI, CAT Scan and X-ray M/Cs	300 kW
Angiography and Gamma Camera, etc.	175 kW
Pathology and microbiology labs	150 kW
CSSR	200 kW
Surgical suites (4–5)	150 kW
Servers, PCs	100 kW
Elevators and Dumbwaiters	125 kW
Laundary and kitchen	250 kW
Water supply and treatment plus	180 kW
Miscellaneous	100 kW
Total	3600 kW
	4500 kVA at 0.8 power factor.

the circulation routes on the hospital site and within buildings. There are two types of circulation:

1. Internal circulation
2. External circulation

Internal circulation: Internal traffic routed are required for linking major clinical departments for use by patients and staff, and for delivery of supplies to these departments. The circulation space involves corridors, stairs and lifts. Corridors with less than 8 feet width are not desirable in hospitals. A large volume of internal traffic in hospital involves use of patient trolleys. Supplies and stores also move on trolleys. In multistoreyed buildings, provisioning for vertical movement of patient trolleys has, therefore, to be catered for. It may be economical to concentrate lifts at one place than distribute at the different parts of the building. Two lifts are minimum for any multistoreyed building. In not so high buildings, planning for ramps for trolley traffic (rampwell) must also be considered in addition to the stairwell. The point to remember is that there should not be an undue criss-crossing of the patient, staff, supplies and visitors. Use of multistoreyed buildings is more economical than low buildings connected by long corridors and scattered lifts. If linear spine concept of building is followed, it will be better for the proper internal circulation. In the linear spine concept of building, the additional departments are entered from the central spine, which may have several levels. It steers the circulation and takes the hospital growth easily and labyrinthine patterns, so common in large buildings, are avoided. An example of the linear spine concept is depicted (Fig. 4.2) for efficient internal circulation, there should be a central main artery serving the whole complex.

Ramps, steps, stairs: Handrails must be provided on both sides of steps and stairs, and should extend beyond the first and the last steps on at least one side. Hard, level, non-skid surfaces are essential for steps and stairs, and handrails must not be of slippery material.

86 Hospital Management

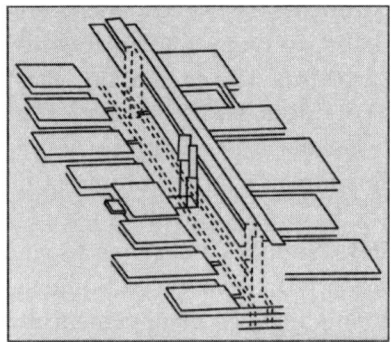

Fig.4.2: Illustration of the linear spine

2. *External circulation:* Only one entrance to the hospital for the vehicular traffic from the main road is desirable. Provided the entrance and exit points are wide enough to take two lanes of traffic, one entry has the advantage of clarity for all visiting traffic, and one exit the advantage of security from administrative viewpoint. Parking area for different types of vehicles should be separately allotted. Parking area should be distinct for patients, staff and visitors.

DISTANCES, COMPACTNESS, PARKING, LANDSCAPING AND VISUAL IMPACT

Distances: Must be minimized for all movement of patients, medical, nursing, and other staff and for supplies, aiming at minimum of time and motion.

Compactness: From the angle of compactness multistoried buildings have the advantage of being convenient when compared with horizontal development as it demands more land involving extra costs in development and installation of services, roads, water supply sewage, electric lines and so on.

Parking: For each inpatient bed, 1–2 visitors will be there per day. For each inpatient bed there will be about 3 outpatients, many of them coming in vehicles. One car parking

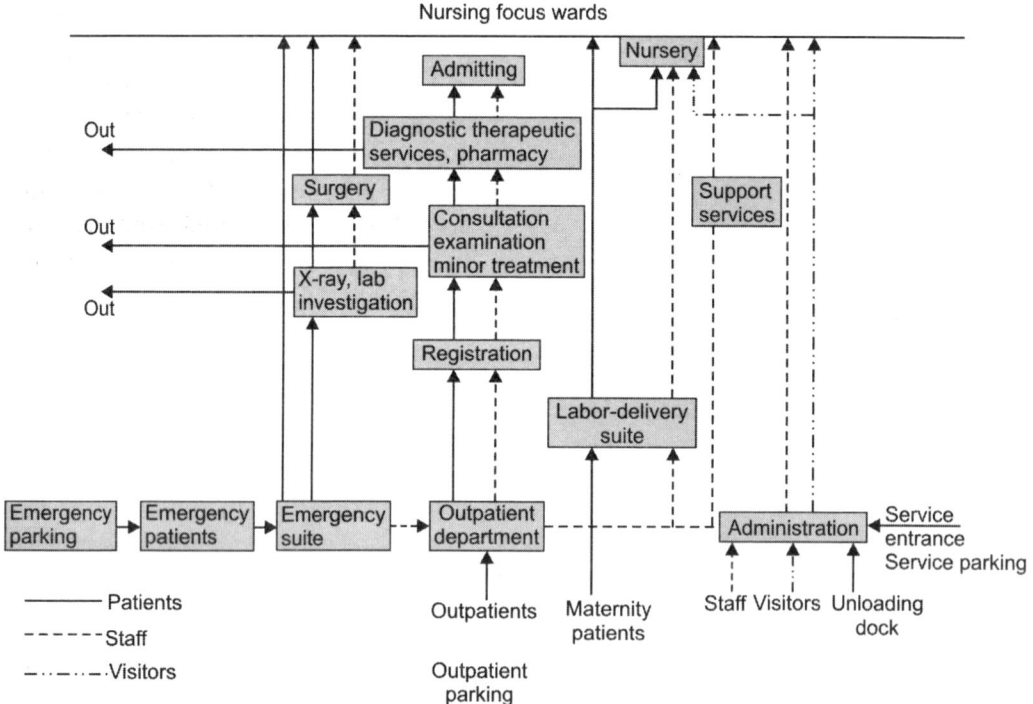

Fig. 4.3: Key flow chart of a general hospital

space per 2 beds is desirable in metro cities, whereas lesser is required in semi-urban and rural areas. Additional parking area for three-wheelers and two wheelers should be considered. Employees staff parking areas should be separated from public parking.

Landscaping: There is a psychological effect of the visual impact of attractive grounds, buildings and surroundings on patients visitors and staff. If possible building should be located on a relatively high ground, the elevation being not so great to be a handicap for those approaching on foot. The building should be built in such a way that it gets maximum natural light and natural wind. In the tropics, the long sides of buildings occupied by patients should face north and south as much as possible. Deft use of sloping sites can be made by the architect for car parking, temporary refuse storage, and recreational activities.

Visual impact: Architectural handling of the design determines the visual impact of the hospital. Here innovations and creativity should come together.

Linearity: It exhibits high degree of stability with reasonable adaptability. The image of a hospital designed linearly will be low and not monumental. The challenge for the architect is to create a unique institution.

ZONAL DISTRIBUTION AND INTER-RELATIONSHIPS OF DEPARTMENT

Each major department clinical area, supportive area and administrative units have to be distributed over the site in appropriate zones to group them in a manner that they are related to each other in continuity. Departments such as outpatient department, accident and emergency or casualty which are in close contact with the public should be isolated from the inpatient area and should be closer to the main entrance of the site. The supportive service departments, viz. the X-ray and laboratory services are extensively used by outpatients and need to be located as near the outpatient department as possible, at the same time integrated with the main inpatient wards. At the main entrance, there should be the main inpatient zone which will consist of ICU, wards, operation theatres and delivery suites. This should be as far away and isolated from the hubbub of activity that takes place in areas proximate to the main entrance. Central services especially the heavy duty service departments such as CSSD, laundry, hospital stores, pharmacy, kitchen and cafeteria are better located on ground floor and grouped around a service core area.

The other factors which should be considered for the zonal distribution include

1. Medical gases: The patient care activities in hospital include medical oxygen, nitrous oxide, carbon dioxide, medical grade air and vacuum for suction. All these except suction are provided in metal storage cylinders. Manifold system should be located on the ground floor. It is a network of pumps, compressors, pressure regulators, cylinders manifold and a maze of pipes. Pipelines carrying medical gases/air and vacuum for suction are colored in different colors as per internationally accepted color coding standard.

Color coding of gas pipelines distribution system:

Item	Color of pipeline
Oxygen	Yellow
Nitrous oxide	Dark blue
Compressed air	Sky blue
Vacuum	Sky blue

2. Size and location of water tanks whether underground, overhead or roof mounted. Storage capacity should be at least three times the total daily requirements.
3. Location of the incinerator where trash and infected material will be burned.
4. Boiler house for the supply of steam to laundry C.S.S.D and kitchen.
5. Mortuary for storage of dead bodies and postmortem room.

6. Accommodation facilities for doctors, nurses and other essential staff.
7. Community centre with grocery and fruit shop, barbers shop, newspaper and bookstall, flower shop, chemist shop and a community hall.
8. Accommodation facilities like dharamshala or choultry for attendants and relatives.

GROSS SPACE REQUIREMENTS

Till few years ago 500–600 sq ft/bed was the space requirement. But with the development of technology, the space requirement has gone up to 700–1200 sq ft/bed (Table 4.3).

Table 4.3: Distribution of floor space by wards and departments

Wards	OPD	Diagnostic and therapeutic department	Administrative	Service Departments
37–45%	12–18%	18–22%	8–12%	15–20%

For inpatients functionally 100 sq ft/bed of 9.29 sq m in general hospital has been accepted as area occupied per bed. With 75 sq ft/bed located in rooms with 4 beds or more. The total hospital area works to be approximately 8–10 times. Approximate breakup of hospital space is given in Table 4.4.

Indian standards institution in their standard IS 10905 part-I have recommended an area of one hectare for every 25 beds.

CLIMATIC CONSIDERATION IN DESIGN

India has a predominantly tropical climate ranging from the hot and humid climate in the east and north eastern states, hot and dry climate of the central and western Indian plains, to the cold climate in the northern regions. In certain climates buildings have to be heated or cooled in winter or summer and in some areas building may need both heating or cooling at different times of year. By concentrating the building as

Table 4.4: Breakup of space requirements General hospitals

Area	Sq.ft bed
Nursing units	250–280
Nursery	12–18
Delivery suites	15–20
Operation theatres	30–50
Physical medicine	12–18
Radiology	25–35
Laboratory	25–35
Pharmacy	4–6
CSSD	8–25
Dietary	25–35
Medical records	8–15
Housekeeping	4–5
Laundry	12–8
Mechanical installations	50–75
Maintenance workshops	4–6
Stores	25–35
Public areas	8–10
Staff facilities	10–15
Administration	40–50
Total	561–751
Circulation	115–40
Total net area	682–891
Add walls, partition	95–125 Sq.ft
Gross total area (Building gross)	~ 780–1005 (72.5-93.46 sq m)

possible, the surface area available for heat loss or heat gain can be reduced. If air conditioning is required, the buildings or the rooms requiring A.C must be made as compact as possible, by using low ceilings and restricting the size of the building to the absolute minimum. The buildings are to be oriented to face their long sides north and south or north east and south west, so that it helps in getting the natural light. In hot humid climate, the building should be open and oriented in such way that even a slight breeze can enter the building and cool its insides. In this climate the building should be reasonably spread out. In hot dry climate building should have thick walls and small windows, as thick walls will absorb heat during day and dissipate at night.

Planning for energy conservation and saving: A colossal amount of energy is used in hospitals for various engineering services like lighting, heating, ventilation, air-conditioning, boilers for CSSD, kitchen and laundry, pumps, lifts, and incinerators. The energy costs are a substantial percentage of the cost of running a hospital. In air-conditioning systems, design criteria gearing comfort levels and air changes per hour are factors influencing the energy consumption. The bifurcation of areas according to their period of AC requirements, say 8 hours, 12 hours, etc. during the design stage can result in energy saving, similarly, solar water heating systems can be installed for pre-heating water used in laundry and kitchen.

PREPARATION OF THE FUNCTIONAL BRIEF OR ARCHITECTURAL BRIEF

The fourth task of the planning team is the preparation of the functional brief or architectural brief or small scale drawings. Analysis of functional needs, definition of operational policies, architectural programmes in relation to the needs of the hospital, inter-relationships of departments, the grouping of accommodation and the main outline of traffic flow, engineering services and communication provide a firm basis for the designers work. Before an architect can develop a hospital design has to be provided with a written programme explaining hospitals operational policy, particularly with reference to the clinical areas. To enable a hospital to serve its purpose, "design must follow function".

Architects brief is a written document which explains the types of services to be provided, operational policies and inter-relationships of facilities with one another.

Contents of the Brief

1. *Introduction:* General introduction, mission, and philosophy of the proposed hospital.
2. *Site information:* To include topography of the area/site, boundaries, surface area-existing public utilities, nearest city, airport, railway station, weather.
3. ***Workload projection and functional content:*** Specifying expected workload, functions and contents of department, to include number of beds and bed mix, work flow, traffic flow.
4. *Equipment:* Type of items of medical equipment and quantities.
5. *Zoning:* Specific grouping and zoning of departments and facilities.
6. *Policies and procedures:* It is related to patient and staff movement services—CSSD, laundry, catering, etc. mains and standby electric supply, HVAC, fire protection, infection control, pollution control and further expansion plans.
7. ***Schedules of accommodation:*** These include description of functions and spaces, number of personnel working at each duty station, list of all other spaces listing the activities performed in each of them, the functional relationship within a department and also between the departments.
8. *Phasing:* If the whole project is considered for breaking up into phases, the activities/work/schedules will have to be suitably divided into appropriate phases.
9. *Financial aspects:* These include construction cost, equipment cost, furniture cost, total project cost, sources of funds.

Determination of the services to be provided in quantitative terms requires consideration of the following for each of the several units ranging from an operation theatre and delivery suite to a utility room: functions, location, relationship, utilization, staffing pattern, space requirements, work flow, communication, traffic flow, equipment, finishes and special requirements.

Preliminary Drawings, Working Drawings and Estimate

From the 'architects brief' and schematic drawings, sketch plans will be prepared. At this stage the services of a structural engineer, electrical engineer, plumbing engineer and mechanical engineer can be taken. At this stage the issues related to structural framing, foundations, plumbing, ventilation, internal circulation, electricity and other engineering problems will be considered. After this an approximate estimate of the cost of the project will be made.

Prelimimanry drawings: Drawing, outline specifications and other material which define in specific detail all the systems, materials and components of a project sufficient to make an accurate cost estimate.

Schematic drawings: Drawing indicating the overall scope of the project in broad detail, usually showing only general functional relationships among its elements.

Working drawings: The final plans and specifications from which a building is actually constructed. This is to be conveyed to the builders regarding the construction of the building. It usually consists of:

1. *Architectural drawings:* It shows the plan of site, roads and path, floor and roof plans, elevations, schedules of doors and windows, finishes of exteriors and interiors.
2. *Structural drawings:* It shows location and size of foundation, footings, columns, beams girders and slabs.
3. *Mechanical drawings:* It shows the details of piping both concealed and exposed, plumbing, ventilating and air-conditioning work. Incoming water supply service, fire hydrant, underground water piping system, storm water, and sewer line networks, medical gas systems, hot and cold water piping system, equipment schedules, and system and fixture schedules.
4. *Electrical drawings:* It shows the details of electric feeders, location of electric panels, plans of lighting, power and special systems, fixtures, items of electrical equipment, requirements of receptacles, nurse call system, intercommunication system, static electricity shielding, special grounding and fire alarms.

There are other essential drawing which the architect needs to prepare are:

License drawings: These are architectural drawings showing the plan of all the floors, heights, details of rooms, exits, doors and windows, tentative details of plant and machinery. These are required for submission to various statutory/regulated bodies to get a no objection certificate and/or commencement certificate before taking the actual construction work. These are also used to appraise the financial institutions in case of external funding of the project.

Tender drawings: These are architectural, structural and other utilities drawings explaining the building and engineering scheme. They also include specifications and typical details of work. The tendering firms make their bids based on these documents. On award of work, these drawings form part of the agreement between the owners and the contractor. Architects and engineers attach great importances to these drawings.

Specifications: These are written instructions describing in detail the construction work to be undertaken. It expresses in writing the quality, performance standards and the ultimate result that is expected from proper assembly of materials and equipment identified in the drawings. Specifications supplement the working drawings and furnish the information not shown in them.

Modular grids: It is advisable to have a standard space module throughout the building for the efficient use of space. To rationalize floor space for various facilities, the use of a functionally optimal planning grid is made to arrive at a space planning module. A 1.6 m grid has been found to be ideal.

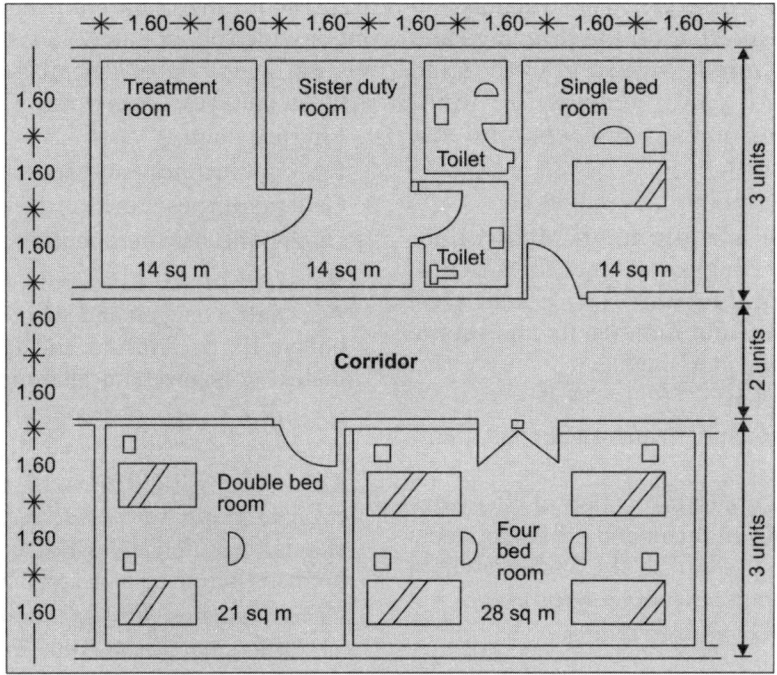

Fig. 4.4: Modular grid: Space-Planning module

Multiples of this grid in varying combinations give standardized areas (Fig. 4.4).

An example is shown below. Five such grid 3.2m × 4.8m) will give a carpet area of about 14.0 sq m, which is adequate for a single bed room. The use of uniform planning grid allows for the applications of standard building components.

Design efficiency: Means the ratio of usable area to plinth area. It is suggested that the built up area may be split into four categories: usable area, service area, circulation area and wall and column area.

Project cost: The project cost is estimated on a per bed basis. Keeping the current level of costs, approximately for a primary care ₹ 5–10 lakhs, for secondary care ₹ 15–20 lakhs and for tertiary care ₹ 40–50 lakhs per bed is estimated. The actual figure may vary highly, depending on the variety of considerations—78–81% of total cost is for construction together with built in equipment, 12–15% for depreciable and non-depreciable equipment and 6–8% for fees and salaries. Depending upon the kind of hospital and how hi-tech it is, the cost of depreciable equipment in today's hospitals may be more than 12–15% of the total cost (Table 4.5).

Direct project cost = Base cost of building + Escalation factor + Fees + Site acquisition

Typical Units of Cost of a Hospital Facility
1. Acquisition of site (Table 4.5)
2. Land development and landscaping
3. Off-site improvements
4. Legal fees and expenses
5. Expenditure connected with:
    a. Preliminary survey/feasibility study
    b. Setting up of a permanent organizations
    c. Fund raising campaign, community and public relations exercise, and promotional activities.

6. Work to be covered by construction contracts (as specified in the drawings and specifications): building with fixed equipment, contingencies for minor alterations, extra work, etc. and site improvement.
7. Site survey and soil investigations.
8. Depreciable equipment: Medical equipment, diagnostic and therapeutic equipment, furniture, office machines, kitchenware and utensils, linen, hospital supplies and store items.
9. Architects fee.
10. Hospital consultant and other consultants fees.
11. Supervision and inspection at site. (superintending engineer and other engineers and personnel at the site and elsewhere who are on the owners payroll).
12. Payment to statutory bodies.

EQUIPPING A HOSPITAL

Mechanical and electrical installations and the plant and the equipment have been estimated to cost about 40% of the entire hospital project out of which about half (20%) is required for medical equipment of general use. Equipment in the hospital can be classified into:

1. Physical plant
2. Hospital furniture and appliances
3. General purpose furniture and appliances
4. Diagnostic and therapeutic equipment

1. *Physical plant:* Lifts, refrigeration and AC, central oxygen and suction, generator, boilers, fixed sterilizers, kitchen equipment, incinerators, mechanical laundry.

2. *Hospital furniture and appliances:* Beds, stretchers, trolleys, wheel chairs, bedside lockers, dressing drums, kitchen utensils, bedside lamps, movable screens, hand wash stands, operation tables, instrument trolleys, bedpans, waste bins, hospital linen.

3. *General purpose furniture and appliances.*
   I. Office machines—Intercom sets, type writers, calculators, cash registers, filing systems, electronic exchange, computer
   II. Office furniture
   III. Crockery and cutlery

Table 4.5: Project cost

• Cost per bed (excluding cost of land)	
• General bed	5–10 lakhs
• Specialty bed	15–20 lakhs
• Superspecialty bed	40–50 lakhs
• Development of land includes topographical survey, site clearance, landscaping, compound wall and fencing, internal road, soil and storm water drainage.	1–3% of total project cost
• Cost of civil construction does not include costs of residential buildings.	30–40% of total project cost
• Cost of hospital building utility includes services equipment (communications, electric substation, generators, UPS and allied electric services, fire protection services, HVAC, lifts, escalators, signage, waste management, interiors, furniture and fittings).	15–20% of cost of construction
• Cost of hospital equipment	40–50% of project cost
• Consultancy charges	5–8% of total project cost.

4. *Diagnostic and Therapeutic Equipment:*
   I. *Equipment for general use* — Surgical instruments, physiotherapy department equipment, clinical laboratory equipment, BP instruments, suction machines, rehabilitation department equipment, sterilisers, glassware washers, voltage stabilizers, refrigerators, chemical analysers-microscopes.
   II. Equipment interacting with patients during diagnostic and therapeutic procedures—Short-way diathermy machines, electric cautery machine, defibrillators, X-ray machines, monitoring equipment, respirators, incubators, ECG machines, USG machines.

While equipping the hospital, cost as well quality should be given due considerations. While going in for costly equipment, their feasibility should be properly studied.

CONSTRUCTION AND COMMISSIONING

Based on the working drawings and specifications, contract bidders prepare their proposal and estimate for the building and submit their tenders when invited bid competitively. Tender document usually consists of notice inviting tenders, special instruction to tenderers, articles of agreement, tender form, general and special conditions of contract, technical specifications, bills of quantities, tender drawing and an appendix which consist of date of commencement, date of completion, EMD mobilization advance payable, rate of recovery of mobilization advance, defects liability period, value interim bills, penalty and bonus clause, retention amount and release amount. The award of contract is made to a bidder, considering cost, quality and experience of the bidder. The architect supervises the construction to ensure that work is carried out according to contract and correct materials are used. An agreement is drawn between the owners and the contractor on time schedule, method and periodicity of payment, terms of penalty and bonus, penalty in case of fault, etc. Sometimes due to unforeseen circumstances, a need may arise to change the construction plan, once the work has started. At this time drawings and specification may have to be changed, which will alter the contract with contractor.

Different Stages in the Construction of a Hospital Building

1. Commencement certificate
2. Demolition (if necessary)
3. Site preparation/gardomg
4. Layout and marking
5. Footings
6. Structure
7. Foundation
8. Structure
9. Floor and decks
10. Walls
11. Window/doors
12. Plumbing
13. Water supply and sanitation
14. HVSC
15. Fire detection and protection
16. False ceilings
17. Interior walls
18. Waterproofing
19. Hard interior
20. Floorings
21. Paint and finish
22. Built-in (fixed) equipment
23. Depreciable equipment
24. External services
25. Landscaping
26. Testing and commissioning
27. Trial run
28. Takeover by the owners
29. Move in

GENERAL CONSIDERATIONS FOR PLANNING AND DESIGNING HOSPITAL

- Orientation of the hospital should be such that maximum natural light and maximum breeze enter the hospital.
- Windows should be screened as far as possible.
- As far as possible there should be only one entrance for general public.
- The service entrance should be adjacent to kitchen and storage areas.
- The main entrance and the lobby should be attractive.
- Great care should be given for planning and development of traffic flow.
- Proper care should be given while planning the floors.
- Corridors of 8 feet/2.4384 meters width with a finished ceiling height of 8 feet/2.4384 meters are the most widely accepted pattern. Corridors in areas not commonly used for patient transportation in beds of stretchers may be reduced by 5–6 feet/1.524–1.82 meters. In general corridors should be as straight as possible, but their long smooth walls should be broken by projections for the sake of appearance as well as to prevent the reverberation of sound.
- Ceilings should be acoustically treated.
- Walls should be smooth so as not to collect dust and dirt and should be easily washable. It should be tiled up to 5 feet. Angles and sharp corners should be eliminated as far as possible. Corners can be rounded in the plaster finish and they should be provided with corner beading as protection for bumping.
- Electrical outlets should be provided on the walls of the corridor for cleaning equipment and for use of mobile X-ray. They should be spaced conveniently to reach every room without the need to use unduly long extension cords. Outlets may also be utilized for food trolleys that need to be plugged on to an electrical outlet to keep the food warm.
- Nursing unit's corridors should have general illumination with provision for reduction of light levels at night.
- It is desirable to place nurses signal lights in the corridor above the doors of patient rooms.
- Stairways are hardly used but they are mandatory and necessary in case of fire. There should be two stairways from the top floor to the ground level exit two separate areas of the building. The minimum width should be 3 feet 8 inches/1.2 meters and with wide landings to handle and negotiate stretchers in an emergency such as evacuations height of approximately 3 feet should be provided with clearance of 3.81 cm (1.5") between the handrail and the wall. Ends should be returned to the wall or otherwise traditional closed dull looking staircase.
- Recessed spaces for fire extinguishers and hose must be provided. They should follow the codes of local and state governments.
- Acoustical treatment of ceiling is strongly recommended to reduce sound transmission.
- Telephone booths, drinking water facilities, vending machines and portable equipment should not be located on the corridors as they will restrict corridor traffic or reduce their usable width.
- Floor should not be hard type. Soft and smooth floor like that of vinyl or linoleum is resilient and makes walking easy, noiseless and non-slippery.
- Hospitals with 125–200 beds should have three or more elevators with one or two being hospital type elevators of larger dimensions to accommodate hospital beds with attendants and separate patient, visitors and staff and service elevators. They are best utilized in a bank and not at separated locations and the door should not

open and unload patients into the main lobby but preferably to an alcove or a side corridor. Safety devices such as dual controls, self-levelling features telephone and alarms should be provided. Elevator call buttons and controls should of material that will not be activated by heat or smoke.
- The minimum width of doors to patient rooms should be 1.2 meters (3'8") preferably 1.16 meters (3'10") and door that may admit a patient in a bed should be 1.21 meters (4'0") and its height 2.13 meters (7'0"). The greater width also reduces damage to doors and frames where frequent movement of beds and large equipment occurs.
- Doors of patient rooms should open outward with an outside lock only and toilets should have doors and hardware that will permit emergency access from outside. Expansion joints and thresholds should be made flush with the floor to facilitate smooth movement of stretchers, wheelchairs and carts.
- Patient toilets should be provided with grab bars and panic button with a pull cord. Bars should have strength and anchorage to sustain a load of about 110 at 120 kg.
- Wash basins should be firmly fixed to withstand a vertical load of about 100 to 120 kg on the frame fixture.
- Mirrors should not be provided in places such as handwashing facilities in food preparation area, nurseries, clean and sterile supply areas, scrub sinks.
- The minimum ceiling height should be 2.43 meters (8'00") except in radiographic, operating and delivery rooms and rooms that have ceiling mounted equipment or surgical light fixtures.
- Boiler rooms should have ceiling clearance of not less than 6.35 cm (2'6") above the main boiler header and connecting piping.
- Ceiling height in toilet rooms, storage rooms, corridor and minor spaces that are normally unoccupied should be 2.13 meters (7'0").
- Recreation rooms, exercise rooms and equipment rooms should be away from patient areas or provisions should be made to minimize noise.
- Laundries, CSSD and boiler rooms should be insulated and ventilated to prevent areas above and adjacent to them from receiving or affected by excessive heat.
- Wall bases in kitchen, OT, delivery rooms and soiled work rooms that are subjected to wet cleaning several times everyday should be made integral with floor, tightly sealed and constructed without voids.
- Ceilings and walls in OT, delivery rooms, isolation rooms, nurseries and CSSD should be monolithic from wall to wall without open joints, crevices or fissures.
- Entering public toilets directly from waiting areas should be avoided. Water closets should be separated from wash basin areas by stall partitions wherever possible.
- High windowsills should be avoided in administrative offices and waiting areas for better ventilation and visual contract outside.
- Provision for disasters.
- The envelope (includes wall materials, colors, insulations, sealing, roofing, etc.) should be carefully planned and designed.
- Environmental impact analysis.
- Ventilation should be achieved by either natural supply and natural exhaust of air, or natural supply and mechanical supply and mechanical exhaust of air (Fig. 4.5).

Commissioning

Hospital is ready to be commissioned, when its building is ready, all equipment installed and manpower engaged. At this time, a commissioning team should be formed, which will have hospital consultant, administrator, other senior managers, heads of clinical services and nursing superintendents. The team has the

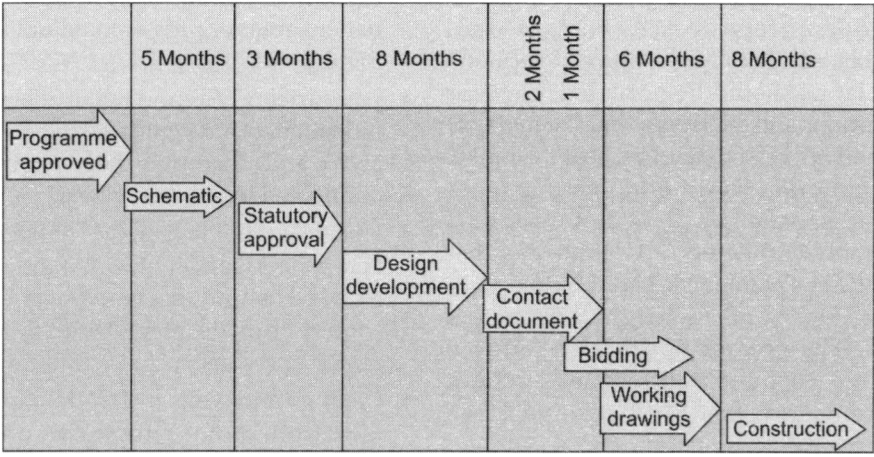

Fig. 4.5: Project time schedule

task of bringing the hospital building plant and equipment to a state of readiness. They should also train the employees.

Scheduling the Sequence of Service

Some services need to be ready, whereas others may take ample time. Services like telephone, stores, etc. need to be started immediately, whereas services like C.S.S.D and O.T require a long preparation.

Categorisation of Services

Group 1: Services required immediately are telephones, domestic services, central line service, stores, work department.

Group 2: Requiring lengthy period of preparation such as CSSD (for trail runs), X-ray (for trail runs), OT (for trail runs), Pharmacy.

Group 3: May be partially open before patients admitted like Paramedical service, OPD.

Group 4: Will not be opened until all the above departments are opened like wards.

Shake-down Period

The period from the time of the commissioning of the hospital till it settles down into a satisfactorily functioning entity is the shake-down period. If proper planning is done, this period can be considerably reduced.

OUTPATIENT SERVICES

OPD is defined as part of the hospital with allotted physical facilities and employees with regularly scheduled working hours to provide care for patients who are not registered as inpatients.

It is estimated that per hospital bed 1.5–3 patients attend the outpatient department of a hospital per day.

It should be close to the main lobby of the hospital and should be adjacent to registration, medical records, emergency, etc. If the laboratory is located at a different place or different block, a sample collection center should be located in the O.P.D.

A hospital expecting 500 outpatients per day over 300 normal working days in a year would require nearly 75,000 sq feet (6975 sq m) of space for its outpatients department.

The main facilities to be planned are
- Public areas
- Clinical areas
- Consultation rooms

- Special examination rooms
- Administrative area
- Circulation area
- Ancillary and auxiliary facilities

Subsidiary/ancillary facilities include
- Injection rooms
- Treatment and dressing rooms
- Pharmacy
- Medical records room (exclusive or combined with IP)

Additional/auxiliary facilities include
- Laboratory
- Medical imaging services
- Screening clinic
- Medico-social services
- Health education facilities.

Administrative area: It includes offices and counters for hospital administrator, nursing superintendent and medico-social workers. This may include storage facilities.

Functional zones: These include
- Public zones
- Joint use zones
- Staff zones

Public zones: These include:
- Main entrance
- Foyer, which includes: Reception, signboards, layout plans and touch screens.
- Bays for trolleys and wheel chairs.
- Public telephone booths.
- Public conveniences.
- Value added services such as vending machines for beverages and snacks and bookstore.
- Registration area which includes:
  - Centralized counter for new, repeat patients.
  - Control desk for monitoring sub-registration at the respective service areas.
- Cash counter
- Health education facilities that include: posters, pamphlets, audio-visuals aids.
- Waiting areas in the foyer as well as each tier of consultation and treatment rooms.

Joint use zone: It includes areas jointly utilized by the staff and the patients such as the consultation and examination rooms.
- Two consultation rooms with one examination cubicle.
- Combined consultation, examination cubicle.
- Rooms should be designed to accommodate multiple medical specialties.

A room of about 12.5 sq m is adequate for consultation and examination. It includes space for examination tables, washbasin, instrument trolley, an X-ray viewing screen, desk and chair for consultant/ doctor as well as 2 chairs for patients/visitors. If examination room is separate then 8 sq m is sufficient.

Depending on the facilities special examination rooms are planned
- Refraction, perimetry, tonography, and slit lamp.
- Audiometry
- EEG
- Dental examination
- Plaster room.

Clinical laboratory: It includes a centralized sample collection area for urine, stool, blood, a washroom and toilets (male and female) and a blood collection room. A large OPD should have side room adjacent to collection station for routine blood, urine and stool examination.

Pharmacy: Nearly 70–75% of the patient will attend the hospital pharmacy. The minimum area should be at least 250 sq ft even for a small hospital. It should be so located so as to serve both inpatients and OPD. They should have multiple dispensing windows, drug storage cabinets and shelves.

Specialized OPD services may include the following

- Gastrointestinal endoscopy lab, sigmoidoscopy and colonoscopy.
- Pulmonary function lab, including spirometry.
- Cardiac OPD with ECG, echo cardiography, TMT and Holter monitoring lab.
- Staff zone—Staff cloak rooms and toilets.
- Seminar room.

Parking and Entrance

- Main entrance should have sloping ramps with slip/skid free surface.
- Double door with a width of 1500 mm.
- Storage area for wheel chairs and stretches should be conveniently located without obstructing the traffic.
- Staff and patient entrance should be separate.
- Parking should be close to entrance.
- Barrier free movement for disabled should be provided.

Enquiry Desk, Reception Station

- A reception and enquiry counter in OPD is necessary at the entrance lobby, where patient seeks information about the location of various clinics, registration procedures, etc.
- The height of counter should be adapted to the needs of wheel chair patients.
- The reception should have counters to ensure patients privacy.
- Sufficient number of drawers and shelving space should be provided.

Minor O.T

An area of 20 sq m is needed for minor O.T, with recovery room for the ambulatory surgeries. Besides a patient preparation room, scrub area and staff room will also be needed.

Waiting Area

- The area of main waiting area ranges from 1 sq ft per outpatient attendance to 8–10 sq ft per daily patient visit in western countries.
- For subsidiary waiting area 8 sq ft/patient or 0.75 m² for 1/3 rd of the attendance at each department.
- A call system should be provided to direct patient to rooms.
- Distance between waiting area and consultation room should be short and clearly marked.
- A scale of 1–2 water closets for every 100 patients and at least 1 urinal for every 50 patients are recommended separate for male and females (Fig. 4.6).

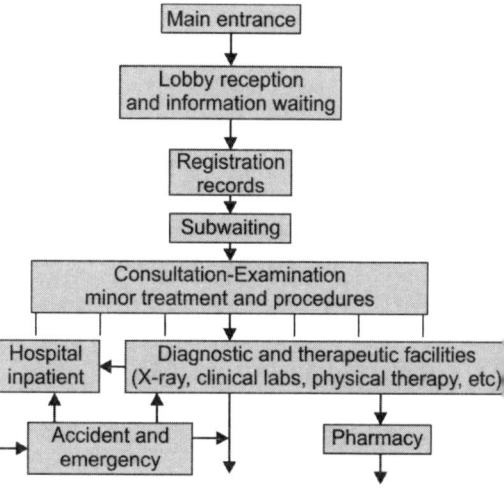

Fig. 4.6: Flow chart of outpatient department

NURSING UNIT OR INPATIENT UNIT

Nursing unit or ward is the grouping of accommodation for the patients with services facilities which enables a team of nurses to care for inpatients under the best possible conditions and includes under one roof patient beds, nursing stations, service area, storage area, work area and sanitary area.

An inpatient area is that part of the hospital which includes the nursing station, the beds it serves, storage and public areas needed to carry out nursing care. It requires holistic planning and designing to suit the requirements of seekers and providers of patient care.

Nursing units include

- General wards
- Isolation wards
- Pediatric wards
- Cardiology wards
- Neurology wards
- Geriatric wards
- Preoperative and Post-operative wards.
- Private wards
- Emergency wards
- Maternity wards
- Psychiatric wards
- Neonatology wards
- Orthopedic wards

Key Planning and Design Parameters

Objectives

- Design should follow the function.
- Ensure privacy and safety for patients.
- Efficient nursing care should be provided with minimum nursing fatigue factor.
- It should maximize usage of shared support services.
- It should be planned on a standardized modular grid.
- It should provide a humanized environment to the healing process.
- A view of the outside including those of elements of nature should be planned and designed for.
- It should harmonize with the functional requirements of treatment and technology as well as patients physical and emotional needs.

SPECIFICATIONS

- The doors of patient rooms should open outward into the corridor with an outside lock only.
- The toilet attached to the patient's room should be provided with a grab bar and an emergency call button. Door of the toilet should open outwards into the patients room.
- In the infectious disease ward, each cubicle should have one sanitary facility and a utensil sterilizer in pantry. It should also have a larger dirty utility room for disinfecting the linen prior to dispatching to laundry.
- Use of natural light through atrium in waiting area may be done.
- The minimum distance between the center of beds should be 2.25 m, space at the foot-end should be 0.90 m and recommended space at the head end 0.25 m.
- Pediatric wards should have additional facility for accommodating family members.
- Electrical outlet should include reading light, nurses call button and night light. Additional outlet for cleaning equipment and portable X-ray should also be provided.
- The nurses station should be located as centrally as possible to the activities of the unit and provide optimal visibility of the patients.

Layout Design of Wards

The arrangement of beds in a ward is determined by various factors such as:

- Size of the hospital.
- Type of services provided such as intensive care/rehabilitation.
- Demands of the community.

Nightingale/Pavilion Type

In such wards beds are arranged perpendicular to longitudinal walls. The nursing station is placed in the center of the hall and beds are placed at rows facing each other. Such wards are economical to construct, and facilitate adequate patient visibility and cross ventilation. No privacy is provided to the patient in such a ward. It is a self-contained unit for 35–40 patients.

Riggs' Ward

This is so named since it was first made in Riggs Hospital in Denmark. Such wards are in the form of cubicles of 4–6 beds. Beds are arranged parallel to the longitudinal walls. It provides privacy to patients and it is possible to segregate patients according to severity/type of sickness. In a unilateral Riggs' ward, beds are placed in each bay, and bays are separated by a common corridor, whereas in the bilateral ward two unilateral Riggs' wards are located on either side of a central nursing station. In this type of ward the nurses walking distance for patient care activities is also minimized.

T Shaped Ward

In this type of design, bed bays are placed in front of the nursing station. Isolation rooms are at both sides. Ancillary and other services are behind the nursing station.

Rack Track or Double Corridor

These beds are arranged in single/double bed rooms.

Courtyard

In this type of plan, courtyard of varying sizes are inserted into the core areas to provide natural light and ventilation.

Cruciform

This has a cruciform shape with the nursing station in the center.

Circular

These beds are placed around a nursing station.

Water

The water requirement in a hospital is 450–500 liters per bed per day. This excludes water required for fire fighting. There should be a separate storage tank for fire fighting purposes. It is recommended that three days requirement of water should be available at all times as reserve.

Electricity

The requirements of electricity is 2 kW /bed / day (5 kW/bed/day for superspecialty hospital). This should ideally be from 2–3 grids.

Specific Requirements

The specific requirements for various specialty inpatient units are as follows:

Pediatric Nursing Unit

- Provision must be made for toilets/sleeping facilities for parents who may be allowed to stay with their children.
- Isolation room along with ante room should be provided.
- Approximately 20–25% beds should be single rooms for the critically ill.
- A play room should be provided for group activities.
- A formula room should be provided with a counter and sink.
- The decor and color of walls should contribute to a cheerful physical environment.

Obstetrical Nursing Unit /Birthing Center

This should preferably be located on the same floor and close proximity to the labor delivery units. It should have an ultrasound scanning room. A day room should also be provided.

Psychiatric Nursing Unit

This should be a single unit, equipped with tamper proof fittings/accessories.

Isolation Room

The entry should be through an ante room with various facilities for hand washing, gowning and storage of cleaned and soiled material.

Single Bed Per Room

The main advantage of the layout is that the patient can rest undisturbed. The location of independent toilets also help to make the patients become ambulatory earlier.

Windows: Window opening should be 20% of the floor area if windows are located only in one wall. It should not be less than 15% of the floor area if the window openings are located on the opposite walls.

Doors: Width should not be less than 1.20 m as a bed measures 1 m breadth and 2.15 m in length.

Dado: From hygienic point of view, dado should be extended up to 1.20 m in all rooms and corridors.

Noise reduction: Use of acoustical structure for ceiling in corridors is preferable to minimize noise.

Bedside lockers and built in cupboards: For each bed, one bed side lockers and one built in cupboard should be given. Besides a chair can also be provided for each bed.

Nursing station: It should be located centrally as far as possible. Nurse should travel only a maximum of 25 feet to reach a patient. Nursing station usually consists of sisters room with attached toilet. Nursing station should have a table for preparing medicine and infection trays. It should have separate cupboard for the storage of drugs, instruments, etc. If feasible separate refrigerator should be provided at nursing station for keeping antibiotics and separate infections.

Dirt utility room and janitors closet: Dirty utility room is to be cleaned bedpan, urinals, sputum mugs, etc. and keep dirty linen. Janitors' closet is to keep janitors like bucket, brooms, brushes, mops and other cleaning materials.

Treatment and dressing room: It is the room where minor treatments and procedures which cannot be done inpatient beds are carried out. For 25–30 beds, one such room is ideal.

Ward pantry: It is desirable to have a ward pantry where food can be received, distributed to the patients and utensils cleaned. The size of the ward pantry of the dining room should not be less than 25 sq m

Clean utility room: Where sterile supplies and equipment are kept.

Day room: For ambulant patients, it is advisable to have a day room, with facilities for recreation. In West this room is called solarium.

Miscellaneous facilities: Facilities for supply of hot water arrangement for piped oxygen and suction and nurses call system, intercom telecom facilities are some of the miscellaneous facilities required in the nursing care units.

LABOR AND DELIVERY SUITES

It should be located in a convenient but segregated area. If possible there should be a separate entrance into the labor and delivery suites.

Reception and Admission

There should be a registration and admission counter which should be open into the entrance lobby, as persons often arrive in a state of imminent delivery.

Examination and Preparation Room

The room should accommodate one or two beds and provide space for the doctor, work table, here the patient undergoes cleansing bath, enema, shaving. Lockers for keeping personal articles should be provided.

Labor Room

This is the room in which the patient remains during the first stage of labor. It should preferably be in the form of cubicles of size 18 ft × 18 ft. On an average there should be two labor rooms for 10 maternity beds. The bed must be furnished with oxygen, suction and compressed air outlets, nurse call system, lighting controls. Piped in music is desirable. Bedpan flushing facility, wash basin and clock with a second timer are required.

Delivery Room

Delivery room should be similar to operating rooms with maximum aseptic conditions. The minimum size should be 18 ft × 18 ft. There should be scrub areas, facility of oxygen, suction and air, a clock with a second timer. There should be separate delivery room for septic cases. It is advisable to have a caesarian section room close to the delivery rooms. It should have an area to receive the newborn babies with baby receiving tray, warmer, suction, oxygen, ambu bag. Each delivery room should have foot or elbow operated emergency call system with a dome light and buzzer on the corridor.

Scrub Facilities

Should be provided near the entrance of each delivery room.

Recovery Rooms

For the observation of the mother after delivery, recovery rooms are provided. In the modern obstetric units, post-partum patients are observed for 6 hours.

LDRP

A single suite for Labor, Delivery, Recovery and Post-partum (LDRP), the LDRP birthing suite blends traditional obstetrics with comfortable atmosphere for expectant mother.

LDRP Suites

Labor, delivery, recovery or post-partum suites are elegantly designed suites which accommodates the entire birthing procedure. It combines the comforts of home and the security of the hospital. A stylish bed opens to become a birthing bed. Examination lights are neatly placed in position; if they are portable, they are readily available. Sophisticated equipment is discreetly hidden behind screens. Each LDRP suite is cheerfully decorated with comfortable furniture, bed, drapes and spread, and has cradle, telephone, music and TV to provide the warmth and convenience of home.

Pre-natal or Lamaze Classes

Hospital must conduct pre-natal classes for expectant mothers to learn about the development of the fetus, labor, delivery, nutrition, parenting and common problems facing new parents. Lamaze classes are conducted in which breathing or relaxation techniques are taught.

Service Areas

- Control/nursing station.
- Supervisor's office.
- Fathers' waiting room.
- Sterilizing facilities.
- Recessed scrub area with sink equipped with gooseneck spouts, foot-operated controls, thermostatically controlled temperature valves, space for nail brushes, sterile caps, masks, an easily visible clock with a second timer.
- Controlled storage for drugs.
- Enclosed soiled work room/storage room with sink, counter, etc.
- Clean work room/supply room.
- Anaesthesia storage facilities.
- Equipment storage.
- Staff clothing change area.
- Lounge and toilet facilities for obstetrical staff.
- Janitor's closet.
- Alcove for stretchers.
- A recessed place for film illuminator, and a desk and chair for chart work.
- Duty rooms with sleeping accommodation, toilet, shower, for resident duty and on call doctors, separate for men and women. Bunk beds may be provided to accommodate more doctors.

ACCIDENT AND EMERGENCY DEPARTMENT

Accident is an unexpected, unplanned occurrence, which may involve injury or unpremeditated event resulting in recognizable damage.

Emergency has been defined by WHO as a condition determined clinically or considered by the patient or his/her relatives as requiring urgent medical services, failing which, it could result in loss of life or limb.

Medical emergency is a situation when patient requires urgent and high quality medical care to prevent loss of life or limb and to initiate action for the restoration of normal healthy life.

Key Planning and Design Parameters

- The design and planning should be done so as not to impede the movement of patients and staff and equipment. The equipment should be located in designated spaces to be readily accessible when needed.
- It should provide privacy during management of patients.
- There should be minimum criss-crossing of patient traffic with separate entrance and exit.
- There should be distinct, ideally separate, access for ambulances and ambulant cases.
- The entrance should be easily identifiable, protected from inclement weather and accessible to disabled patients.
- Depending on the type and location of hospital, a helipad may be planned.
- Ground level location is the best.
- It should ideally be situated near ICU and operating room(s).
- Patient waiting area should be welcoming, visually appealing and comfortable.
- There should be a readily identifiable triage area with expansion facilities.
- It should have multiple walled in rooms or multi-bed bays.
- It should have acute care rooms arranged around the main nursing work area.
- It should have trauma rooms in proximity to the entrance.
- There should be effective day and night sign posting.
- The non-patient care areas should be located peripherally in the floor plan.
- Door should be wide enough to accommodate stretcher, trolleys and portable X-ray machine. A door of width 1.6 m is desirable.
- Clinical care areas should have exposure to maximum feasible daylight.
- An office for security personnel near the entrance should be considered. Duress alarms should also be positioned at suitable places.
- All patient spaces and clinical areas should have access to emergency call facility.
- Departments using telemedicine facilities should have a dedicated room with appropriate power and communication cabling.
- Emergency department must have provision for round-the-clock emergency, X-ray, ultrasound examination and imaging investigations.
- A laboratory medicine department should provide round-the-clock services.
- Blood bank facilities should be available.
- The floor finishes inpatient care areas and corridors should have non-slip surface impermeable to water and body fluids and easy to clean.
- It will be ideal to provide a separate fracture treatment and plaster room.
- The emergency operation room should be self-contained.

The following areas must be planned:
- **Public areas**
  - Entrance for patients.
  - Control station.
  - Public waiting space with appropriate amenities.
- **Treatment facilities**
  - Patients observation area examination and treatment cubicles.
  - Critical care rooms.
- **Supportive services**
  - Staff rooms along with amenities.

Components

The following should be included in an accident and emergency department:
- 'May I help you' desk
- Reception and information area

- Trolley bay
- Resuscitation/major trauma room
- Acute patient care room (with cardiac monitoring).
- Isolation room
- Observation rooms
- Registration/clerical area
- Triage area /room
- Nursing work area
- Doctors work station
- Toilets
- Patient waiting room
- Bereavement /counseling room
- Medico-social worker room
- Conference room
- Lounge and/or locker room for staff
- Doctors duty room
- Office/station
- Radio imaging room having facility of X-ray imaging and CT scan
- Laboratory services
- Dirty utility room
- Clean utility room
- Equipment storage area
- Administrative offices
- Pharmacy
- Orthopedic and plaster cast room
- Room for brought-in-dead
- Obstetric room
- Operation room
- In addition, it may have specially designed areas for management of pediatric patients, psychiatric patients and of patients following sexual assault.

Entrance

- It should be separate and located adjacent to the outpatient.
- The department should be accessible by two separate entrances, one for the ambulant patients and the other for patients coming by ambulance.
- The entrance should be well-marked and illuminated.
- It should open into a spacious lobby.
- There should be a porch outside the lobby and the approach to the lobby should be in the form of ramp and steps.

Reception and Information Area

The following parameters are recommended:
- It should be adjacent to triage area.
- It should be close to the waiting area.
- It should have communication links such as telephones, pagers.
- It may also be utilized for storage of records.

Waiting Area

- It should provide sufficient and comfortable space for waiting patients and relatives/escorts.
- The area should be easily observed from reception and triage areas.
- It should be appropriately furnished with visual displays on health education and hospital related information.
- It should have public telephone booth, coffee/tea vending machine, toilet facilities separately for men and women.

Nursing Work Station

- It should be centrally located to enable staff to monitor patient care areas.
- It should include central cardiac monitor station.
- It should have communication links to triage and resuscitation areas.
- It should have desks that will enable staff to work from either side.

Doctors Work Area

- It should be centrally located for facilitating response to an emergency.
- It should provide privacy.
- The location should be such that doctors and nurses are able to view central cardiac monitoring station.

Acute Treatment Areas

It should have standard mobile bed with ample storage and usage space for essential equipment. It should have service panel, examination light, wall mounted sphygmomanometer, emergency call facilities. Treatment area requires space of 15 m^2 and 2.4 m clear floor space between beds.

Resuscitation Room

- The patient is to be stabilized in resuscitation room.
- It should have space to accommodate specialized resuscitation bed, allow 360 degrees access to all parts of the patient.
- It should include overhead X-ray, lead lining of walls and partitions between beds, radiolucent resuscitation trolley with cassette trays, X-ray viewing/digital electronic imaging system and stand-by circuits.
- An OT light should be made available.
- Ceiling arrangement needs to be carefully planned so that surgical lights, X-ray tracks, curtains and IV racks do not interfere with each other.
- It should have alarm line to the nursing work area.
- Storage cabinets should have glass or plexiglass panels.
- It should have oxygen and suction outlets.
- An area of about 30 m^2 is suggested.

Observation Ward

This is utilized for patients who have been evaluated and need extended treatment, observation, re-evaluation or time-consuming procedures. A 6–8 bedded ward is recommended.

Special Treatment Rooms

- *Obstetric rooms:* This should be equipped for pelvic examination, evaluation of patients in labor and emergency delivery.
- *Ophthalmology and ENT rooms:* These should be equipped with a silt lamp and other necessary equipment.
- *Dental room:* This should have a dental chair.
- *Decontamination room:* This should have a flexible hose shower.

Doctors Duty Room

The doctors on duty must be available for all the 24 hours. For their convenience a retiring room with amenities along with bath and toilet should be provided.

OPERATING UNIT / OPERATION THEATER

An OT is that specialized facility of the hospital where life saving or life improving procedures are carried out on the human body by invasive methods under strict aseptic conditions in a controlled environment by specially trained personnel to promote healing and cure with maximum safety, comfort and economy.

Size: Operating room must have a clear minimum area of 360 sq ft (18 × 20) excluding fixed cabinets and built in shelves. Some surgeons recommend 480 sq ft (20 × 24). For orthopedics operation theater of 42 sq m and for cardiovascular surgery 50 sq m areas are required.

Location: It is better to group all operating rooms in one central location as it results in:
- Efficient use of staff and facilities.
- Efficient maintenance of hygiene and ventilation.
- Improved utilization.
- Economy in terms of engineering maintenance.
- Problem of supplies of materials simplified.
- Improved supervision.

Location of the surgical suite should be such that it permits a convenient and uncomplicated flow of patients, staff and supplies. It should have accessibility to elevators, emergency department, radiology, ICUs, CSSD, etc (Fig. 4.7).

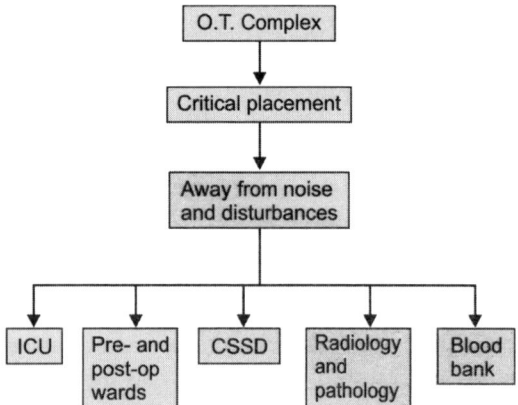

Fig. 4.7: Design of operation theatre

DESIGN PARAMETERS

OTs should be planned so as to ensure:
- Avoidance of unrelated hospital traffic flow in the area.
- Convenient functional relationship and communication with the surgical ward, ICU, CSSD, blood bank, medical imaging and laboratory services.
- Avoidance of any outdoor source of noise.
- Provision for future expansion or alterations.
- In modular theatre, the wall cladding should be galvanized iron/stainless steel panels, joined filled with epoxy and grinded. The final prepared surface should be treated with anti-bacterial paint.
- Doors should be of sliding type with a minimum of 1.2 m width in areas. It should be electrically operated, hermetically sealed sliding doors to ensure sterilization and correct air pressure.
- Corridors should not be less than 2.85 m in width to facilitate the movement of trolley and stretchers.
- Walls and ceilings should be aesthetically pleasing, non-porous, fire-resistant, water and stain proof, seamless, non-reflective and easy to clean. They should not cause a build up of static electrical charge. They should be joint less or have joints that can be thermosealed.
- Floors should be smooth, non-slip, and made of impervious material that is conductive enough to dissipate static electricity but not conductive enough to endanger personnel from shock. The flooring should either be inset mosaic with the least possible number of joints and copper strips. Conductive copper mesh and self-leveling epoxy flooring may be done.
- The ceiling should be painted with washable paint and corners of the rooms should be rounded off to prevent any collection dirt and dust.
- Taps in the scrub room should be knee/elbow operated or preferably electronically controlled, activated by infrared sensor.
- There should be a power back-up with provision for stand-by generating sets.
- In operating rooms, anesthetic room(s), recovery room, holding area, the color of the walls and ceilings should be such that they do not alter the observers perception of skin color.
- An OT should have facility for high speed autoclaves/ sterilizers to meet the immediate/emergency requirements of sterilizing equipment.
- Essential pharmaceutical storage including refrigeration facilities should be available.
- There should be a waiting room with toilet facilities for the patients attendants.
- Pass through cabinets which allow the transfer of supplies from outside to the OT. They help ensure the rotation of supplies in storage and can be used only for passing supplies as needed from a clean center core.
- X-ray film illuminators should preferably be recessed into the wall.
- There should be emergency communication system that can be activated without the use of hands.

Preoperative Patient Holding Area

This should facilitate the movement of both stretchers and ambulatory patients not requiring stretchers. Each stretcher station should be of 7.43 m² (80 sq ft) and should have a clearance of 1.22 m (4 feet) on the sides as well as foot of the stretcher to facilitate monitoring and therapeutic management of patients.

Post-anesthetic Care Units

These should contain a medication station, handwashing station, nurse station, storage space for stretchers, supplies and equipment. Additionally, there should be 7.43 m² (80 sq ft) space for each patient bed. Clearance of 1.6 m (5 feet) between the beds, and 1.22 m (4 feet) between the patient bed sides and adjacent walls should be present.

Service Area

This area should include control station so as to permit observation of all units into the suite.
- A sub-sterile area between two or more operating areas for flash sterilizer, sterile supply storage area and handwashing station.
- Scrub facilities near the entrance of each operating room.
- Dirty utility for collection and disposal of soiled material.
- Clean (sterile) supply room.
- Operation room.
- Medical gas storage facilities.
- Anesthesia workroom for cleaning, testing and storing anesthesia equipment.

Staff Amenities

Separate areas/rooms should be provided for male and female staff containing lockers, showers, toilets, and space for donning surgical attire. These areas should be designed to allow one-way traffic, i.e. personnel entering from outside the surgical suite to change and move inside. Duty rooms should be provided for nurses and doctors.

Medical Gases

The main storage area for medical gases should be outside the facility and there should be provision for additional separate storage of reserve gas cylinders to meet at least one extra day requirement.

Anesthetic Work Room

This should provide space for anesthetic trolleys and equipment and should have direct access to the circulation corridors and ready access to the operating room. It should be designed to facilitate cleaning, testing and storing of anesthesia equipment. It should contain work benches, sink(s) and racks for cylinders. It should also have sufficient power outlets and medical gas panels for the testing of equipment.

Blood storage: There should be provision for adequate refrigerated blood storage.

Set-up Room

This is the clean workroom where clean/sterile materials are stored and arranged prior to their use in the operating room. Its functions include the storage of instruments and materials holding of sterile supplies and packs, preparation of dressing and instrument trolley and storage of drugs. If theater sterile supply unit (TSSU) is not available, flash sterilization of unsterile specialized instruments is also carried out here.

Laboratory

An area for the preparation and examination of frozen section may be provided. Depending on the operational policy, this may be a part of the main laboratory.

Storage

Adequate store rooms for equipment and supplies utilized in the operating unit should be provided. The design should allow ease of access to the storage areas for the delivery of consumables. Controlled access from an external corridor is recommended. Store rooms are best designed in an elongated rectangular shape to allow easy access to all items. Part of the room may be utilized as an area for testing operating equipment. For this purpose, a separate room (bio-medical engineering room) may also be planned. Storage bays that are preferably recessed into the corridor walls should be provided for equipment such as stretchers and portable X-ray machines.

ZONING

Zones are areas of varying degrees of cleanliness in which the bacteriological count progressively diminishes from the outer to the inner zones (operating area) and is maintained by a differential decreasing positive pressure ventilation gradient from the inner zone to the outer zone (Fig. 4.8).

Principles for Zoning

- Clean and dirty traffic flows should be segregated as best as possible. Spaces in the suites should be arranged in such a manner that while moving from one space to another, there is continuous progression of cleanliness from the entrance of OT suite to operating room.
- Staff working in OT should be able to move from one clean area to the other without having to pass through unprotected area.
- Soiled materials and wastes should be removed from OTs without passing through clean areas.

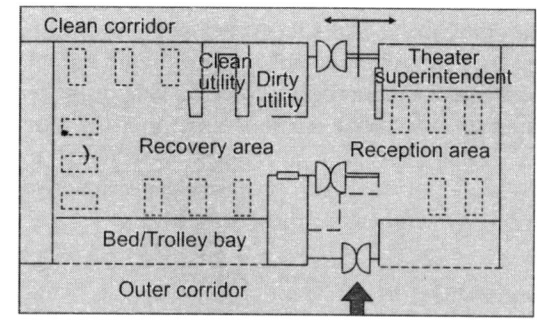

Fig. 4.8: Zoning

- OT ventilation should be independent of the air flow from the rest of the hospital (Fig. 4.9).
- These are of the following types:

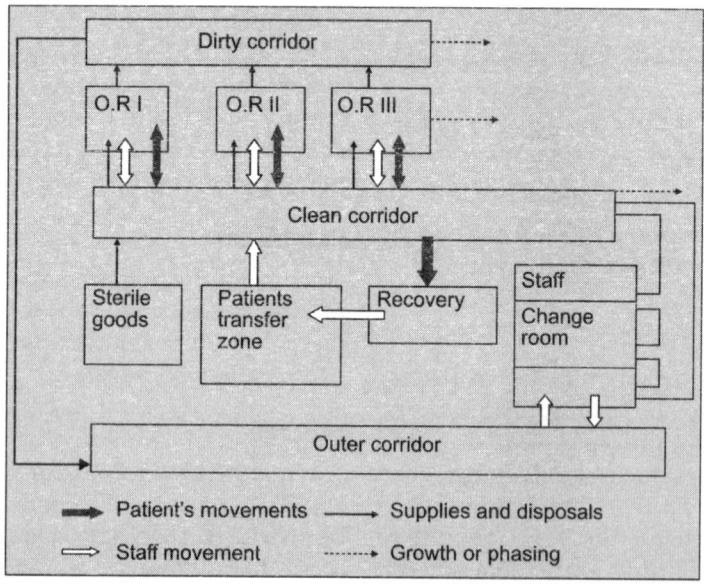

Fig. 4.9: OT circulation pattern

Protective Zone: Areas included in this zone are:
- Reception
- Waiting area
- Trolley bay and
- Changing room

Clean Zone: Areas included in this zone are:
- Preoperative room
- Recovery room
- Plaster room
- Staff room and
- Store

Sterile Zone: Areas included in this zone are:
- Operating suite
- Scrub room
- Anesthesia induction room
- Set-up room

Disposal Zone: Areas included in this zone are:
- Dirty utility
- Disposal corridor

SUPPLY AIR

Supply air to operating rooms should be delivered at high level in a way that

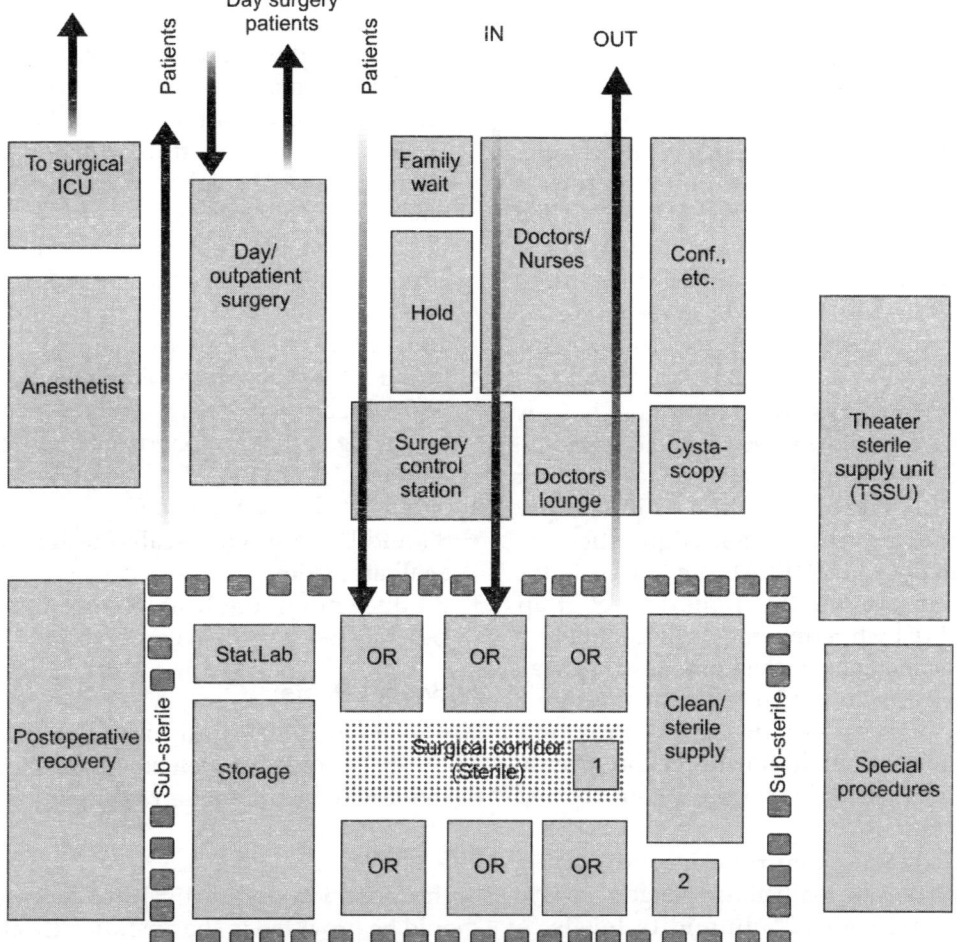

Fig. 4.10: Flow chart of surgical suite

minimizes recirculation of potentially contaminated room air and provides the cleanest practical air supply over the operating table area. Graduated negative pressurization relative to pressure in areas adjacent to the operating unit is recommended. It should range from 10 Pascal's positive in the operating room(s) to slightly negative pressure in areas like entrance foyer, recovery and change rooms and slightly more negative in clean-up room(s). This should be achieved by using carefully balanced supply air and exhaust air systems. Operating room relative humidity should be maintained within the range of 45 to 60%. The operating room temperature should be adjustable. Range is recommended to be 21–24°C.

Air Flow

- *Down flow system:* The air flow at one meter from the supply air outlet must have a minimum average velocity of 0.35 m/s and at working height, not less than 0.3 m/s.
- Operating rooms where lasers are being used should have adequate suction/evacuation controls for the plume generated.
- In modern hospitals laminar air flow system is followed. Air velocity varies at 50 feet per minute at foot level to 75 feet per minute at table height to 150 feet per minute at ceiling level. High efficiency particulate air (HEPA) filters used in the system provide the highest level of air sterility by filtering out particle matter up to 0.3 microns which eliminates almost all known size of micro organisms. A down flow of operating air system, provide a comfortable environment for the surgical team in terms of thermal, acoustics and lighting.
- **Ventilation:** Central air conditioning should ensure temperature range of 21°C to 24°C. with 45–60% humidity levels. A minimum of 15 air changes per hour should be ensured. It is preferred to have 100% fresh air. The theater should maintain positive pressure. Controlling of pressure is adhered to by providing pressure release dampers at the time of opening and closing of the door.
- **Lighting:** Electrical wiring should be in concealed conduit. Lighting, both natural and artificial should be of appropriate illumination. Ground fault, circuit interrupters (GFCIs) may be utilized which are designed to shut-off the electric power within a few milliseconds of the occurrence of a ground fault, thereby preventing serious electric shock. To minimize eye fatigue, the ratio of intensity of room lighting to that at the surgical suite should not exceed 1:5, preferably 1:3. Color and hue of the lights should be consistent. The overhead operating light must provide an intense light, within a range of 50,000–125000 Lux, into the incision without glare on the surface. The light may be equipped with an intensity control.
- Provide a circular light pattern and focus appropriately for size of the incision.
- Be shadow less. Multiple light sources and/or reflectors decrease shadows.
- Produce the blue-white color of daylight.
- Be freely adjustable to any position or angle by having vertical and horizontal range of motion.
- Should enable easy cleaning.
- Should be aerodynamically designed to facilitate airflow.
- Produce minimum heat. Halogen bulbs generate less heat than other types.

Auditory Effects

Sound level in OT should be limited to 25–35 db. The reverberation time in OT should be reduced to below one second.

Fire Safety

Both ionization and optical fire detectors should be provided in the operation theaters instead of heat detectors, since equipment-oriented operation theaters are likely to create more smoke than heat in the eventuality of fire. Hydrants and fire extinguishers should be provided. The fire exit route should be clearly identified, earmarked and well-illuminated.

Modular Systems are increasing with the number of hospitals coming up. These consist of factory made components for operating suites, complete with integrated mechanical and electrical engineering services including air-conditioning. The advantage of these modular theaters is that they are pre-designed and engineered with guaranteed performance and shorter construction time. The vertical laminar flow system with the operating enclosure are specially designed operating theaters to reduce the air-borne infection to an exceptionally low degree.

Integrated Operating Room

In an integrated OT technology, it is possible to control everything from medical devices, lighting cameras and teleconferencing from a central station, which may be inside or outside the sterile area. (Table 4.6)

INTENSIVE CARE UNIT

ICU is a specially equipped place for the management of critically ill patients and those requiring specialized care/monitoring.

Types of ICU

- Cardiac care unit
- Neonatal ICU
- Pediatric ICU
- Neurology ICU
- Neurosurgery ICU
- Burn care center/unit ICU
- Organ transplantation unit.

Key Planning and Design Parameters

Location: It is preferable to have the ICU in close proximity to the operation theaters, accident and emergency department and medical imaging departments.

Number of ICU beds: The number of beds required depends on the type of hospital and services it provides. It is recommended that at least 5% of total hospital bed may be designated ICU beds. In cardiac and neuro-surgical centers, about 10–15% beds may be ICU beds.

Size of units: Depending on the requirement, an ICU of 6 to 12 beds is recommended. A unit of less than 6 beds is economically not viable. Where the requirement is more than 12 beds, multiple units may be planned. The ICU may be planned as large single room having multiple beds or individual single bed accommodation.

Separate cubicles/bedrooms should have dimension of 4.0 m × 4.0 m.

Bed space: 22 m^2 floor area for single bed accommodation which is exclusive of service areas and 20 m^2 for multiple bed accommodation is recommended.

Lighting: It is recommended to have a 300 lux light illumination for patient areas with anti-glare arrangement, 100 lux for corridor, 150 lux for staff area and floor lights for monitoring drainage seal and suction equipment. Provision of natural light should be maximum. The color of walls and ceiling should not affect perception of skin color by the staff.

Environmental control: Rooms in the ICU should be sound proof and air conditioned

Table 4.6: OPD operation theater

Total number of beds	OPD Operation theater		OPD Operation theater	
	Major	Minor	Major	Minor
50	1	–	–	1
75	1	1	–	1
100	1	1	–	1
300	3	1	–	1
500	5	1	1	1
750	8	2	1	1

with facilities of environmental control for each room. Air-conditioning should ensure 50 ± 5% humidity, and 20–25°C temperature. Ceilings, flooring and walls should be constructed of materials with high sound absorption capabilities. The recommended noise level should be in the range of 35–50 decibels. There should be 8–10 air changes per hour and air pressure maintained. Special provision of exhaust to eliminate any odour and as and when required.

Doors: Having width of 1.25 m are recommended.

Beds: Mechanically or electrically operated beds should be provided in the ICU. These should be readily adjustable to therapeutic positions and should have X-ray transparent bedstead bottoms. The base of the beds should be firm to enable cardiac compression during resuscitative procedures. There should be detachable rails at the head end of the bed to facilitate tracheal intubation.

Bed head panel: It should have a minimum of two oxygen outlets, two inlets for suction, one compressed air outlet per bed, nurse call button and wall mounted blood pressure equipment.

Electrical requirements (minimum 6): It is recommended that multi sockets and one power socket (15 amp) for mobile X-ray unit should be provided per bed. There should be backup source of power.

Toilets: These should enable entry of wheel chairs and should have grab bars and panic buttons. They should have doors that slide or open outwards. They should have two way operable latches.

Minimum space to allow resuscitation and other procedures: The minimum space requirement is 0.9 m between the head end and the wall and 1.2 m between the foot end and the wall. And minimum distance of 38 m between centers of two adjacent beds. These are required to facilitate resuscitative procedures, endotracheal intubation and use of radiography equipment.

Visibility of patients: Patients should be visible from the nursing station. There should be individual rooms with full height glass walls between the room and the corridor. Curtains may be drawn over the glass walls as and when required. Patient privacy should be an essential consideration.

Windows: To maintain visual contact with the outside world. Windows should approximately constitute 15% of floor area.

Walls: These should be easily washable.

Equipment installation: Wall or ceiling installation of equipment should be done to facilitate easy accessibility, personnel movement and necessary cleaning procedures.

Storage/utility area: Alcoves should be provided for the storage and rapid retrieval of resuscitation trolleys and portable monitors/defibrillation equipment. There should be storage space for janitors closet, sink and bedpan flushing facilities. There should be lockable storage for controlled drugs.

Laboratory services: Round-the-clock available either through central hospital laboratory or a satellite laboratory.

Isolation rooms: At least one isolation room per ICU should be provided.

Visitors waiting room: This should be provided outside the entry to the ICU. It should have comfortable seating arrangements along with toilet facilities. There should be an overnight room facility for relatives/friends along with areas for the storage of clean gowns and masks.

Nursing station: It should provide optimum visual observation of patients. There should be provision for computerized individual monitors at the bed side with facilities for automatic communication to the computer located at the nursing station. U-shape or semicircular layouts minimizes the nurses fatigue factor.

- A treatment room should have provision of medical gas outlets.

- It should have provision for procedure room for conducting emergency invasive procedures. It should be designed for fluoroscopy.
- There should be duty rooms for doctors with sleeping accommodation, and toilet facilities. Briefing room for doctors to talk to the relatives/friends of the patients in privacy.
- Handwashing facilities for staff should be provided.
- Staff changing rooms and toilets should be separate for male and female staff.
- ICU bed may be equipped with wall mounted dialysis unit.

DAY CARE SERVICES

A day care unit is where operative procedures are performed and/or treatment provided in a manner which allows the patients to return home on the same day. The procedures may be diagnostic and/or therapeutic. The unit may be stand alone, attached or shared service. Emergency cases generally should not be handled in the surgical day care units. Some of the other terms used for surgical day care units include 'ambulatory surgery', 'day stay surgery', 'in and out surgery', and 'day care surgery'.

Key Planning and Design Parameters

The following are the main planning and design considerations:

- The facilities and standards of care should be comparable to those provided to inpatients.
- The waiting areas should be separate from recovery and procedure area.
- Patient bed spaces should be provided with suction, oxygen and nurse call facilities.
- All door widths should allow easy access for trolley bed/ trolley transfer.
- The fittings and fixtures such as bed screens should ensure privacy and dignity to the patients.
- Arrangements must be made for about 10% of the patients to spend the night after the procedure/treatment under medical supervision.
- If the day care unit is part of or attached to a hospital, the general clinical records facility may be used in lieu of a dedicated and separate room or a separate room should be provided for the storage, documentation and retrieval of clinical records.
- Floors and wall finishes should be seamless, impervious. Flooring should be non-slip. The intersections of walls and floors should be covered in continuous materials. Joints, if any, should be thermosealed.
- General and individual offices should be provided for administrative and professional staff, which should be away from public and patient areas.
- *Entry area:* This should include convenient access to wheel chair storage, reception and information counter, waiting area and a convenient access to public toilet facilities.
- *Holding area:* This should be provided where gowned patients enter after changing and wait for their procedure.
- *Pre-operative holding area:* This area should have facilities/area for patient trolley/patient seating, privacy screening, hand basin, patient nurse call buttons, medical gases including oxygen and suction at each bed.
- *Operating/procedure rooms:* The design of these must allow for adequate space, ready access, free movement and demarcation of sterile and non-sterile areas.
- *Patient change area:* This is the area where patients can change into hospital clothes and be prepared for surgery. It should include waiting rooms and lockers.
- *Treatment rooms/area:* In a medical day care unit (e.g. hematology, medical oncology), treatment rooms/area should be provided for supervised administration of drugs. Facilities should be similar to preoperative holding or recovery area.

- *Preparation room:* This may be required for patients undergoing procedures, such as endoscopy. The room should have adequate space for procedures, equipment trolleys, bench and cupboards for set and an examination couch with privacy screening to ensure patient privacy.
- *Recovery areas:* In larger facilities it is desirable to have a three-stage recovery area. The first stage involves intensive supervision, the second stage is for patients who have either local anesthesia or patients who have regained consciousness after anesthesia but require further observation. The second stage should have changing facilities. In the third stage the patient is fully mobile and may be allowed to meet visitors.

Endoscopy Service

In cases where the endoscopic service is attached to an operating unit, the recovery area and support services may be shared. The room size varies as per the equipment installed. The minimum ceiling height should be 3 m.

Day care units provide facilities which are effective, safe and decrease risk of hospital acquired infections. It permits more efficient use of hospital facilities and minimises the psychological burden of hospitalization.

LABORATORY SERVICES

Laboratory services helps in prevention, diagnosis and control of diseases. Medical laboratory services generate patient related information that enhances delivery of healthcare and constitutes an important link. Laboratories are process intensive centers and are vital for patient care delivery.

Key Planning and Design Parameters

Areas

- Waiting area, examination cubicles and toilets for patients.
- Specimen and blood collection area having a work bench space for patient seating; handwashing facilities and a urine and faeces collection room equipped with a toilet and hand basin.
- Chemistry including urine analysis and toxicology
- Photometry
- Hematology
- Microbiology
- Immunology
- Virology
- Gross tissue
- Histology and cytology
- Autopsy (in specific hospitals)
- Specimen disposal, sluice room
- Staff lockers/toilets
- Storage facilities for reagents, supplies, stained specimen microscope slides.
- Office
- Report center
- Other areas must also be considered while planning include the culture media preparation room, sterilizing area, storage areas for surgical specimens, chemicals and flammable liquids, reagents, supplies and stained specimen microscopic slides.

Number of Laboratory Units

The nature and type of healthcare facility determines whether a central laboratory is sufficient or sub-units are required in the acute and ambulatory patient care units.

Location

It should preferably be situated on the ground floor/first floor in close proximity to the ambulatory and acute patient care areas as well as inpatient areas. Collection point for specimens must be conveniently located for ambulatory patients. The collection point must have space for patient reception, registration, waiting area and toilet facility. Provision should be made for pneumatic tube systems, either for the present or for future installations.

Space Requirements

The main determinants of space in a laboratory are the extent of automation and type of technology used in it. A standing human body requires 4 sq ft space, whereas a sitting posture requires 6 sq ft. The working space should be adequate with equipment and materials within easy reach of the worker.

Specimen Collection Area

There should be adequate specimen collection area for blood, urine and faeces. In the blood collection area, there should be work counter providing space for patients seating and for urine and faeces collection. There should be separate toilets for men and women with washbasins and counter tops to place the specimen. Hatch windows may be provided through which the specimens may be passed through.

Storage

Facilities include those for refrigeration, reagents and supplies, maintenance of patients records and water purification. Appropriate and separate storage for flammable liquids should be provided. Separate facilities should be provided for incompatible materials, such as acids and bases. Vented storage for volatile solvents should be provided.

Safety

There should be provision for safety, including eye flushing devices, emergency shower and fire extinguishers.

Work Station

Work counters with space for equipment, microscopes, incubators, centrifuge, under the counter and overhead cabinets should be provided. They should be equipped with vacuum gas, electrical services, sinks and water supply. The drainage system of work areas where highly corrosive liquids used should consist of glass lined iron traps and pipes. Counter sinks for handwashing should be provided. Chemical and stain resistant materials should be used for laboratory work and case work finishes. One of the work benches should be planned as a service station for use for equipment commonly by staff such as centrifuges, water baths and colorimeters.

Lighting

Natural light should be utilized. Reception areas and stores require 200 lux, offices require 300 lux, while at working places, the requirement is of 500 lux. Essential equipment should be on emergency power backup systems and UPS. Dedicated earthing should be provided for laboratory equipment.

Fume Hoods

These are particularly required in laboratories where radioactive substances are used. Forced ventilation should be accompanied by an extraction system. The fume hoods should be located away from the traffic areas and doorways.

Floors

They should be acid, alkaline and salt-resistant. The use of seamless or self-leveling epoxy flooring is desirable. Floor materials should be cleaned and disinfected easily and requires a high load bearing capacity. The load bearing capacity of the floor should not be less than 500 kg/m^2. The requirement may be as high as 2000 kg/m^2 in laboratories having heavy.

Doors

Laboratory doors should not be less than 1 m wide. Some doors of total width of 1.50 m should be constructed. (One of the doors in these may be of 1.0 m width and the other of 0.50 m). There should be easy and distinct routes for disposal of laboratory waste from the principal work area. Air lock should be provided at the entrance to the laboratory.

Corridors

Width of corridors is recommended to be of 2 to 2.5 m to facilitate movement of patients including those on wheel chairs.

Benches

Countertop heights (750–900 mm) vary depending on whether work is to be conducted sitting or standing. For sitting it should be 750 mm and for standing 900 mm. Depth of wall tables should be 700 mm. The height of conveniently reached overhead table cupboards should be 1500 mm from floor level. Length of bench needed for each technician ranges from 1.6 m to 1.8 m. Each laboratory bench should have a sink with swan neck fittings with facility of cold and hot water supply. In planning the under bench units, adequate knee space should be left at intervals for the convenience of workers. The bench tops are to be seamless and acid/alkali resistant.

Ventilation

Mechanical ventilation system is required with 10–15 air changes per hour in areas where fumes are expected, and 8–10 air changes in other areas.

Pathology, Autopsy and Body Holding

It is important that systems serving pathology areas be independent of other systems. Exhaust from these areas must be designed not to create any harmful effect to occupants or contamination to any adjacent areas. Facilities that conduct autopsies must include the following:

- Air-conditioning that utilizes 100% exhaust of all air.
- Exhaust intakes arranged to provide maximum fume and odour removal with protection of personnel.
- Room operation at negative pressure relative to adjacent areas.

BLOOD BANK

Blood Bank means a place or organization or unit or institution or other arrangement made by such organization/unit/institution for carrying out all or any of the operations for collection, apheresis, storage, procuring and distribution of blood drawn from donors and/or preparation, storage and distribution of blood components.

Location

The ideal location for the blood transfusion services is on the ground floor with prominent signage's for donors and patients/attendants. It should be close to accident and emergency services and hematology department. Proximity to operation theater complex is desirable. A proper access with ample parking space adds more appeal to donors.

Physical Layout

- **Public access areas**, *i.e.* donor reception office, counseling room, medical examination room, bleeding room and refreshment/rest room (including toilet and pantry).
- **Laboratory areas** are broadly sub-divided into those areas/rooms which process donor samples; and those which are used for component separation. Proper facilities for management and disposal of biomedical waste as per statutory requirements is essential.
- **Storage and issue counter:** Adequate and appropriate storage facility is required and it should have proximity to the issue counter. The issue counter should be prominently displayed and open on a hospital corridor close to accident and emergency and the hospital vertical transportation system (in multi-storeyed hospital).
- **Administrative areas:** These include the office of the medical officer in charge of the blood bank, other medical officers, paramedical staff, technicians rest room, stores, departmental library, study/research presentation room, etc.

Key Planning and Design Parameters

The following factors must be considered while planning a BTS:
- Number of beds; including surgical discipline beds.
- Types of surgeries done in hospital (trauma; general; specialized; superspecialized).
- Whether a regional blood transfusion service exists or not.
- Number of ICUs, especially surgical-super specialty.
- Whether hospital has separate department of hematology, oncology where the requirement of blood is likely to be on a regular basis.

The general planning considerations include
- Should be situated away from public lavatories, restrooms, crowded areas, and other unhygienic surroundings.
- Building should have proper construction to prevent entry of insects, rodents and flies.
- Premises should be well-lighted (minimum 200 lux), ventilated and mesh screened or have air curtains to prevent entry of flies and other insects.
- Walls and floors should be smooth, washable and capable of being kept clean easily.
- Walls should not have dust-collecting projections.
- Drains should be of adequate size and if connected directly to a sewer, should have traps to prevent back siphonage.
- Adequate clean and hygienic toilet, handwashing facilities should be provided.
- Minimum movement of persons in the corridors.
- Limiting entry of patients and attendants into the laboratory areas.
- Clear demarcation of public access and other areas with proper and adequate signages.
- Laboratories should be contiguous, with minimal criss-crossing of traffic to eliminate/reduce chances of mixing up of samples/specimen.
- Doors should be wide (1800 mm) and rooms in the BTS area spacious enough for proper installation of mandatory equipment.
- Adequate provision should be made for power points and power backup.
- Adequate space should be provided for proper storage of blood units in designated rooms/areas and should not encroach on corridors and common spaces.
- As far as possible furniture should be modular, with provision for future expansion.
- Sinks of adequate size should be provided in rooms processing specimen for cleaning and disinfection.
- Central air-conditioning is recommended in large BTS, smaller units individual air conditioners is sufficient for maintaining temperature between 20 and 25°C.
- Recommended air changes should be 10–15/hour.
- Furniture in public access and administrative areas should be comfortable, provision for health education messages should exist.
- The donor couches in bleeding room should be comfortable and ergonomically designed for comfort.

Space Requirements

According to the existing statutory provisions, the blood bank should have an area of 100 m^2 for its operations, and an additional area of 50 m^2 for preparation of blood components. It should consist of at least a room each for registration and medical examination, blood collection, component preparation/laboratory for transfusion transmissible infections, sterilization-cum-washing, refreshment-cum-rest room and store-cum-records.

CAFETERIA UNIT

Location

The unit should preferably be located on the ground floor. The storage area should be close to the unloading dock and in proximity to the inpatient wards with easy access to vertical transportation system. The cafeteria, dining room(s) should have convenient access to the preparation room as well as to the patients, attendants, visitors and staff. In case steam is utilized in the unit, the kitchen and boiler facility should have facilitating locations to optimise the steam utilization (Fig. 4.11).

Design

Receiving area: It should have easy outside access for receiving of supplies, loading and unloading platforms. It should be equipped with scales to weigh materials and supplies.

Storage area: Storage for crockery, cutlery, utensils, dry storage area for staples and refrigerated storage for perishables should be planned. It should have walk-in coolers and refrigerators for meat products, dairy products and vegetables. Walk-in coolers and freezers may be lockable from outside but must have a release mechanism for exit from inside. An automatically operated lighting should be installed to be switched on when the door is open.

Preparation area: In this area sorting, peeling, slicing, chopping, mincing and kneading is done. It should be located between the storage and cooking areas. A double sink with draining board, worktops, peelers and grinders are the required facilities/equipment.

Production/cooking: This area requires cooking ranges, bulk cookers, chapatti puffers, baking ovens and frying equipment. The area is required to be located between the preparation area and the service area.

Service area: Here prepared food is received and assembled into food trays. Refrigerators, table tops and cupboards for storing trays, prepared food, cutlery and other items for assembling trays are some of the equipment/facilities required in the service area.

Food distribution: A cart distribution system should be provided with spaces for storage,

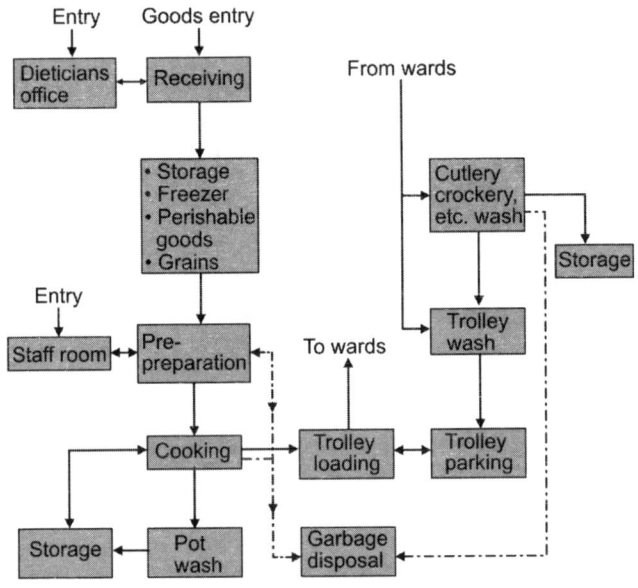

Fig. 4.11: Cafeteria

loading, distribution, receiving and sanitizing of the food service carts. Trolley washing area should also be provided.

Dishwashing area: Automated dishwashing machines, storage racks, stainless steel sinks and drainers should be installed as per workload.

The area should also provide space for receiving, scraping, rinsing sorting and stocking of soiled tableware.

Floors and Walls

Floors should be impervious and non-slip, walls and ceilings should be smooth, impervious and easily cleanable.

Garbage Disposal

It should have regular wet and dry garbage storage, removal and disposal. Grease trap should be provided before connecting the drain with main sewer line.

Offices

Manager, dieticians and supervisors offices, staff change rooms, locker for workers, toilets and rest room for staff and a clerk room are required.

Other Considerations

- There should be proper ventilation and lighting.
- LPG cylinder bank should be available.
- There should be provision for adequate steam supply.
- Fire protection devices should be provided.
- Hot and cold water outlets should be provided.
- Air lock should be provided between the kitchen and the outside.
- All tables, benches and other surfaces on which food is prepared or handled should be covered by a smooth impervious material.
- To prevent accidents, all internal kitchen doors should have clear glazing on the top half to allow view of the other side of the door.

HOUSEKEEPING AND WASTE MANAGEMENT

Housekeeping refers to the cleaning and upkeep of the hospital premises which renders the environment surfaces safe to handle by removing organic matter, salts and visible soils.

Sanitation is defined as "the science of safeguarding health", and refers to the entire gamut of activities in the environment with a view of reducing diseases and improve health.

Bio-medical waste is defined as "any solid, fluid, or liquids waste, including its container and any intermediate product, which is generated during the diagnosis, treatment or immunization of human-beings or animals, in research pertaining there to, or in the production or testing of biologicals, and the animal waste from slaughter houses or any other like establishments" (Table 4.7).

Location

Chief housekeeper's office should be near the hospital management in the business area; and the housekeeping office near the patient care areas adjacent to the vertical transportation system for easy carriage of materials. A smaller sub-stores for sanitation between couple of floors/buildings. A dedicated area for interim storage of bio-medical waste (for a few hours) before being sent for treatment and final disposal.

Functions

- Daily cleaning activities include mopping of floors and other horizontal surface, wet dusting of furniture and fixtures used in direct patient care.
- Frequent cleaning and disinfection of high touch surfaces like doorknobs, bedrails, light switches.
- Periodic cleaning of doors, windows, window frames, sills ceilings, walls, etc. on a weekly/fortnightly basis.
- Washing of corridors, staircases, toilets and bathrooms, cubicles, rooms with water and detergents.

- Garbage and bio-medical waste removal. It should be segregated into color coded containers (yellow, blue/red, white and black).
- Periodic cleaning of fans, tube lights, exhaust fans, geysers, refrigerators by adequately trained staff.
- Pest and rodent control by regular use of chemicals and sprays.
- Control of stray animals, bat infestations also fall within this responsibility.
- Cleaning and maintenance of nebulizer, ventilator, suction machine.
- Transportation of items to and from patient care areas to support service.

Key Planning and Design Parameters

- The design and planning considerations for all patient care areas housekeeping activities, should receive due consideration.
- Regular washing of patient care areas, toilets and corridors require adequate sewerage system for exit of water, soil and detergents and also electrical points (especially in corridors) where sanitation equipment is used.

SCHEDULE I

Table 4.7: Categories of bio-medical waste

Category	Waste category	Treatment and Disposal option
Category No. 1	Human anatomical	Incineration@/deep burial*
Category No. 2	Animal waste	Incineration@/deep burial*
Category No. 3	Microbiology and biotechnology waste	Local autoclaving/ microwaving/ incineration@
Category No. 4	Waste sharps	Disinfection (2 chemical treatment@@/ autoclaving/microwaving and mutilation/shredding##)
Category No. 5	Discarded medicines and cytotoxic drugs	Incineration 2/destruction and drugs disposal in secured landfills
Category No. 6	Solid waste (non-plastic)	Incineration@/autoclaving/ microwaving
Category No. 7	Solid waste (plastics, etc.)	Disinfection by chemical treatment@@/ autoclaving/microwaving and mutilation/shredding##
Category No. 8	Liquid waste	Disinfection by chemical treatment@@ and discharge into drains
Category No. 9	Incineration ash	Disposal in municipal landfill
Category No. 10	Chemical waste	Chemical treatment@@ and discharge into drains for liquids and secured landfill for solids

@@ Chemical treatment using 1 per cent hypochlorite solution or any other equivalent chemicals reagent. It must be ensured that chemical treatment ensures disinfection.
Mutilations/shredding must be such so as to prevent unauthorized reuse.
@ There will be no chemical pretreatment before incineration. Chlorinated plastics shall not be incinerated.
* Deep burial shall be option available only in towns with population less than five lakhs.

SCHEDULE II

Table 4.8: Color coding and type of container for disposal of biomedical wastes

Color coding	Type of container	Waste category	Treatment options per Schedule I
Yellow	Plastic bag	Cat. 1, Cat. 2, and Cat. 3, Cat. 6	Incineration/deep burial
Red	Disinfected container/plastic bag	Cat. 3, Cat. 6, Cat. 7	Autoclaving microwaving/chemical treatment
Blue/white	Plastic bag/puncture proof translucent container	Cat. 4, Cat. 7	Autoclaving/microwaving/chemical treatment and destruction/shredding
Black	Plastic bag	Cat. 5, Cat. 9, and Cat. 10 (solid)	Disposal and secured landfill

Table 4.9: Guidelines of ministry of environment and forests for BMW

The healthcare facility should:
- Ensure **segregation** of waste of **different categories** at the **point** it is generated.
- Bio-medical waste should be **stored** and **transported** in specially designed **trolleys, color-coded labeled bags, covered bins,** etc.
- Submerge sharps like **forceps, scissors,** and **blades** into container having chemical disinfectant for minimum 30 minutes.
- **Change solution** when **bin is 3/4** full or periodically as and when required.
- **Label** and **seal** garbage bags containing waste indicating the ward, etc.
- Have bags replaced regularly and maintain cleanliness and hygiene in their work areas.
- Take **precautionary** measures by **wearing gloves, apron,** etc. while handling a **bleeding patient** or while **dressing wounds**.

- A janitor's closet or room with sinks, spaces and shelters for stores. Separate sanitation sub-stores in critical and semi-critical areas.
- Proper color coded plastic bins lined by (color coded) plastic bags for collection of segregated bio-medical waste. Proper display system with clear indication regarding sorting of waste, so that inter-mixing is prevented. These bins should be placed in the dirty utility (sluice) room and smaller bins in the treatment room/cabin/isolation rooms.
- There should be intramural transportation system (push cart; garbage trolley) with designated lifts/vertical transportation systems.
- It should have separate cubicles for chief housekeeper and assistant housekeeper, a store room for current stores; distant bulk store room for bulk supplies, a space/room for sanitation equipment, pest and rodent control activities.
- Access to the storage spaces/areas should be based on need, so as to prevent theft and pilferage.
- To ensure presence of housekeeping staff in the patient care areas, a supervisor is a must.
- The interim storage site of BMW should be located at place which is accessible and have facility for locking. There should be clear warning sign with proper labels.

- There should be provision of specially designed floor drain traps.
- Provision of hand and eye wash station should also be present.
- If in-house bio-medical waste treatment facility is available it should be sited away from hospital premises, with proper access, and necessary equipment for treating BMW, depending on available resources.
- A **vaporised hydrogen peroxide** (VHP) may be installed in places conducting research and biological safety applications. VHP is a low temperature sterilliant used for bio-decontamination of sealed enclosures such as isolators, work stations, pass through rooms in research and biological safety applications. VHP cycle operates in four phases:
- Dehumidication—Reduction of relative humidity occurs;
- Condition—Rapid increase of desired hydrogen peroxide vapour concentration;
- Biocontamination—Maintenance of desired hydrogen peroxide concentration and
- Aeration—Rapid reduction of hydrogen peroxide vapour.

Space Requirement

The space requirement is entirely dependent upon the type of service provided (in-house/contractual); degree of mechanization and automation and whether BMW is treated in-house or not.

LINEN AND LAUNDRY SERVICES

The activities/services pertaining to the washing/cleaning of linen come under the ambit of *laundry services.*

Linen Classification

General purpose linen: This includes curtains, drapes, table cloths, counter panes and similar items commonly used in all parts of the hospital. This is not used for direct or indirect patient care.

Patient linen: This consists of patient clothing such as pyjamas, shirts, gown, coats, etc. worn by patients.

Bed linen: This consists of patient bed clothing such as bed sheets, pillows, blankets, etc. used by the patients.

OT, labor room and procedure room linen: This includes clothing such as pyjamas, shirts, petticoats and tops worn by surgeons, anesthetist and OT personnel and also surgical gowns, caps, masks, trolley covers, OT towels, DL wrappers, leggings, etc. required in operating room, labor rooms or procedure rooms, etc.

Linen Requirement for Hospitals

Linen requirements for general hospitals vary from 3.5 to 7 kg per bed per day in western countries. The average for general hospitals in India is about 3.5 kg per day. The above figures are for the purpose of laundering processes and are for dry weight. On an average the percentage by weight of different types of linen are as follows:

1. Flatwork (sheets): 70 per cent
2. Rough finish (towels, OT and labor room linens): 22 per cent
3. Hand finished: 8 per cent.

Norms for linen per bed (bed linen and patient linen).

A hospital should have 6 sets of bed linen per bed; one in use, one ready for use, one being processed in laundary, one in transit, and two as reserve for weekends, holidays and unforeseen requirements.

The suggested norms are:

1. Bed sheet (54" × 90"): 6 per bed.
2. Draw sheet (44" × 60"): 3 per bed (Not all patients require draw sheets)
3. Pillow cover: 6 per bed

Table 4.10: Weight of items of hospital line

Items	Weight
Surgeons shirt	200 gm
Surgeons pyjama	200 gm
Surgeons gown	500 gm
Cap	15 gm
Mask	15 gm
Ladies head wear	30 gm
Patients shirt	250 gm
Patients pyjama	250 gm
Patients petticoat	200 gm
Pillow cover	150 gm
Bed sheet	700 gm
Draw sheet	350 gm
Abdominal sheet	500 gm
Trolley cove	350 gm
Blanket	1000 gm
Baby blanket	350 gm
OT towel	400 gm
Mackintosh cover	350 gm
Bath towel	700 gm
Hand towel	250 gm

Note: These are weights of cotton fabric. The actual weight will depend on the quality, thickness and blending of fabric with polyester yarn.

4. a. Shirt and pyjama for males: per bed (20% extra)
   b. Blouse and petticoat for females: 3 per bed (20% extra)
5. Patient towel: 3 per bed
6. Blanket: 1 per bed (20% extra)

This scale is adequate for a daily change of bed linen and alternate day change of patient body linen. If the hospital policy required daily change of patient body linen also, the requirement of such items will increase accordingly. This scale is also based on the assumption that the hospital has its own functioning mechanical laundary. OT linen, labor room and procedure room linen should be determined based on anticipated workload.

Classification of Linen for Laundering Purpose

1. **Dirty (used) linen:** Ordinary washable linen.
2. **Soiled linen:** Soiled linen with crusts of body fluids and smelling foul. Foul linen is not necessarily infected.
3. **Foul linen:** Soiled linen with crusts of body fluids and smelling foul. Foul linen is not necessarily infected.
4. **Infected linen:** Lined which is considered by clinicians as infected.
5. **Foul and infected linen:** Foul linen lying untented for more than six hours can be considered as infected.

The above classification assumes significance because all linen received by the laundary will require segregation at the point of receipt accordingly. The soiled foul, infected linen has to be pretreated before it is subjected to the usual laundering process.

Location

The location of a laundry should be convenient to the user units and close to the service elevator. It may be located in the basement with proper drainage system. If possible, it should be in close proximity to the CSSD and dietary services due to the common requirement of steam from the boiler plant by these services.

Physical Layout

A mechanized laundry service is not only convenient but also safe and dependable as compared to other methods. The design of the laundry should facilitate the following laundering processes:
- Reception of soiled laundry
- Sorting
- Sluicing
- Washing
- Hydroextraction
- Drying

- Calendering and pressing
  - Packing, storage and distribution of clean laundry.
- A separate room should be provided for receiving and holding soiled linen until it is ready for pick up or processing.
- There should be a barrier separating the soiled linen and infected linen.
- There should be a physical separation between the clean and soiled areas.
- Laundry should generally have a separate entry and exit.
- The ceiling height should be approximately 4.5 m.
- The floor should be smooth, washable, non-slippery and water impervious.
- The walls should have a smooth and washable surface without dust collecting projections.
- The door should be wide enough (minimum 1500 mm).
- The room should have effective ventilation. The recommended air changes are 10 per hour.
- The boiler room should be appropriately located and there should be separate exhaust pipes, for letting off steam.
- The recommended water supply is 15 liters of hot water and 10 liters of cold water for every kilogram of linen. Utilization of solar thermal system is recommended.
- If the water is excessively hard, a water softening plant should be installed.
- Provision must be made for fire safety.
- Separate trolley storage areas of clean and soiled linen should be provided.
- The equipment installed should be able to process at least a seven days supply within the regular scheduled work week.
- Appropriate placement and space should be available for the equipment in the laundry.
- The arrangement of equipment should permit an orderly workflow with a minimum of cross traffic that ought mix clean and soiled operations.
- The following facilities should also be planned and designed for:
  - Sewing room.
  - Laundry manager's office.
  - Toilet facilities, resting room and shower facilities for workers.
- The drains especially in the sorting and washing area should have sediment and lint trays.
- Laundry should be planned and designed for the present with adequate capacity for future expansion.

MEDICAL IMAGING SERVICES

Medical Imaging Unit assist the clinician in the diagnosis and treatment of diseases.

Depending on the type and size of the healthcare facility, the medical imaging unit may provide for X-ray diagnostic investigations, PACS (picture archiving communication system), diagnostic screening (fluoroscopy), ultrasonography, mammography, computerized tomography or interventional radiographic procedures (Fig. 4.12).

Organization

In large hospitals, the unit may be organized as three separate sections, viz. diagnostic radiology, interventional radiology and nuclear medicine, whereas in other hospitals, services of only diagnostic radiology may be made available.

Key Planning and Design Parameters

- Flexibility in design is essential and it is necessary to provide for future expansion. Rooms should also be sized larger to allow upgrading of equipment and augmentation of services in the future.

- Provision for mobile X-ray units should be available.
- The imaging unit may consist of the following functional areas:
  - Reception and waiting areas.

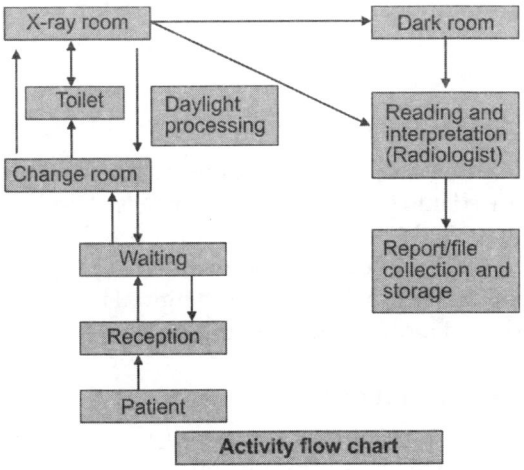

Fig. 4.12: Medical imaging unit

- X-ray and screening room with access to patient change areas and toilets.
- Support areas including preparation, storage, disposal and utility room.
- Film processing areas—both daylight and darkroom areas.
- Film storage areas—with cabinets and shelves for easy retrieval.
- Viewing and reporting areas.
- Administrative and office areas.
- Staff amenities including staff room, staff change rooms and toilets.

Location

Should ideally be located on ground floor and conveniently accessible to:
- Inpatient services
- Outpatient department and
- Accident and emergency department.

Entrance

There should be a separate entrance for accident and emergency cases.

Waiting Area

Main waiting space may be located at the entrance of the department. A separate waiting area, should be provided for wheel chair and stretcher patients. A special enclosed area for the injured or seriously ill should be provided. The receptionists desk is recommended to be centrally located in front of the entrance between the waiting room and administrative area. The floor area of about 13 m^2 is recommended for each waiting patient.

Corridors

These are recommended to be 2.4 m wide to facilitate patient movement, including those on stretches/wheel chairs.

X-ray Room

Optimum size of an X-ray room is 5.5 m x 6 m. Ceiling height of 3 m is recommended. A control booth with adequate radiation exposure protection should be located in the room. There should be a lead glass window to enable the operator to see and communicate with the patient. The room will also require provision of cassette changer.

Dressing Rooms

To enable staff and equipment to function efficiently, it is recommended that 2 to 4 well-lit and ventilated cubicles for each X-ray machine should be provided. Each dressing room should be equipped with a mirror, clothes hook and a bench. For the convenience of patients in wheel chairs, a larger-sized dressing room should be provided. It should have curtains instead of a door. A toilet with change facility may also be provided.

Dark Room

If more than one X-ray room is planned, it is preferable to have a dark room located between the two X-ray rooms. The dark room should have utility suite with drain board for mixing clinical solutions and handwashing. A light lock between the dark room and light room, equipped with interlocking doors, is necessary.

Film Processing Area

The processing of film begins at the developing tank in the dark room. In daylight processing, use is made of self-contained film developing units. Cassettes are loaded into the unit from the X-ray room side, pass through the processor unit and emerge developed from the opposite side.

Storage

Storage should be planned for bulk supplies such as films, linen, gowns, janitors closet, developing and contrast solutions, and office supplies.

Toilets

It is recommended that for each X-ray room, two toilets should be provided. Toilets should also be conveniently available for waiting patients and immediately available for patients undergoing fluoroscopy. For wheel chair patients toilets should be larger. Grab bars should also be provided. Sufficient toilets and lockers should be provided for staff.

Room Lighting

Dimmer controls on lights are recommended particularly in procedure and fluoroscopic rooms.

Dark Rooms and Rim Processing Areas

It must be ensured that air spill does not occur from the dark room to adjacent spaces. Daylight processing equipment must be provided with adequate local exhaust ventilation to prevent the uncontrolled escape of chemical emissions. Fumes or potentially contaminated air must be exhausted to outside air and not recirculated. Special ventilation requirements are dependent upon the type of film processor (automatic or manual) to be installed in an X-ray dark room, processing and viewing areas.

Fluoroscopy Room

In fluoroscopy, radio opaque media is introduced into the body to create images of tissues that would not otherwise show up well on an X-ray. The room is recommended to be 5.5 m x 6 m with a 3 m ceiling height The room should have an attached toilet.

Mammography Room

In this procedure, low level radiation is utilized to identify tumors calcifications, cysts and/or lumps in breast tissue. The room should be of 10 m^2. Visual and acoustic privacy should be provided.

Ultrasound Room

Ultrasound waves are of frequency between 2.2 and 10 MHz and not audible to human ear. Diagnostic sonography may be utilized to demonstrate soft tissue structures and to study physiological movements. The room should be minimum of 12 m^2. Facility for patient reception, registration and sub-waiting should be provided based on workload. It should have patient toilet facilities from within the room.

Nuclear Medicine Room

In nuclear medicine diagnostic procedures, low strength, short-lived, radiation emitting isotopes are introduced into the human body. The emissions are captured by the camera and translated into images. SPECT (Single photon emission computed tomography) combines a gamma camera inter-digital image acquisition and interpretation capabilities to generate tomographic portrayals of blood flow to the brain and heart.

Key Planning and Design Parameters

- Special provision must be adhered to as per recommendations of regulatory authorities for storage and disposal of radioactive substances.
- Supporting spaces have to be planned such as:
  - 'Hot' lab where radio-pharmaceuticals are prepared having lead lined containers and refrigerators, exhaust radio isotope and approved system for radioactive waste collection and disposal.
  - Dose room where patients are injected with radio-pharmaceuticals.
- Flooring should meet load requirements for equipment.
- Floors and walls should be constructed of materials that are easily decontaminated in case of accidental radioactive spills.
- Walls should have provision of vents of radioactive gases as well as medical gases and vacuum.
- Provision for wiring, ducts or conduits should be made in floors, walls and ceilings.

CT SCANNING (COMPUTERISED TOMOGRAPHY)

In CT scanning the transmission is picked up by a detector and is reconstructed by the computer on a video screen. CT examinations involve cross sectional imaging of the body.

Functional Areas

CT imaging room: Area requirement is in the range of 38–42 m^2. The room should be located adjacent to the CT control room. There should be clinical scrub facilities adjacent to the room.

CT console room: It accommodates the computer and other controls for the equipment. A viewing window permitting full view of the patient should be provided. The room should be located with direct access to the CT imaging room and ready access to film processing areas. Area requirement is 6–8 m^2.

CT computer room: It provides area for the computer and generator modules associated with the CT scanning equipment and should be located adjacent to the CT scanning and console room. The area required is about 6 m^2.

Scrub up/gowning area: An area of about 6–8 m^2 is required.

Patient holding areas: A patient bay of approx 9 m^2 is required for holding/recovery. Two bays per scanning room are recommended.

Patient toilet and change facilities: An approximate area of 4 m^2 is required. Other areas which should be planned include staff change and toilet facilities and storage.

Circulation area: The area of about 35% should be provided.

MRI (MAGNETIC RESONANCE IMAGING)

The mechanism is based on the individual electromagnetic properties of the atoms within tissues. Conversion of information contrast scan is done by disturbing the individual magnetic field of various tissues with radio frequency waves. A copper fabric is often utilized to shield the room. It should be located with ready access to the emergency unit, operating unit and critical care area. Ground floor is the preferred location for a MRI unit.

Functional Areas

MRI computer room: Recommended space is of 35 m^2. The room should be located adjacent to the MRI scanning and console room.

MRI console room: This is required to accommodate the computer and other controls of the equipment. There should be a window to provide full view of the MRI room. A minimum space of 10 m^2 is recommended. It should be located with direct access to the MRI scanning room.

MRI room: This provides the area and equipment for MRI scanning procedures. It should be located with direct access to the console room. Power conditioning and voltage regulation equipment as well as direct current (DC) may be required. Magnetic shielding to restrict magnetic field plot and radio frequency shielding to attenuate stray radio frequencies are required.

Cryogen facilities: These may be required in areas where service to replenish supplies is not readily available. If facilities are provided cryogen venting will be required.

Circulation space: The space of 35% should also be provisioned for.

ANGIOGRAPHY

The angiography unit may be located within the medical imaging unit or a separate unit, which provides facilities for diagnostic X-ray investigation of the heart and blood vessels. The unit should be located with ready access to the emergency unit, operating unit and intensive care/coronary care units.

Angiography room: It provides an area and equipment for angiography examination. The minimum space recommended is 40 m². It should be located adjacent to the control room and should have ready access to patient holding areas and staff change facilities. A scrub suite for staff should be located outside the staff entry to the angiography room.

Control room: It provides for remote operation of the angiography. A viewing window to permit full view of the patient should be provided. This should have a direct access to the angiography procedure room. A space of 8 m² is recommended for the control room.

Computer equipment room: A space of 6 m² is recommended.

Circulation space: The space of about 35% is allotted.

PET ROOM

- In positron emission tomography, isotopes after being injected/inhaled attach to body's own molecules and become a tracer as it moves throughout the body. The isotope is generated on-site with the aid of cyclotron.
- Ceiling height recommended is 3 m.
- The unit should be located with close access to nuclear medicine unit, emergency unit, intensive care unit and operating unit. It would require a ground level location due to the weight of the equipment and for ease of installation and replacement.

PET Camera Room

This provides area and equipment for PET camera scanning procedures. It should be located with ready access to patient waiting areas, holding and anesthetic room if provided as well as preparation room and laboratories. The room should have direct access to the control room. A size of approximately 40 m² is recommended.

The following design parameters should be considered

- Room lighting should be controllable and glare-free.
- Floor should be antistatic.
- Floor should be structurally suited to bear the weight of the equipment which may exceed 3000 kg.
- Provision should be made for medical gases, medical air and suction.
- Visibility between camera and control rooms should be ensured.

PET Control Room

It provides for the computer and control for the PET equipment. It should be minimum of 10 m².

Preparation Room

It is required for preparing radio-pharmaceuticals and injecting patients. It should have ready access to patient waiting areas and laboratories. It should be minimum of 12 m². The room would require working benches and hand basin. The toilet used by patients injected with radio-pharmaceuticals should have a radiation shielding.

Waiting Areas

A patient bay area is required for patients on beds/trolleys who have received an injection of imaging agent and are awaiting the scanning procedure. Radiation protection screening will be required since the imaging agents emit low level radiation. Area recommended is 10–12 m².

Hot Laboratory

It is used for preparation and storage of radio-pharmaceuticals. It should be located with ready access to the quality control laboratory, the preparation room and the PET camera room. It would require laboratory benches and also radiation protection. An area of 20 m² is recommended. The storage and disposal from this room to another should be as per the recommendation of concerned statutory authority.

Quality Control Laboratory

This is required for preparation of radionucleides, quality control procedures involved in the production process. It should have ready access to the hot laboratory and preparation room. It would require laboratory work stations, sink and radiation protection. An area of 10 m² is recommended.

CYCLOTRON

It is a device that is used to produce beam of charged particles that can be directed at a specific target. They are used for radio-isotope production and cancer treatment. The cyclotron should be located with ready access to the PET camera room, hot laboratory/radio-chemistry and quality control laboratory. The room size is dependent on the equipment to be installed, the minimum room size being 47 m².

Key Planning and Design Parameters

- Radiation protection
- Sink and floor drain
- Dedicated three phase power supply
- Chilled water supply
- Compressed air supply
- Gas bottle storage
- Air conditioning with filtered exhaust system and negative pressure selective to the surrounding area.
- Structural requirements for weight bearing, i.e. 40000 kg (40 tons).

CENTRAL STERILE SUPPLY DEPARTMENT

A central sterile supply department (CSSD) is a hospital support service, which is entrusted with processing and issue of supplies including sterile instruments and equipment used in various departments of a hospital.

Functions and Activities

- *Receipt:* This includes receiving the materials, supplies and equipment, dressings, and specialized surgical items for processing.
- *Cleaning*: This includes cleaning of used equipment/materials, and plastic goods either manually or by machines, e.g. ultrasonic cleaner, jet glove washing machines, washer disinfectors, anesthetic washers and dryers. This function may also include the cleaning of the delivery trolleys.
- *Checking, assembling and packaging:* This entails the checking of glass items for breakages, needles and instruments for sharpness and breakages, assembling of the equipment after washing and drying, making sets and packaging for sterilization.
- *Sterilization*
- *Labeling*
- *Storage:* This function includes the storage of sterilized packs, and disposables, dressing materials, spare parts of machines or

sterilizers for routine maintenance and broken/ unserviceable items for condemnation. Space for storing distribution trolleys.
- *Issue and distribution:* This includes the issue of sterilized, packages, dressings, linen, instruments and disposables to various departments of the hospital.

Key Planning and Design Parameters
- There should be no back tracking of sterile goods.
- Materials/items from contaminated and sterile areas should be separated from each other.
- There should be separate receipt and dispatch areas.
- The clean and dirty areas should be separated by a physical barrier.
- The floor surface should be smooth, impervious, non-skid and robust.
- Light fittings should be recessed.
- Relative humidity should be maintained at 45 ± 5 %.
- The clean area should be provided with air locks and maintained at positive pressures relative to the adjoining spaces. The minimum rate should be 6 to 10 air changes per hour.
- Facilities must be planned for at least one high speed autoclave preferably in the OT complex. Flash sterilization is performed in the user departments to sterilize instruments that are required immediately.
- The preparation and assembly of gauze packs should be confined to a separate, enclosed ventilated work area wherein gauze cutting machine with table and storage racks of gauze packs should be provided.
- There should be no exposed light fixtures, pipes, ducts or cables to collect lint and dust.
- The walls and ceilings should be of a smooth surface to facilitate easy cleaning.
- The work area should be made of marble/granite/stainless steel.
- The sterilization must be planned for autoclaving by steam as well as by gas.
- Plasma sterilization system: It is a low temperature hydrogen peroxide gas plasma sterilization system. It sterilizes metal and non-metal instruments, endoscopes, electronic and optical equipment as well as plastic and rubber products. Its main advantages are:
    - Fast instrument turnaround
    - Cycle time is short
    - Safe and easy to use
    - Process is gentle on instruments since sterilization is at temperatures below 55°C under dry conditions.
- It eliminates instrument stress related to heat, rapid temperature change and humidity.

Location: It should be close to accident and emergency department, operation theaters and wards. In a multistoreyed building, the CSSD may be situated in the lowest floor. The OT suite and CSSD may be connected by means of two dedicated dumb waiters, one utilized for transportation of sterile and the other for soiled material.

Physical Layout
- Area for receipt of materials/items.
- Areas for storing sterilized material/items.
- Cleaning, washing and decontamination area.
- **Assembling area:** This requires workstations for assembling medical/surgical treatment packs, sets and trays. Work benches with multiple drawers should be provided. In the linen pack area, an inspection table must be provided for detecting holes in the linen.
- Glove processing area
- Gauze cutting area
- **Storage area** for packed sets waiting for autoclaving.
- **Sterilizers room:** This should be equipped with double door pass-through autoclaves

which are built into the wall between the clean and sterile areas. Materials are loaded on the clean side and unloaded after sterilization on the sterile side.

- Sterile store
- Supervisors room
- Issue counter
- Office
- Change room
- Trolley washing and packing area.
- Area for storage and supply of steam, hot and cold water.

Space

Depends on total beds of the hospital and other factors such as number and type of sterilizers installed. It varies from 0.7 to 1 m^2 per bed. The higher the number of beds, the lesser is the space requirement per bed.

HEATING VENTILATION AND AIR CONDITIONING

Hospitals have a multi-dimensional role of providing a safe and comfortable environment to the patients, visitors and staff. Various areas of the hospital require different air pressures, temperatures, humidity, filtration and circulation. Specified range of temperature and humidity is also required for effective functioning of hospital equipment. It is thus essential that heating, ventilation and air conditioning (HVAC) of the hospital is done scientifically.

Components of HVAC System

- Outside air inlet or intake filters
- Humidity modification mechanism
- Heating and cooling equipment
- Fans
- Ductwork
- Air exhaust
- Diffuser or grills for proper distribution of air
- Controls and switches
- Electricity supply system with DG set backup.

Process

The outdoor air enters the system where low efficiency or coarse filters remove large particulate matters and micro-organisms. The air then enters the distribution system for conditioning to appropriate temperature and humidity levels, passes through another bank of filters for further cleaning and is delivered to each zone of the building. After the conditioned air is distributed to the designated space, it is returned through a return duct system and delivered back to air handling unit. A portion of the return air is exhausted outside, while the remainder is mixed with outside air for dilution and filtered for removal of contaminants. Total fresh air (100%) system is used in ultra clean operation theaters with high efficiency particulate air filter (HEPA) and well supported by the heat recovery devices.

Air Conditioning Plant

The essential components of an air conditioning plant are the condensing unit and air handling unit (AHU). The cool air produced in the refrigeration unit is transferred either directly to circulating air or to circulating water, which in turn cools the circulating air. These are called direct expansion system and chilled water system respectively. The cooling of circulatory air occurs in the air handling unit (AHU). It has the air filters, cooling coils and air blowers. Air ducts convey the air to and from the AHU. The direct expansion system can handle one AHU as compared to many by the chilled water system. The capacity of an air conditioning unit is expressed in tones of refrigeration (TR), which is the heat extraction capacity of the plant. 1 TR is equal to heat extraction rate of 12,000 British Thermal Unit (BTU) per hour.

Fire Dampers

The ducts offer an easy propagatory passage to fire hence fire dampers should be inserted in the air ducts. The fire dampers are actuated to close the passage by fire detectors. They could also be closed by fuse links, which melt when the fire heat reaches them.

Air Filtration

There are three types of air filters:

Coarse filters to prevent large particles and insects from entering AHU. These are also called prefilters. Efficiency is 90% down to 5–10 microns.

Micro fine filters which filters out particles up to 5 microns (1 micron is one thousand of a millimeter). Efficiency is 99.9%.

High efficiency particulate air filters (HEPA filters) which filter up to 0.3 microns with 99.97% efficiency.

Key Planning and Design Parameters

Heating

- Furnaces or boilers are the two selected heating units for central heating plants, which act as standby in the event of failure or maintenance of one heating unit.
- To provide both normal and standby service, boiler accessories including feed pumps, heat circulating pumps, condensate return pumps, fuel oil pumps, and waste heat boilers should be connected and installed.
- The heating systems should be thermostatically controlled.
- Operation of heat exchangers may be supplemented by cogeneration unit and heat recovery equipment of engine drive chiller.

Cooling

- For removal of solids from the circulating water system in the cooling towers and evaporative condenser, a cyclonic separator or side stream filter should be used.
- The kitchens and workshops and some other non-critical areas, where suitable evaporative cooling may be used for comfort.
- Selection of central cooling plant chiller sets should ensure that in the event of failure of a compressor, adequate standby capacity is made available for important critical areas.

Ventilation—Exhaust Air

- Hazardous exhaust should be discharged from the highest point possible in order to expel contaminants above building recirculation flow pattern.
- Toilet, dirty utility and similar spaces should be segregated from clinical areas and exhaust duct should be discharged outside and not in the internal courtyards.
- High velocity discharge stack increases effective stack height.
- MRI emergency exhaust fans are activated by oxygen sensors where a helium leak could displace breathing air.
- Scavenging systems to be used to vent waste gases in the space used for administering inhalation anesthesia and inhalation analgesia which can be exhausted directly to the atmosphere.
- Contaminated exhaust systems, including those serving toilets, and those necessary to attain positive airflow from clean to dirty areas should be provided with duplex fans or fan motors and automatic change-over from duty to standby in the event of a failure of the fan or motor. Provide remote alarm indicating fan failure.

Ventilation—Outdoor Air

Each mechanical ventilation system or exhaust is recommended to be equipped with a readily accessible means of either shut off or volume reduction.

Air Handling Systems

Conditions to Meet

- Location of plant and components should be easily accessible for routine maintenance.

- Technical expertise should be available on site to operate and adjust the system.
- Systems should be simple, cost effective and easy to maintain.
- Critical patient care areas should have separate duct for supply and return air.
- Plant room ventilation supply air should be filtered.
- Non-corrodible material should be used for ducting and grills.
- For humidification, low-pressure steam into the supply air stream should be used failing which an electrode type humidifier may be used.
- Avoid using evaporative pan humidifiers or reservoir type water spray.
- Fire prevention methods should be adhered to wherever heating coils are used.
- Ducts should be well insulated acoustically and thermally and should be devoid of any fibers in supply route.
- All AHUs should have easy accessibility, enough area for inspection of unit and internal surfaces hygienic and easily cleanable.
- Design should provide right air pressure, air filtration and air flow controls.
- Control systems should be adjusted to suit patient needs.
- Regulatory mechanism should exist in terms of shut down or control of flow rate, or operation of HVAC when partial area is not in use, such as operation theater, etc.
- Utilization of non conventional energy in design and execution should be encouraged.
- Ultra clean air (UCA) systems may be required for operating rooms for specialized procedures.

Air Quality Indicator

These include viable and non-viable airborne particle analysis. Non-viable airborne particles may be assessed with particle counter either optical or laser type. Particles more than 0.5 microns are used to assess facility air quality status. Counting of particles is done where there are no persons in the room. Viable airborne particle analysis may be done by micro biological air sampling. Sedimentation methods using settle plates and volumetric methods are utilized. Settle plates rely on gravity during sampling and hence smaller airborne particles may be missed leading to erroneous readings.

Outdoor Intakes

The bottom of outdoor air intake serving central system should be located not less than 1.8 meters above ground level but ideally at 3.6 meters. If installed above the roof of the building, they should be located 0.9 meters above the finished roof level.

Exhaust Outlets

The general exhaust should be located at a minimum of 3 meters above the ground level and away from doors, occupied areas and openable windows.

Direction of Air Flow

The direction should be from clean to less clean area. Air flow rate of 0.28 to 0.47 meters per second is desirable across an open door to prevent back flow into clean area. Average air velocity in the room must be between 0.1 and 0.15 meter per second (Table 4.11).

Power Supply

Reliable power supply should be ensured to critical areas. Regulatory methods should be adopted to control the fluctuation of power. Low voltage cannot operate the equipment, hence to ensure proper supply, voltage correction devices may be used. Generators should be utilised as power backup devices particularly in critical care areas.

Air-conditioned Rooms/Areas

Minimum recommended areas which should be air-conditioned are:
- Operation theaters and procedure areas

Hospital Management

Table 4.11: Recommended air changes

Space/area	Air changes per hour	Temp oc +2	RH%
Hospital store, patient corridors.	6–8	24	50
Pharmacy, clean work room, storage (of diagnostic, treatment and sterilization areas).	6–8	23	45
Anesthesia gas storage.	8	24	50
Recovery rooms (surgery), ICUs, labor rooms, patient rooms, newborn nursery.			
Examination rooms, treatment rooms, X-ray rooms, biochemistry, cytology, histology, microbiology, nuclear medicine, pathology, serology, soiled or decontamination rooms, laboratory services.	10	23	50
Toilet room of wards, bathrooms, darkroom of imaging unit, glass washing and sterilization room, ETO and sterilize equipment room of sterilizing and supply unit, soiled work room, soiled holding of diagnostic and treatment room, laundry, janitors closet.	10	24	50
Food preparation center.	10	25	50
Operating room, delivery room, trauma room, procedure room, endoscopy, bronchoscopy room, isolation room, protective environment room, autopsy room.	15–20	22 / 22	45 / 45

- Recovery area
- ICU, CCU, NICU
- Laboratories
- Imaging areas
- High dependency units in any departments
- Dialysis rooms/facility
- Delivery suites/labor rooms
- Therapeutic facilities, endoscopy suite, radiotherapy facility, path labs, treatment room
- Blood transfusion service (BTS)
- Stores—walk in coolers, cold room
- Mortuary services
- General wards isolation rooms (optional)
- Private wards

Humidifier System

- Humidification should be achieved by the direct injection of low-pressure steam into the supply air stream. Where reticulated steam is not available, an electrode type humidifier may be used.
- Ductwork with duct mounted humidifier should have adequate means of water removal. The other essential conditions recommended for ductwork module are as follows:
  – No internal lining.
  – Reasonable access for cleaning without need for major works.
  – Attenuators must have impervious lining between facing and acoustic lining.
  – Attenuators must be readily removed and located within plant rooms and other accessible areas that facilitates easy removal.
- *Bronchoscopy and sputum induction units:* The supply air to these units should be delivered at high level in a way that

minimizes recirculation of potentially contaminated room air. Total circulated air quantity should not be less than 1.2 ACHR when the supply air filters are at their maximum pressure drop. Rooms or booths used for bronchoscopy, sputum induction and other high risk cough-inducing procedures should be provided with local exhaust ventilation.

- *Cardiac catheterization unit:* The important considerations are that direction of air flows within the procedure room must always be from clean to less clean areas. Supply air to these units should be delivered at high level in a way that minimizes circulation of potentially contaminated room air and provides the cleanest air supply over the procedure area. Total circulated air quantity should not be less than 15 ACHR.
- *Endoscopy units:* Ventilation in work rooms where endoscopes are cleaned should achieve a minimum of 15 ACHR.
    - Where manual endoscopes disinfection with glutaraldehyde occurs, the endoscopes and disinfection trays should be contained by a system of local exhaust ventilation.
    - Where automatic or semi-automatic disinfectors are used, a localized exhaust system should be provided to achieve appropriate capture and removal of contaminated air.
    - Fumes must be drawn away from the operator's work.

CARDIAC CATHETERIZATION LABORATORY

Cardiac catheterization laboratory or cath-lab is one of the advanced facilities in the modern day hospitals. With the increased incidence of coronary heart diseases, cath-lab has become indispensable for hospitals specializing in cardiology. Diagnostic and therapeutic procedures such as angiogram, catheterization, angioplasty, stent and pacemaker implantation, etc. are performed in cath-lab.

Location

Cath-lab can be set up as an independent unit or within the diagnostic radiology suite. Since asepsis condition is a critical factor, the same considerations that apply to surgical suites hold with regard to location, circulation and infection control. Some hospitals locate their cath labs close to but separate from the surgical suite.

Space requirement: The optimum space requirement for the procedure room is 24×30 or 720 sq ft., 10×15 or 150 sq.ft for control room, 100 sq ft for clean preparation/store.

Design Elements

- Procedure room should be air conditioned
- Control/Console room
- Centralized arrangement of patient holding spaces or rooms usable for pre-procedure preparation, as well as post-procedural recovery.
- Patient holding room, preferably equipped with ECG monitors.
- Technicians work room
- Dark room for 35 mm film, if necessary
- X-ray protection and structural stress
- Film viewing areas for cardiologists
- Desirable: A small chemistry lab. Advanced cath-labs have full scale electrophysiology labs.
- Scrub facilities
- Storage space for case carts
- Alcove for wheel chairs and stretchers
- Clean and soiled utility rooms
- Toilet(s)

Dialysis Unit

Dialysis is required for patients who are in the end-stage diseases. Two dialysis techniques are available—Hemodialysis and Peritoneal dialysis. Hemodialysis is the popular mode of dialysis. In this, patient's blood flows through an extracorporeal dialysis, a device which exposes a minimum volume of blood to the maximum possible area of a semi-permeable membrane, as the blood flows across one side of membrane tends to come into diffusion equilibrium with a stream of dialysate, a balanced electrolyte solution, flowing across the other. Fluid removal is by varying dialyzer blood pressure.

Hemodialysis System

It consists of the following components
- Circulatory access
- Blood pump
- Dialyzer or the artificial kidney
- Method for anticoagulation
- Dialysate delivery system
- Water treatment—Two processes to treat water are reverse osmosis and deionization.

Dialysis Monitors: Factors monitored include arterials venous pressure concentration of dialysate, dialysate flow rate temperature, pressure, and blood in the dialysate.

Design Elements of Dialysis Unit

20 station dialysis facility will require between 540 and 756 m² or 6000 and 8500 sq ft of gross floor area or about 27 and 38.25 m² or 300–425 sq ft per patient.

Patient Areas
- Individual cubicles separated by curtains, partitions or movable screen units.
- Bed cubicles should have at least 150 sq ft/bed and dialysis chairs should 120 sq ft/chair.
- Scrub sinks at the station, 1 sink for 10 patients should be provided.
- A toilet should be provided.
- Handwashing facility for staff.

Service Areas
- Nursing station
- Toilet
- Clean utility room
- Store room
- Refrigerator
- Office space

Water supply pipes to dialysis machines shall be larger than regular water supply pipes to ensure rapid water supply.

MEDICAL GASES

Medical gases refer to those gases which are required in hospital for patient care activity. These include medical oxygen, nitrous oxide, dioxide, medical grade air, (at different pressures) and vacuum suction; some of which can be provided from cylinders and also as a part of centralized supply.

Manifold is a device which is used for connecting the outlets of one or more gas cylinders to the central piping system through a control panel. Generally, there are two banks of cylinders which depend on the requirement (for that medical gas); and the cylinders are connected through tail pipes to ensure continuity. At times the entire pipeline system is referred to as "manifold system".

Objectives

The main objective of the medical gas pipeline services is to provide adequate quantity of safe, reliable, pure medical gases (oxygen, nitrous oxide, carbon dioxide, medical grade air) at the appropriate pressure at all outlet points. It also provides vacuum suction at required pressure at the outlet points, besides anesthetic gases scavenging system (AGSS) in the operation theaters.

Location
- Designated area should have proper ventilation.
- Location should be chosen in such a manner so as to permit access by delivery

vehicles and transportation of cylinders (e.g. proximity to loading docks, access to elevators, passage of cylinders through public areas).
- If the gases are planned to be located indoors then care must be taken to avoid the following areas:
  - areas involved in critical patient care.
  - anesthetizing locations.
  - locations storing flammables.
  - rooms containing open electrical contacts or transformers.
  - kitchens.
  - areas with open flames.
- Temperature in areas where cylinders are used or stored should not reach in excess of 540°C (130°F), as there are chances of fire and explosion.

Design and construction

- Provision for lockable doors or gates to prevent unauthorized entry.
- If the facility is planned outdoors, an enclosures (wall or fencing) must be constructed of non-combustible materials.
- If it planned indoors, it should be constructed while using interior finishes of non-combustible or limited-combustible materials so that all walls, floors, ceilings and doors can withstand a minimum of one-hour fire.
- Electrical devices must be located at or above 1520 mm (5 ft) above finished floor to avoid physical damage.
- Indirect means of heating (e.g. steam, not water) need to be provided, if heat is required.
- Racks, chains, or other fastening should be provided to secure individually all cylinders, whether connected, unconnected, full, or empty, from falling.

Physical Layout

- Source of supply includes bulk liquid systems (tanks), cylinder manifolds (banks), medical air compressor, medical-surgical vacuum producers, AGSS.
- Pipeline distribution system comprises alarms, zonal control boxes, line pressure gauges, risers.
- Point use delivery connections, including panel support boxes, outlet points, pendants, etc.
- Monitoring and control equipment for ensuring safety.

Key Planning and Design Parameters

The medical gas pipeline system, being a critical lifeline in the hospital, should conform to the international standards and the existing rules and regulations. The standards developed in other countries are:

- National Fire Protection Association (NFPA), USA-99C (revised-2002 and 2005).
- Hospital Technical Memorandum (HM)-2002 in the UK.
- EN-737 (European Union).
- Canadian Standards 1169.
- German Standards.
- As standards for medical gas pipeline system do not exist in India, relevant portions of the following Acts, rules and regulation must be complied:
- Indian Explosives Act, 1884 (4 of 1.884), and rules framed thereunder, viz.
  - Gas Cylinder Rules, 1981.
  - The Static and Mobile Pressure Vessels (unfiled) Rules, 1981. The designing and installation should also conform to relevant codes by ANSI, ASMS, ASTM, AWS, CGA and NEMA for various parts of the system if it is according to NEPA standards.

Hospital Categories

According to NFPA (99), standards which were revised in 2002 healthcare facilities are divided into there categories on the basis of effects in case of disruption of gas supply, viz.

Level 1: Facilities where an interruption of the piped systems would place the patients in immediate danger of morbidity or mortality. This is usually limited to hospital, where patients are dependent for life on the gases, or where mechanical ventilation is utilized at anytime.

Level 2: Facilities where an interruption in the piped systems would place the patients at manageable risk of mortality. This is limited to facilities that stand apart from hospitals, are not interconnected to hospital medical gases, and the patients do not require mechanical ventilation or assisted mechanical ventilation, during anesthesia.

Level 3: Facilities where interruptions in the piped systems would terminate procedures but would not place the patients at risk of morbidity or mortality. The facility of total quantity of the gases, excepts nitrogen, does not exceed 3,000 cubic feet, and only cylinders are used to supply oxygen and nitrous oxide to the facility (except for cryogenic oxygen). This is usually limited to dental officers.

Requirement of various services in a particular healthcare facility will determine the type of centralized services to be provided; whether it is required in a centralized or decentralized manner. As a general rule, it will be economical and cost-effective for decentralized medical gas supply system in all healthcare facilities with more than 200 beds.

The following factors must be kept in mind while planning and designing for the central source of medical gases.

Ventilation of Location138s for Manifold

All relief valves must be vented of indoor supply systems. Where the total volume of medical gases connected and in storage is greater than 84,950 L (3000 cu) at STP, indoor supply locations should be provided with dedicated mechanical ventilation systems that draw air from within 300 mm (1 ft.) of the floor and operate continuously. If the total volume is less than 84,950 L at STP or the only compressed gas in the room is medical air, natural ventilation may be employed. This should consist of two louvered openings each having a minimum free area of 46,500 mm^2, one within 1 foot from floor and other within 1 foot of ceiling. These should not be located in an exit access corridor.

Signages

Doors of the locations containing central supply systems of cylinders containing only oxygen or medical air may be marked for easy recognition and safety compliance.

Fire Safety

According to the provisions of static and mobile pressure vessel rules, 1961; provision should be made for adequate water supply in storage area as per local fire service regulations, the hydrants should be accessible and control of water pressure should be possible from outside the danger area. Sufficient hose length should be provided, with outlet equipped with combination jet and for module.

Bulk Liquid Systems

Bulk liquid oxygen tanks are economical, especially for tertiary level, superspecialty hospitals with more than 200 beds, if the weekly consumption is likely to exceed 10,000 liters. This comprises the vacuum insulated evaporator (VIE), vaporizer system, oxygen delivery control panel assembly and remote alarm system. Liquid oxygen tanks should be installed as per the Static and Mobile Pressure Vessels (unfired) Rules, 1981 in India and certified by Chief Controller of Explosives, Nagpur, in accordance with Indian Explosives Act, 1884. The liquid oxygen tank should have capacity for at least six days, and preferably located outdoor with easy access. While

installing, the following guiding principles should be observed:
- The supply system should be anchored firmly to a poured concrete pad, appropriate for the weight, surface load and complying with local seismic requirements.
- The site should be completely enclosed with the poured concrete pad (equipment pad) completely filling the enclosed space.
- Drainage from the equipment pad and vehicle pad should be away from any building parked vehicles, or other potential sources of ignition.
- No sunken areas, trenches, manholes, pits or drains should be located within the pad or closer than 2450 mm (8 ft) from the edge of the pad.
- It should have proper fencing of 2 m height with double gates for filling to vessel and single rear emergency gate.

Source of the bulk supply should consist of one or more supply vessels, whose capacity should be determined after considering delivery schedules, proximity to alternate supplies, when there are multiple bulk liquid vessels, they should be categorized as primary, secondary and reserve and the operating cascade should be *primary* ⟶ *secondary* ⟶ *reserve* at all times. When the main supply fails or falls to a critical point, the reserve supply should get automatically switched on.

Emergency Oxygen Supply (EOS)

Generally in hospitals having liquid oxygen tank this is planned through a secondary manifold comprising of two banks of oxygen cylinders. The number of oxygen cylinders will depend upon the daily oxygen requirement, flow rates required (usually at 10 psi) in case the primary supply is through a lesser capacity secondary manifold.

Ideally this should be located at the exterior of the building being served, in a location accessible by emergency supply vehicle at all times, in all weather conditions. It should be connected to the main supply line immediately downstream of the main shutoff valve.

While planning the emergency oxygen supply, following tampering and theft can happen.
- Physical protection to prevent unauthorized tempering and theft.
- A female DN (NPS) inlet for connection of the emergency source gas pressure.
- A manual shutoff valve to isolate the EOS when not in use.
- Two check valves, one downstream of the EOS and one downstream of the main line shutoff valve, with both upstream from the tee connection for the two pipelines.
- A relief valves sized to protect the downstream piping system and related equipment from exposure to pressures in excess of 50% higher than normal line pressure.
- Any valve necessary to allow connection of an emergency supply of oxygen in isolation of the piping to the normal source of supply.

Medical-Surgical Vacuum Supply System

Vacuum or suction is considered as a vital life support therapy and treatment. Types of suction vary from oral/tracheal to remove fluid, irrigation liquids, blood and related debris. Vacuum systems are dry by design. They consist of the source of supply (vacuum pumps) distribution piping, terminal inlets and alarms. Fluids suctioned from a patient are collected in volume and viscosity of the liquid being suctioned.

Vacuum Systems Comprise
- Two or more vacuum pumps sufficient to serve peak calculated demand with the largest single vacuum pump out of service.

- An automatic means to prevent backflow from any on-cycle vacuum pumps to any off-cycle vacuum pumps.
- A shutoff valve or other isolation means to isolate each vacuum pump from the centrally piped system and other vacuum pumps for maintenance or repair without loss of vacuum in the system.
- A vacuum receiver vessel, which should be floor mounted, with inspection access panel.
- Piping between the vacuum pump and the source shutoff valve should be hard drawn seamless copper.
- Bacterial filter assemblies for proper infection control. These should be installed on a sturdy supporting base, in a well-lighted and ventilated room.

Medical Compressed Air

The medical compressed air plant provides air at two pressures, viz. 4-bar and 7-bar. The machinery comprises compressors of adequate capacity, with air inlet filter, silencer and auto/manual drains, receiver vessels, filter dryer assembly consisting of four level filters and a control panel for each compressor.

Anesthesia Gas Scavenging System (AGSS)

Anesthesia gas scavenging system (AGSS) is responsible for removal of residual anesthesia gases from the OTs. The AGSS comprises the exhauster unit which is a two-stage lateral channel vacuum pump unit with an impeller mounted on the master shaft.

Table 4.12: Medical gas outlets for oxygen, vacuum, (suction) and air

Location	Oxygen	Vacuum	Air
Patient rooms in medical, surgical, obstetric and pediatric wards	x	x	x[4]
Examination/treatment rooms in nursing units	x	x	–
Intensive care, coronary care unit	xx[3]	xxx	x
Nursery	x	x	x
General operating room, emergency trauma room	xx	xxx	xx
Cyctoscopic and special procedure rooms	x	xxx	xx
Recovery room	x[2]	xxx	xx
Labor room	x[2]	x[2]	x[2]
Deliver and birth room	xx	xxx	x
Emergency	x[2]	x[2]	x[2]
Anesthesia work room	x	–	x
Autopsy	–	x	x

[1]One outlet accessible to each bed (one outlet may serve two beds)
[2]Separate outlet for each bed.
[3]Two outlets for each bed.
[4]One outlet for air is required in the pediatric unit
Nitrous oxide, which is not shown here, is required only in the operating and special procedure rooms.

SPACE REQUIREMENTS

The space requirement of a hospital will depend upon the capacity of liquid oxygen tank, number of cylinders in each bank of emergency manifold, number of OTs and requirement of nitrous oxide. It will also depend upon capacity of compressors, number of vacuum suction units and AGSS system. The most important factor to be kept in mind is adhering to the minimum standards prescribed for distances from other buildings and between pressure vessels vide Static and Mobile Pressure Vessels (unfired) rules, 1981.

Perimeter should be protected by industrial type fence of two meters high.

Format types: There are four types of formats:

1. *Source oriented medical records: (SOMR)* In this type different records in the medical record are organized according to the department which provides care and initiates data. The forms are arranged according to the data in each section and are usually compiled in reverse chronological order as long as patient is under treatment, so that the most recent information is at the top. After the discharge of the patient, the medical record is rearranged in the normal chronological order.

2. *Problem oriented medical records:* (POMR): This is developed by Lawrence weeds in 1960. This format helps in reflecting the logical thinking of the physician who is giving the treatment. It provides a systematic method of documenting the care given to the patent. POMR has four basic parts:
   (i) Database
   (ii) Problem list
   (iii) Initial plans
   (iv) Progress notes

   (i) **Database:** It includes the main complaint, social data, previous diagnostic reports, history, physical examination, etc.

   (ii) **Problem list:** This list contains specific diagnosis, abnormal investigation findings, suspected condition. The problem list is updated when new problems are identified, changes made as and when needed. Problems in the list are not erased out, they are marked as dropped or resolved and the date is noted.

   (iii) **Initial plan:** Initial plan consists of plans regarding what has to be done to learn more about patients condition, treat the condition and to educate the patient about the condition. Each problem has three plans which falls into one of the three categories:
   a. More data for diagnosis.
   b. Care or therapy (includes list of drugs, procedures)
   c. Patient education.

   (iv) **Progress notes:** It contains the follow up for every problem stated in the problems list. Progress notes contain the following elements:
   - Subjective (symptomatic)
   - Objective (observable and measurable)
   - Assessment
   - Plan.

   The acronym for the process is SOAP.

3. *Integrated medical records:* These forms are arranged in strict chronological order. The main feature of the system is that the forms from various sources are inter-mingled.

4. *Decision directed medical records:* It is a recent model of medical record, which relates patient data to clinical decision, providing information for better care.

Minimum Basic Data Set (MBDS): Originated in the Mayo Clinic Rochester, USA. It refers to the core data which is to be gathered about a patient. It is relevant for clinical and epidemiological studies.

Physical Layout

- Office of medical record officer.
- Office of assistant medical record officer.
- Waiting space/lounge.
- Modular workstations for different functions with scope for expansion.
- A conference/seminar room for doctors—incomplete record control.
- Issue desk/counter with photocopying equipment.
- Storage room/area for active records.
- Storage area/room for inactive records in a contiguous area or remote area with paper communication.

Key Planning and Design Parameters

- Admission and enquiry office (front office) should be spacious, well ventilated, and lighted. Health education posters, CCTV, air cooling and optimal ventilation should be provided.
- Medical record office should be spacious, well ventilated, and have adequate protection from pests and rodents. It should have air-conditioning to control humidity and improve comfort levels.
- The walls, floors and ceiling should be leak and seepage proof.
- Adequate light (200–300 lux) should be provided for office works.
- Work stations should be modular with independent space for computer consoles.
- Compactor system for storage areas to increase the storage space.
- Entry gate should be strategically located to access control to storage area. Fire sprinklers and smoke detector systems must be installed. Sewerage systems from toilets should be away from storage areas.

SPACE REQUIREMENTS

- The admission and enquiry office should be 15–20 m²; with waiting areas @ 0.5 m²/bed.
- The thumb rule for OPD registration space is @ 1.0 m²/bed, but would also depend upon status of computerization of the hospital.
- Storage should be 15–50 m² with compactors to store more number of files in the same space.
- Filing space should be provided adequately and can be calculated by the following formula (Table 4.13):

$$\text{Indoor} = \frac{\text{No. of beds} \times \% \text{ bed occupancy} \times 365 \text{ days} \times \text{year of storage}}{\text{ALS} \times \text{average thickness of file}}$$

$$\text{Outdoor} = \frac{\text{No. of new patients per year} \times \text{year of storage}}{\text{Average thickness of file}}$$

Table 4.13: Space requirement

Hospital	Office no.	Room size	Filing no.	Room size
Up to 30 beds	1	10' × 12"	–	16' × 20'
30–100 beds	1	10' × 12'	1	16' × 20'
100–250 beds	2	10' × 12'	3	16' × 20'
250–600 beds	3	10' × 12'	3	16' × 20'

MORTUARY SERVICES

Mortuary is defined as the facility for the holding of dead bodies, and viewing by authorized persons for identification purpose prior to handing over for last rites.

Morgue is defined as the place where dead bodies are kept in the body store and examined in the postmortem room.

Location

It should be located in a separate building near the pathology laboratory on the ground floor, easily accessible from the wards, accident and emergency department and operating theaters. It should be located in one wing of the hospital away from the general traffic routes used by the public. It must have a separate entrance and exit for relative and for hears vans.

Physical Layout

- *Access / Portico:* A covered access or portico for vehicles should be provided at the entrance which leads to mortuary complex as a protection in wet weather and as a screen from adjoining areas. The exit to a subsidiary road with nearby car and rear van parking area is also desirable.
- *Autospy / Postmortem room:* The autopsy room should be constructed with spacious window of frosted glass, adequate water supply, fluorescent lighting, built in cupboards and fans. Autopsy room should provide accommodation for:
  - Autopsy tables of stainless steel with sink.
  - Sinks with running water for specimen washing and cleaning.
  - Built-in cupboards for keeping instruments and equipment.
  - Room should have a water impervious floors sloping to a drain.
  - Tiled walls so that whole room can be easily washed.
  - Junction between walls and floors should be suitably covered.

Body store room where the bodies can be kept should be close to postmortem room. Refrigerated body storage room is essential. There should be a provision of deep freezers with capacity of two decomposed bodies to be kept for a longer period. The most practical arrangement is to provide chambers averaging about 1–1.5 m. high in which six bodies may be stored in three sets of two tiers. Cabinet doors should open through 180 degrees to allow the attendant to approach either side of the trolley. Depending upon layout, a depth of 3–6 m for the body store and depth of 2.2 m for cold cabinets are usually satisfactory.

Doctor's Office

Stores: It is preferable to have the following stores:

- *Clean store:* This is for clean gowns, aprons, robber gloves, gumboots, towels, linen items like shrouds, drapes, and towels may be stored here. It should be adjacent to the doctor's room and outside the postmortem room.
- *Instruments and equipment store:* This should open directly into the postmortem room. In this area all the instruments, equipment and reserve stock instruments, electric saw, portable trolley mounted spot light are kept.
- *Chemical store:* This is utilized for storing chemical solutions for preserving the viscera, specimen jars and packing material. Room for technicians/attendant — suitable room of size 10–12 m^2 is required for staff on duty.

Seminar room: This is required in teaching hospitals.

Waiting area: These should be in the form of enclosed covered space or open verandah (corridors) with seating arrangements. The internal finishing should be pleasantly furnished and soberly decorated where one can pay last respect with dignity. It may also be prudent to have a well-ventilated prayer room.

Key Planning and Design Parameters

- Type of hospital; acute care, specialty or superspecialty.
- Whether medico-legal cases (trauma, poisoning, etc.) are admitted in the hospital.
- Numbers of OTs, ICUs and HDUs.
- Whether forensic medicine and toxicology and/or pathology exist in hospital.

Orientation of the complex: It is preferable to have natural daylight through windows.

Engineering Works

- It should be designed in such a way that there is minimum interruption of services during repair and maintenance activities.
- Floors should be durable. It should be made up of material which is moisture resistant and easily cleanable.
- Walls should be permanent, durable construction with impermeable and washable finish.
- Ceiling should be made up of materials that are easily cleanable. Height should be more than 3 m in the waiting, autopsy rooms, doctors, technical and staff room. In other ancillary rooms it can be up to 2.5 m.
- Doors should be sliding double doors with (min 150 mm) width in the main rooms to allow easy access of trolleys, portable X-ray machine.
- Windows should be adequately provided to obtain maximum natural light, and daylight factor should be one. These windows should be provided with opaque glass and fly-proof mesh screens on the outside.

Corridors

Corridors should be minimum of 2400 mm wide for easy passage of trolleys.

Lighting

Tungsten or fluorescent lighting may be used. In postmortem room, special lighting should be provided. The light fittings should be glare free, easy to clean and maintain. Switchers in wet areas should be of the hose proof type. Sufficient hose proof 15 ampere sockets outlets mounted on the walls at a height of 1500 mm are desirable in damp areas such as post-mortem room and body store.

Heating and Ventilation

The temperature required in various areas of mortuary is 10°C to 19°C. Natural ventilation by fly screened windows and fresh air inlet grills should be adequate, except in postmortem rooms where mechanical exhaust system is necessary. The fans should be of the variable speed type designed to produce up to 10 air changes per hour. Deodorizing equipment may be provided in the postmortem room.

Air-conditioning

In large settings it is preferable to have air-conditioning with 100% fresh air.

Refrigeration

The temperature of cold room is to be maintained between 5.5° C and 6.5° C. A thermostat control will be required.

Hot and Cold Water Supply

Hot and cold water should be supplied to mortuary. Postmortem tables should be fitted with individual water hoses. All tapes in the working area should be provided near waiting operated type.

Toilets and Drinking Water Facilities

Toilets and drinking water facilities should be provided near waiting area and offices.

Communication Facilities

Facilities for internal and external telephone lines should be provided.

Fire Alarms and Fire Fighting Equipment

Fire alarm system should be installed. Fire-fighting equipment should be provided and fire exit routes system should be clearly identified and earmarked with green colored paint and well illuminated.

SPACE REQUIREMENTS

This will vary from hospital to hospital depending upon:
- Type of hospital
- Workload
- Level of care provided and
- Jurisdiction for medico-legal cases.

As a general guideline, an area of 0.6–0.8 m²/bed is recommended. It has been estimated that generally four bodies holding spaces are required for every 100 beds. Similarly, two autopsy tables in a room (40 m² area) required up to 400 beds; with 15 m² space for each additional table (for every 200 beds).

Medical Records Department

Medical records is defined as a "clinical scientific, administrative and legal document related to patient care, in which is recorded sufficient data written in sequence or events, to justify the diagnosis, and warrant the treatment and ends results".

Medical records has been defined as a "clear, concise and accurate history of patients life and illness, written from a medical point of view".

Importance

- It documents the medical problems of the patient.
- Assists in the continuity of care.
- Avoids omissions/repetition or duplication of investigation.
- Helps in settling legal and insurance claims.
- It helps in continuity of care.
- Provides assurance of the adequacy and quality of care.
- Helps in medico-legal cases and evaluation of care.
- It helps in evaluation of quality of care, resource allocation and defence of litigations.
- To create external database of registration of births and deaths, PNDT Act and notifiable disease.
- It provides the basis for the biomedical research in hospital.

Functions

MRD can be divided into three district areas/divisions
1. Admission and enquiry office/counter
2. Indoor wards and OPD including registration counter (ambulatory patients)
3. Medical record office

Admission and Enquiry Office

This deals with reception and registration of patients, initiation of the "face sheet" which includes all demographic parameters, allotment of ward and bed number to the admitted patient and notification of communicable/notifiable diseases to medical record office which is also a part of medical record department.

Indoor Wards/Nursing Units

Here history taking, physical examination, investigations, plan of treatment, consultations,

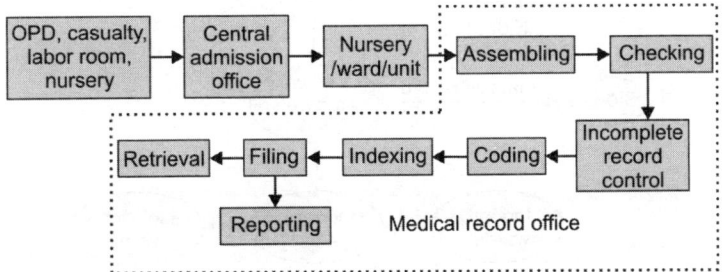

Fig. 4.13: Functional activity flow chart

treatment and progress notes, blood pressure, temperature, pulse respiration charts, input/output charts, consent form, anesthesia notes (wherever applicable), discharge/death reporting, including patients leaving hospital against medical advice (LAMA) is generated.

Medical Record Office

This is responsible for collection of records of discharged patients/deaths in the wards, assembly, deficiency checking, incomplete record control, coding and indexing, analysis and statistical reporting, filing, numbering, storage and retrieval. Other functions include:

- Receipt of summons from courts of law and submission of as desired.
- Maintaining correspondence with insurance agencies for reimbursement purpose.
- Standardization of forms and other documents used in hospital.
- Custodian of patents records taken for medical audit/death revies/peer revies.
- Notification of communicable/notifiable disease cases to appropriate authorities.
- Coordinate issue of medical certificates, estimates for treatment, reimbursement certificates and other documents used by patients.

Location

- The admission and enquiry office should be near the main entrance to the hospital, OPD and accident and emergency department.
- The OPD registration counters should be at the entrance/outside OPD.
- The nursing station/indoor wards should be located in the hospital building in a proper sequence and should have provision for easy entry of information (manual or computerized) in the records.
- The medical record office, should be within the hospital building, near to business office/administration in the records.
- The medical record office, should be within the hospital building near to business office/administration, and not far from the entrance. The inactive records storage office can be located relatively distantly from the hospital building.

Recommended level of illumination for various room of mortuary

Rooms	Required illumination
Postmortem room	300
Postmortem tables and benches	500–750
Pathologist/Forensic specialist room	200
Body store	100
Staff change room/waiting rooms	150–200

Note: Value of illuminations is taken at 900 mm above floor level

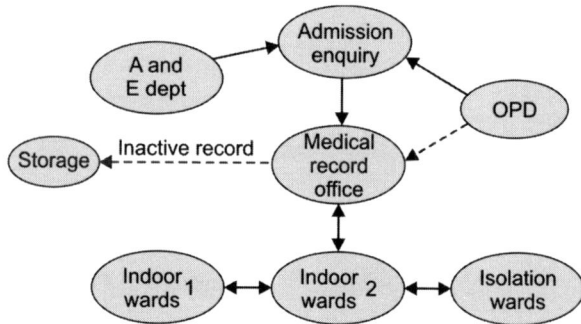

Fig. 4.14: Schematic bubble diagram

Hospital Planning

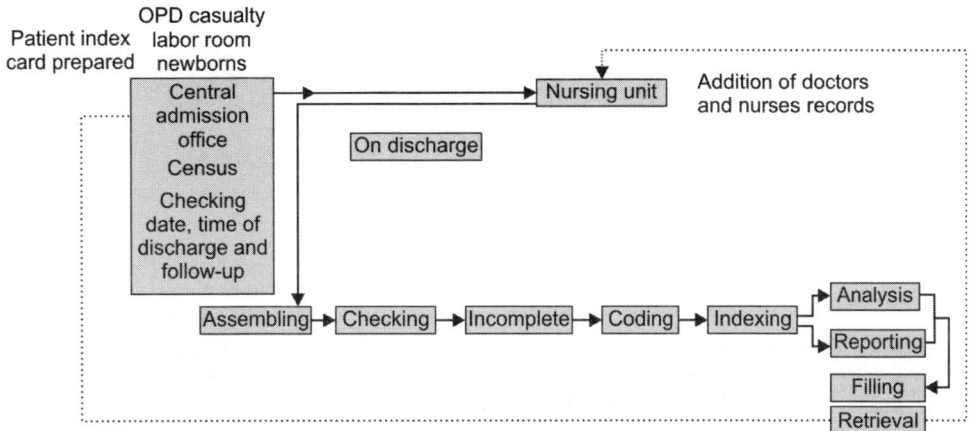

Fig. 4.15: Flow chart of inpatient record

References

Donabedian A: Volume, quality and regionalization of healthcare services, Medical care 22 (2) m: 1984.

Gupta S, Kant S, Chandrashekhar R, Satpathy S: Modern Trends in Planning and Designing of Hospitals—Principles and Practice, Jaypee Brothers, New Delhi, 2007.

Jolly SS; Hospital Statistics. Hospital Administration 17 (1);1980.

Kunders G: Hospitals Facilities Planning and Management, Tata McGraw-Hill, 2004.

Kunders G: Hospitals—Designing for Healing. Prism: 2009.

Kleczowski BM, Pibouleau R: Approaches to Planning and Design of Healthcare Facilities in Developing Areas.3: WHO Geneva, 1979.

Llevelyn-Davis R, Macauley HNC. Hospital Planning and Administration WHO, Geneva, 1966.

McGiboni JR: Principles of Hospital Administration GP Putnam's sons: New York, 1969.

National Building Code. Indian Standards Institution, New Delhi, 1984.

Recommendations for Basic Requirements of General Hospital Buildings (IS: 10905-part 1 to 3). Indian Standards Institution, New Delhi, 1985.

Sakharkar B M: Principles of Hospital Administration and Planning, Jaypee Brothers: New Delhi, 2009.

5
Overview on Hospital Operations Management

V. R. Girija

- Production/operations management can be generalized as the transformation of resources to goods and services.
- The essential function of any organization is to bring together people, machines and material, to provide goods or services and thereby satisfying the wants of the people.
- Hospital as a service organization will bring together the services of human resource (doctors, nurses, paramedics), sophisticated equipment (diagnostic and therapeutic), high quality materials (medicines and disposables) to provide high quality healthcare, which the patient wants.
- Operations either in manufacturing or in service are purposeful activities of an organization. All operations can be said to add value to some object, thereby enhancing its usefulness.
- **Operations** can be defined as the **"process of changing inputs into outputs** and thereby adding value to some entity"; this constitutes the primary function of virtually every organization.
- There are four major ways for value addition:
  1. *Alter:* To change the form or state of inputs through process, e.g. comfort or satisfaction after getting cured from illness.
  2. *Transport:* The entity gets value added through transport because it may have more value if located somewhere else.
  3. *Store:* The value is enhanced if entity is kept in a protected environment, e.g. storing medicines in refrigerator (at right temperature and conditions).
  4. *Inspect:* By inspection, better understanding can be gained which helps in decision making.

SYSTEMS CONCEPT IN OPERATIONS MANAGEMENT

In operations management, the system consists of three basic elements: input, process and output supported by two more elements, feedback and control (Fig. 5.1).

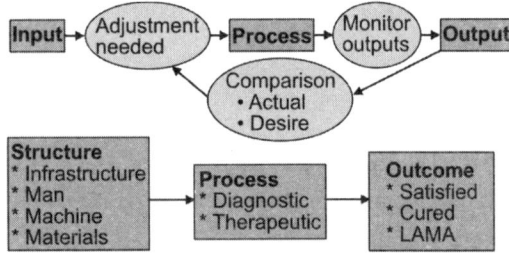

Fig. 5.1: Elements of operations management

This concept of infrastructure, process, output is proposed by Donabedian.

BRIEF HISTORY OF OPERATIONS MANAGEMENT

- Roots of operations management go back to the concept of 'Division of Labor' advocated by Adam Smith in his book "The Wealth of Nations" in 1776.
- In 1832, Charles Babbage, a mathematician extended Smith's work by recommending the use of scientific methods for analyzing factory problems.
- Father of scientific management F.W. Taylor, published the book "Principles of

Scientific Management" which laid the foundation of modern scientific management.
- Henry Ford developed the concept of mass production.
- In 1924, Shewart pioneered the concept of statistical quality control.
- In 1933, famous Hawthorne experiments was conducted by Elton Mayo, which paved the way for behavioral school of management.
- In 1950's the application of operations research in industry was started by L.D. Miles.
- In 1958, the concepts of PERT and CPM were developed for the analysis of larger projects.
- In 1970's systems approach taking a holistic look at the operations management evolved.
- In 1980's Japanese Management Techniques like Just-In-Time (JIT) or Kanban system, quality circles, etc. became a buzzword in operations management.
- In the recent past, information technology began to play a critical role in the operations of organization. The concepts like ERP, CRM, etc. are widely used.

Role of HOM (or Operations Manager)

1. *Planning:* To establish goals, the means of achieving these goals and the time scale.
2. *Organizing:* Structuring the organization in the best way to achieve its goals.
3. *Staffing:* Making sure there are suitable people to do all jobs.
4. *Directing:* Coaching and guiding employees
5. *Motivating:* Empowering and encouraging employees to do their jobs well.
6. *Allocating:* Assigning resources to specific jobs.
7. *Monitoring:* To check progress towards the goals.
8. *Controlling:* To make sure the organization keeps moving towards its goals.
9. *Informing:* Keeping everyone informed of progress.

Scope of Operations Management in Hospital Industry

The main objective of operations management in hospital industry should be to give quality treatment at affordable cost. For this certain long-term strategic decisions and short-term operational decisions regarding operations management needs to be taken.

Some of the *Strategic Decisions* regarding operations are as follows:

1. *Product/service selection and design:* Hospitals will have to decide what all services and specialties they are providing to the patients. They have to design the services in the form of various packages and value-added services, e.g. packages for diagnostic, packages for specific surgeries and diseases.
2. *Process selection and planning:* It involves taking decisions regarding technology, machines and equipment.
3. *Facilities location:* Decision regarding location of hospital and the location of various facilities within the hospital.
4. *Facilities layout:* Facilities should be arranged in such a manner that service can be provided in smooth manner.
5. *Capacity planning:* Regarding total number of beds, outpatients, number of diagnostic tests, etc.

Operational or Short-Term Decisions Include

1. *Production/service planning:* It involves allocating resources at various service areas, e.g. posting nurses at various units, scheduling the surgeries, etc.
2. *Production/service control:* It aims to see that the activities are carried on line with pre-determined standards.
3. Inventory control
4. Quality control
5. *Method study:* Standard methods should be devised for performing the repetitive functions efficiently.

6. Maintenance and replacement
7. Cost reduction and control

Objectives in Operations Management

Two Types of Objectives

I *Performance objectives*
- Efficiency
- Effectiveness
- Quality
- Lead time
- Capacity utilization
- Flexibility

II *Cost objectives*
  A. Explicit (visible) costs
  - Material costs
  - Direct and indirect labor costs
  - Scrap/rework cost
  - Maintenance cost
  B. Implicit (invisible/hidden) cost
  - Inventory carrying cost
  - Cost of stock outs and shortages
  - Cost of delayed deliveries
  - Cost of grievance and dissatisfaction
  - Unity cost

APPLICATION OF COMPUTER AND ADVANCED OPERATIONS TECHNOLOGY

Computers play an important role in today's world. They help in administration, act as clinical and diagnostic aids, and also facilitate in providing better patient care. They carry out different functions and act as an effective tool right from doctors, nurses, administration to management.

Computers help in better operations, helps medical directors to save time in managing routine administrative tasks and concentrate more on medical and clinical problems. The loss of revenue due to wrong billing can be avoided using computers. Inventory control modules, pharmacy modules play an important role in decreasing the wastage of stock and checking the expiry date of drugs, especially the costlier ones. Hospitals can reduce at least 5–10% expenditure by having proper inventory modules. Medical equipment is very costly and needs maintenance which can be monitored easily through usage of computers. Reduction in paper work through computers facilitates easy work, e.g. registration counters, nursing station, accounts, billing, etc. Nurses can do a better job, if drug, test , diet and other data are updated through computers. Nurses can directly place a requisition for patient drugs without really sending any one to pharmacy. Computerization of medical records helps in medical audit, epidemio-logical analysis, community surveys, medical education and research. Computers can act as a communication link between departments and allow the common database to be shared by them. The computers can manage the complex task of securing the data as required. Well-designed, integrated computer systems can be a great tool in the hands of the hospital management in improving services, controlling cost and ensuring optimal utilization of facilities. Computers help in decision making, management, planning and medical research. They are widely used to improve the patient care and improve the quality of patient care.

Bates et al. (1999) evaluated the impact of computerized physician order entry (POE) with decision support in reducing the number of medication errors and found that computerized POE substantially decreased the rate of non-missed-dose medication errors. Picture archiving and communication system (PACS) is a digital image management system in which images can be called and displayed on any computer monitor over the LAN and viewed as well as processed for the diagnosis. PACS is an image archiving and networking system that handles only image data. The knowledge-based system (KBS) is designed to fill in the knowledge gaps of the individual physician with special focus on specific patient problems. KBS and other such expert systems (ES) can prove to be a boon for rural health centers because even the general medical practitioners can operate the systems. KBS are aids supporting medical decision-making in the diagnosis, investigation and treatment of medical and surgical patients. Computer-based patient record (CPR) is a type of computer-based documentation of physician-patient encounters that consists of the patients' personal details, clinical findings, investigations, diagnosis, line of treatment and follow-up. Computer-based patient record (CPR) is an essential technology for healthcare management. The internet has made it possible to connect multiple systems and databases all over the world. Mutually acceptable protocols enable patient information to be transferred between different systems. Better access to data collected at the time of the encounter benefits not only the hospital managers but also payers and regulators. Computer-assisted medical education (CAME) helps to manage information, support patient care decisions, select treatments and develop the abilities of medical and healthcare professionals as life-long learners. Virtual reality, visualization, and simulation technologies have the potential of becoming ideal learning opportunities for surgical education and training. Heinch, et al. (1985) defined computer-assisted learning as "instruction, which is delivered to students by allowing them to interact with lessons programmed into the computer system". Computer-assisted learning is evolving rapidly and provides several advantages over the traditional approaches. Advancements in information technology have made telemedicine an important part of medical practice. This method of distance management in medical and healthcare benefits not only patients but medical practitioners also.

Telemedicine enhances patient access to care, encompasses remote consultation on a doctor-to-doctor level and doctor-to-patient level and includes education and communications between the patient and the health provider. Three-dimensional imaging-virtual endoscopy have immensely helped surgeons in increasing their spatial knowledge of the related anatomy but have some limitations in assisting the surgeon during the operation. VE leads to new possibilities for the examination of hollow structures and vasculature. VE is a promising tool for teaching and training as well as for planning and simulation of minimally invasive surgeries. The interest in computer-assisted surgery is motivated by the prospect of increased intraoperative patient safety. Image guidance assists the surgeon in navigating though the diseased or surgically revised complex anatomy. Through surgical simulations three-dimensional interactive anatomic road map for a particular patient's disease and anatomy is developed enabling the surgeon to make an accurate pre-operative assessment. In this interaction with a real-time performance-intuitive environment, students can study the lessons and practice the procedures in a non-threatening way. Virtual environment (VE) means realistic simulations of interactive scenes. In the simulated world of virtual environments, the surgeon can plan and practice surgical procedures. Computer-generated surgical simulation has a tremendous potential. Virtual reality is valuable wherever the anatomy is complex and the surgical problem is difficult. This advanced technology can become an adjunctive training aid for both the residents in training and the experienced surgeons. Telesurgery will emerge as a low cost yet highly intelligent system to serve the remotely placed and less privileged people

Thus computers help in better patient care, efficient administration of procedures, cost control, better utilization of procedures, elimination of revenue losses, medical audit and research, better nursing care and overall management of resources. There are also different modules developed like registration module, billing module, pharmacy module, patient care module, inventory module, diet module, appointment scheduling, etc. which play an important role in carrying the overall operations of the hospital.

Hospital Information System (HIS) provides lot of benefits like

- Speed and accuracy in billing
- Timely action at various levels
- Storage and record of each and every event
- Saves time and money
- Several statistics of the hospital like average outpatient, average inpatient, bed occupancy rate, total revenue, etc. can be easily found through HIS.
- Reduces the dependence of manpower especially when there is a shortage of human resources like nurses, technicians, skilled doctors, etc.
- Provides way to use the latest technology and helps in decision making.
- The element of human error can be reduced and prompt care to the patients is achieved.
- Patients can be tracked from time to time
- Pilferage is reduced especially in stores, drugs.
- Overall reduction in manpower can be achieved.
- Recording of events at every level helps in quick decision making.
- The efficiency of the system is increased.
- Waiting times of patients can be reduced.
- Performers and non-performers can be traced.
- Hospital costs and patient care costs can be reduced.
- Helps in planning the resources timely.
- Wastage of stationery is reduced and usage of telemedicine and other advanced technology helps to view the test results even from remote locations.
- Automatic check on billing, expiry dates, stock is done.
- All the text, graphic, audio, visual images can be exchanged through network.
- Database can be made to carry out research, epidemiological studies, training, research, etc.
- Data stored is useful for insurance claims, medico-legal cases, medical education.

OPERATIONS STRATEGY

- An operations strategy includes all the strategic decisions made by operations managers.
- Operations strategy is concerned with setting broad policies and plans for using the resources of a firm to best support its long-term competitive strategy.
- A firm's operations strategy is comprehensive through its integration with corporate strategy. The strategy involves a long-term process that must foster inevitable change.
- An operations strategy involves decisions that relate to the design of a process and the infrastructure needed to support the process.
- Process design includes the selection of appropriate technology, sizing the process over time, the role of inventory in the process and locating the process.
- The operations strategy can be viewed as part of a planning process that coordinates operational goals with those of the larger organizations. Since the goals of the larger organization change over time, the operations strategy must be designed to anticipate future needs.
- It defines the overall policies for operations and gives the framework for more detailed operations management decisions.
- The operations strategy is really concerned with matching what the organization is good at, with what the customer wants. Keys to success in operations strategy lie in identifying what the priority choices of a customer are and in understanding the consequences of each choice.
- Operations strategy is based on products that meet customer demands and the

process used to make these. This is a key area for decisions in every organization.
- The operations strategy sets the overall direction for operations within an organization.
- Operational decisions include:
  - **Scheduling** (for appointments, surgeries, OPD consultations, diagnostics, shift of doctors, nurses, D.M.O's, etc.)
  - **Staffing** (doctors, nurses, fourth class staff, etc.)
  - **Inventory** (keeping the required stock)
  - **Reliability** (improving equipment reliability, reliability of treatment protocols and the consistency in results)
  - **Maintenance** (equipment maintenance)
  - **Quality control** (to check whether services are up to the standards)
  - **Job design** (What is the best way to do operations, i.e. giving job description to all the staff)
  - **Work measurement** (How long will operations take, e.g. to know how much time procedure takes, a surgery can be performed, a test takes, etc.)

Operations competitive dimensions include

1. *Cost*—"make it cheap" (offering CT scans at less cost without compromising on quality)
2. *Product quality and reliability* — "make it good" (e.g. reliability in diagnostic reports)
3. *Delivery speed*—"make it fast" (e.g. decrease waiting times)
4. *Deliver reliability*—"deliver it when promised" (doctor coming at appointed time, surgery performed without delay from hospital side)
5. *Coping with changes in demand*—"change its volume" (going for expansion or for starting new units when the patient flow is more, e.g. Apollo, Wockhardt, Care, Yashoda)
6. *Flexibility and new product introduction speed* — "change it" (offering wide variety of products such as home care, evening clinics, Sunday clinics, well women clinics, lifestyle clinics, etc.)

Operations Strategy as a Competitive Tool

All organizations have competitors, those that already offer similar services or others who come up later with the same services. The part of business strategy that deals with competition is referred to as competitive strategy. The competitive strategy will only be successful if it makes products that customers want, and these are better than the competitors.

GENERIC CORPORATE STRATEGY

Michael Porter, a well-known strategic management writer, proposes that an organization may serve the entire market using market wide generic strategies or serve a particular segment of the market using the focus generic strategies. For both market wide and market segment focus, there are two fundamental positioning strategies—cost leadership and differentiation (Fig. 5.2).

Strategic target	Strategic Advantage	
	Uniqueness perceived by the customer	Low Cost
Market wide (Broad)	Differentiation	Overall cost leadership
Particular segment (only narrow)	Differentiation or focus	Cost/focus

Fig. 5.2: Corporate strategy

Market Wide Strategies

- Market wide strategies position the products/services of the organization to appeal to a broad audience (the entire

market), e.g. a community hospital may be positioned to serve all area residents—serve a broad market with a broad range of services. These products and services therefore are not tailored exclusively to the needs of any specialized segment of the population such as children or the aged.
- Market wide positioning strategies can be based on **differentiation or cost leadership**. Thus, the community hospital may try to differentiate itself from other hospitals by emphasizing quality or convenience or may compete as a low-cost provider.

Market Segment Strategies

- Market segment strategies are directed toward the particular needs of a well-defined market segment such as pediatric oncology or women's health and often are called focus strategies.
- Thus, a focus strategy identifies a specific, well-defined "niche" in the total market that the organization will concentrate on or pursue. Because of this attributes, the product or service or the organization itself may appeal to a particular niche within the market, e.g. Heritage, Lotus Children Hospital, Fernandez, etc.
- Similar to market-wide strategies, focus strategies may be based on **Cost leadership (cost/focus) or differentiation (differentiation/focus).**
- Because of the complexity of medicine and the entire healthcare industry, focus strategies are quite common. Just as physicians have specialized, the institutions within the field have tended to focus on specialized segments, e.g. Rehabilitation Hospitals (Sweekar–Upkaar), Psychiatric Hospitals (Erragadda), Ambulatory care Centers, etc.
- These specialty organizations may be further positioned based on cost leadership or differentiation.

Cost Leadership

- Cost leadership is a positioning strategy designed to gain an advantage over competitors by producing a product or providing a service at a lower cost than competitors' offerings.
- The product or service is often highly standardized to keep costs low.
- Cost leadership allows for more flexibility in pricing and relatively greater profit margins.
- Cost leadership is based on **economies of scale** in operations, marketing, administration and the use of the **latest technology**.
- As Porter suggests, "Cost leadership requires aggressive construction of efficient-scale facilities, vigorous pursuit of cost reduction from experience, tight cost and overhead control, cost minimization in the areas of R and D, service, scale forces, advertising and so on.
- In order to use cost leadership effectively, an organization must be able to develop a significant cost advantage and have a reasonably large market share.
- This strategy must be used cautiously within healthcare, as consumers often perceive low price to mean low quality. However, cost leadership allows the organization the greatest flexibility in pricing, e.g. Narayana Hrudayalaya (offering heart surgeries at low costs), Amritha Institute of Medical Sciences (AIMS), etc.

Differentiation

- Differentiation is a strategy to make the product or service different (or appear so in the minds of the buyer) from competitors' products or services. Thus, consumers see the service as unique among a group of similar competing services, e.g. Apollo Life Style Clinics, Evening Clinics, Sunday Clinics, Daycare Surgeries.
- The product or service may be differentiated by emphasizing quality, a high level

of service, ease of access, convenience, reputation, and so on, e.g. Apollo brand name.
- There are a number of ways to differentiate a product or service, but the attributes that are to be viewed as different or unique must be valued by the consumer. Therefore, organizations using differentiation strategies rely on brand loyalty (reputation or image), distinctive products or services, and the lack of good substitutes.

Facility Location and Layout

Reasons for a Firm to Expand

- To establish new venture
- Expansion of the existing business (e.g. from 100 beds to 150 beds)
- Significant changes in the existing demand, supply and market locations (e.g. more OP and cardiac patients are coming)
- Significant changes in cost and availability of inputs such as doctors, nurses, lab technicians, etc.
- Company policy on diversification and change of working climate (e.g. to establish a rehabilitation unit, hospital should get more area which may not be readily available in the center of the city)
- Government policy on expansions, waste disposals, etc.

Options available for expansion
- Make or buy decision
- Sub-contract instead of expansion
- Expand the existing plant instead of buying a new one
- Build a new plant instead of shifting the existing one
- Dispose of the existing plant and build a new one

Importance of location
- Location influences hospital layout and facilities needed (e.g. hospitals in city center have no enough space for parking, waiting area, etc.)
- Location influences capital investment and operating costs (hospitals in cities have more capital investment and operating costs than those located in towns and villages).

Selection of location: This is an integral part of organizational strategies of the business. A good location may reduce the cost of service delivery and transportation to a considerable extent. The success of organization depends on its planning (location, layout and facilities). Hospital facilities planning is based on the following principles or factors:

- *High quality patient care* (competent staff, job description, team work, continuous review of patient care, CME programmes, establishing and enforcing standards in patient care)
- *Effective community orientation* (including persons of community in governing board, extending programmes to community, planning for community programmes, ensuring support from community, inform the services provided in hospital to community)
- *Economic viability* (finances to provide quality patient care, retain competent staff, equipment and facilities, maintenance, etc.)
- *Sound architectural plan* (engaging a good architect, site selection, determining size of the hospital, establishing traffic patterns, no duplication of facilities, attention given to important facilities like emergency, OT, ICU's (Intensive care units, infection control, disaster planning, etc.)

Importance of location: Following factors to be kept in mind for selecting a site

- **Accessibility to transportation and communication lines** (good roads, availability of public transportation)
- **Availability of public utilities** (water, sewerage, electricity, fuel telephone lines, etc.)
- **Proper elevation for good drainage and general sanitary measures**
- **Freedom from noise, smoke, vapors and other annoyances** (away from airports,

main traffic, railroads, children play areas with enough natural lightening and air)
- **Future expansion** (after 10 or 15 years)
- **Cost** (total cost to be considered in making a hospital)

Location of Different Facilities

A. Location of Administrative Services

- *Administrative block:* It should be conveniently accessible to authorized visitors and to the hospitals main entrance as well as to vertical and horizontal communication areas. It should be designed to avoid cross traffic from the main lobby. Units generating more traffic such as the human resource department, financial services and to some extent the nursing administration should be located nearest the lobby, whereas those requiring privacy and generating less traffic such as the executive suite should be at the far end of the lobby.

- *Executive suite:* The executive suite is the pivotal point around which the administrative services and activities of the hospital revolve. In direct charge of the hospital and responsible to the governing board is the CEO who acts for it in an executive capacity. The executive suite should be located at a focal point on the administrative corridor in the administrative block. As some of the activities in the CEO's office are of confidential nature, privacy is important. Because of this and limited staff traffic, the unit should be located at the end of the administrative corridor, and yet it should be accessible to the members of the governing board, medical staff, department heads, patients, community leaders, government and public health officials, leaders of civic organizations and others.

- *Professional service unit:* Under the chief of medical staff or the medical director, the professional service unit directs and coordinates all medical and related activities of the hospital, excluding nursing service, and has overall responsibility for the quality of medical care provided to the patients in the hospital. It is recommended that the unit is located in the administrative block between the executive suite and the nursing administration unit with access from the main administrative corridor.

- *Financial management unit:* The unit generates heavy traffic and many transactions occur. Because the department relates directly with the administrative departments and must have a convenient access to the general public and staff of various departments, it must be located on the administrative corridor adjacent to the administrative block from the main lobby. Nevertheless, much of its work requires a level of concentration demanding privacy and freedom from frequent interruptions. One way of providing this is to have a front office for functions like billing, cashiering, etc. and a back office for work demanding concentration and privacy.

- *Hospital information system:* It can be located in the administrative corridor itself, but never in the cellar to prevent fire, short circuits, etc. The department should be there in a place where it is easy to connect all cables, air conditioning, security and expansion it required in future.

- *Nursing service administrative unit:* The nursing administration unit generates moderate to heavy traffic. It should be clearly located in the administrative block convenient to the executive suite from where it can also improve coordination of nursing services on the floors. With a view to decentralizing nursing administration and to improve patient care, communication and administration staff relationship, many hospitals place supervisory nursing staff in the patient care areas.

- *Human resource department:* The HR department generates relatively light to moderate traffic within the hospital with respect to the hospital personnel. However, there is heavy traffic from job applicants. A street level entrance to the department is recommended so that the department is easily accessible to the job applicants. Such an arrangement will also eliminate the stream of these applicants interfering with the regular hospital traffic. Because of the close working relationship between the director of human resources department and the CEO under whose direction the former works, the department should be in close proximity to the executive site. It should also be centered in the administrative block with convenient access to payroll records of the financial service unit but adjacent to a waiting area directly accessible from outside to accommodate job applicants.

- *Public relations department:* The office of the public relations director should be located in close proximity to the office of the CEO. Proximity to the CEO's office is necessary because generally everything that is of significance emanating from the public relations office requires the approval of the CEO. It also helps the public relations director to have personal consultations with the CEO and accomplish things speedily. In addition, many of the activities of the department such as planning events and programmes, news, releases, etc. must be done in cooperation with the CEO and sometimes other senior administrative officers. The department is subject to a minimum amount of personal traffic.
- *Marketing department:* Location should be preferably in administrative block away from clinical activities.

B. Location of Medical Services

- *Outpatient services:* The outpatient department should be conveniently located adjacent or in close proximity to vital services such as registration, medical records, admitting, emergency and social services. It should also be easily accessible from laboratories, radiology, pharmacy and physical therapy departments since practically all the diagnostic and therapeutic departments are used by patients during every visit. Attention should be paid to circulation, which should result in the smooth flow of the various traffic lines traversing the department.
- *Emergency services:* The emergency department should be located on the ground floor with easy access for patients and ambulances. There should be a separate entrance to the department, which is away from the main hospital, and the outpatient entrance, it should be well marked with proper lighting and signs, and should be easily visible and accessible from the street. Since the emergency department becomes the main entrance for the hospital during night, it must relate to the public and vehicular transportation.

The department should be close to admissions, medical records and cashier's booth. Where possible, admitting functions, cashiering, registration of new patients and creation of their medical records should be done in the department. A good percentage of emergency patients (studies show over 40%) require x-ray. The portable x-ray unit is not satisfactory. So close proximity to the radiology unit is essential to facilitate the movement of accident cases and to save every minute, which is precious. The laboratory services including the blood bank should also be accessible to emergency since a sizable number of patients need this service. In the location of the emergency department, proximity to elevators is also important in order to proceed to surgery without delay.

- *Clinical laboratories:* The laboratory should be conveniently located on the ground floor to serve the outpatient, emergency and admitting departments. It should also be close to or easily accessible to surgery, intensive care, radiology and obstetrics.

In large hospitals which have a large number of outpatients or when the main laboratory is not within walking distance, there may be a laboratory sub-station in the OPD. The autopsy area should be a little away from the emergency and inpatient areas. Access to the autopsy area as well as to the morgue should not be from patient areas and the removal of dead bodies to the outside should be through non-public corridors as this should be protected from patients and visitors view for psychological reasons.

- *Radiology services:* These services include diagnostic radiology, therapeutic radiology and nuclear medicine.
- *Diagnostic radiology:* This department should be located on the ground floor, conveniently accessible to inpatients, outpatients and emergency patients. It is also desirable to locate the department close to the elevators and near other diagnostic and treatment facilities. Functional needs of the department are best served by locating the X-ray rooms at the end off a wing. In this way the activities within the department will not be disturbed by traffic to other parts of the hospital.
- *Radiotherapy department:* The department must be carefully located in view of the need for dense shielding as a protection against radiation as mandatory required by Bhabha Atomic Research Centre (BARC) which is the regulatory body.

The major factors that should be borne in mind in determining the location are the requirement of three-foot-thick walls and ceilings and the required access for the placement or removal of equipment. It should be so located that it does not block future expansion plans. It should be ideally on the ground floor in close proximity to the OPD. Since most patients are outpatients and are ambulatory, proximity to easy accessibility from the OPD is important. The department should also be close to vertical transport facilities.

Radiation therapy is best located where it will adjoin the earth on several sides and has no departments below. From this point of view, a basement floor may be suitable. Although it is desirable to locate the department adjacent to diagnostic radiology, the two departments can be separated, as they are not dependent on each other.

- *Nuclear medicine:* Since the nuclear medicine department caters to the needs of all clinical departments, it should be located at a center place. At the same time, because of radiation hazards associated with the use of radionuclides, planning of the department should be done in such a way that there is no radiation exposure to nonradiation employees and the general public, and also that radiation workers handling radioisotopes receive minimum exposure. A major problem always is the safe and proper disposal of radioactive material.

The department should be close to diagnostic radiology, outpatient services, social services, laboratory, and medical records. In some hospitals, nuclear medicine is a part of diagnostic radiology using the common facilities of the department.

- *Surgical department:* The best location for the surgical department is the one, which permits a convenient and uncomplicated flow of patients, staff and supplies. Surgery receives inpatients from the floors through non-public corridors, elevators, and ramps. In most cases they are returned after the surgery through the same route. Convenient access to elevators is, therefore, essential. In regard to services, ideal adjacencies would be emergency, radiology, clinical laboratories, intensive care units, CSSD and delivery suite, particularly if it does not have a room for caesarean section.
- *Labor and delivery suite:* The clinical section of the obstetrical department should be located in a convenient but segregated area. Within the clinical facilities, the labor and delivery suites should be as remote as practicable but easily accessible from the

entrance to the department so as to avoid non-related and unnecessary traffic through the suites, and to provide privacy to the patients. The facility should be close to the nursery, obstetrical nursing unit and to vertical transport so that access is easy to patients. The department should be in close proximity to operating rooms, this is particularly important if it does not have an operating room of its own.
- *Physical medicine and rehabilitation:* This includes physical therapy, occupational therapy, recreational therapy, speech and hearing therapy and pulmonary medicine.
- *Physical therapy:* Since the department provides therapy services for outpatients, inpatients and emergency patients, it should be carefully located to accommodate all categories of patients. It should be close to the elevators with easy access to both outpatients and inpatients. It should be adjacent to other rehabilitation services such as occupational, recreational, and speech therapy as well as social and outpatient services. The orthopedic surgery, one of the major users of physical therapy, should be as close as possible.
- *Occupational therapy:* It should be located adjacent to physical therapy as occupational therapy department is in one sense an extension of the work of the physical therapy department. Besides, the members of the rehabilitation team need to consult each other and coordinate therapeutic activities of individual patients.
- *Recreational therapy:* It should have close relationship with physical therapy for the continuity of care. Close proximity is also desirable with the psychiatric department, which is one of the major users of recreational therapy.
- *Speech and hearing therapy:* Location should be near ENT and other outpatient services like ambulatory care.
- *Pulmonary medicine:* It should be in close proximity and have vertical access to departments like inpatient areas, ICU's, post-operative areas and emergency rooms.

C. Location of Nursing Services
- *General nursing unit:* Nursing units have a close relationship with the operating rooms, pharmacy, central stores, laboratory and the dietary. In maintaining this relationship, they are highly dependent on vertical transportation and an efficient communication system.
- *Pediatric nursing unit:* It is generally noisy and should be away from mainstream of hospital traffic, adjacent to outside terrace, which can be used as play area and proximity to vertical transportation conveniently accessible to other services.
- *Obstetrical nursing unit:* Located in labor-delivery suite with close proximity to vertical transport.
- *Psychiatric nursing unit:* Located in a floor with a separate entrance from the rest of the hospital.
- *Isolation rooms:* They may be located within the individual nursing units and placed at the end of the corridor. They should be available for normal acute care when not required for isolation cases. Isolation rooms may be grouped as a separate isolation unit.
- *Intensive care units:* Located close to emergency department, operating rooms, recovery rooms, respiratory therapy, laboratory and radiology and so located that the specialized cardiac team is able to respond promptly to the ICU emergency calls with a minimum travel time. They should not be too far from the general nursing units, and should be close to vertical transportation to facilitate rapid transport of patients and personnel. Location should be away from traffic and noise. All ICU's can be combined at one location or they can be adjacent to respective operating rooms like surgical ICU.
- *Newborn nurseries:* The nurseries should be located in the obstetrical nursing unit as

close to the mothers as possible. It should also be close to the labor-delivery suites so as to minimize travel distance and exposure of the newborn infants. It is desirable that they are in close proximity to the pediatric service, particularly if premature nursery and neonatal intensive care units are also located there.

D. Location of Supportive Services

- *Admitting department:* It should be there on the same level as the hospital main entrance, readily identifiable, provided with a sign that can be seen without difficulty from the hospital's main entrance, reception area and the main desk. The department should be adjacent to emergency service, OPD, medical records, laboratory, radiology and the cashier's booth. It must have convenient access to business office, operating rooms, elevators and the administration.
- *Medical records department:* It should be close to admitting area, OPD, emergency room and the business office.
- *CSSD (Central Sterilization and supply department):* It should be centrally located in relation to the surgical departments, recovery room, nursing units close to elevators, stairs, and ramps. Ideal location is adjoining the departments from which it receives materials such as general store, linen store and laundry.
- *Pharmacy:* A ground floor location close to the outpatient department and to elevators servicing the inpatient areas. It should be conveniently accessible to OP, IP and Bulk pharmacy store.
- *Materials department:* Ideally located in the ground floor, far away from other hospital traffic, conveniently accessible for unloading goods and supplies from trucks.
- *Food service department:* The department should be close to the materials department. The storage area should be in close proximity to the unloading dock. Easy access to the vertical transportation system serving patient care units to facilitate delivery of patient meals and return of used trays and utensils. The cafeteria and dining room should be close to food preparation and production area, and within convenient access to the hospital staff.
- *Laundry and linen service:* The laundry should be so located to have ample daylight and natural ventilation. Ideally it should be on the ground floor of an isolated building connected to or adjacent to the power plant. The traffic flow line should be as short as possible in vertical and horizontal transportation to reduce costs.
- *Housekeeping:* It should be centrally located and close to vertical transport system for easy movement of housekeeping materials and equipment.
- *Volunteer department:* It should be centrally located, easily accessible to the administrative services, particularly to the public or community relations department.

E. Location of Public Areas and Staff Facilities

- *Entrance and lobby area:* Close to main entrance.
- *Gift, book, florist shops:* Close to main lobby accessible to patients and their attendants.
- *Coffee shop cum snacks bar:* Easily accessible to patients and their attendants.
- *Meditation room:* Location should be at a quiet place away from generator and other sounds where it acts as a prayer hall for patients as well as staff.
- *Staff facilities:* The facilities include locker rooms, staff toilets, staff lounges, library.

F. Location of Engineering Facilities

The ideal location for the engineering and maintenance department is on the ground floor in a non-prime area. Convenient access to elevators, unloading dock, mechanical areas, and the boiler plant is essential. The main shop area should preferably have an outside wall on one side for ventilation as well as future expansion. The storage area for grounds maintenance equipment should have an outside entrance.

It includes maintenance management, biomedical engineering, electrical system, air-conditioning system, water supply and sanitary system, centralized gas system, telecommunication system, fire safety, alarm system, etc.

Types of Layout

1. *Product layout:* A product layout groups together all the operations used to make a particular product, e.g. gynic and obstetrics preparation room, labor room, OT, etc. for gynic patients); treating cardiac patients in cardiology department using the processes like TMT, cath-lab, 2D-ECHO, etc. In hospitals product means "cured/ satisfied/ dissatisfied/LAMA/dead patients".
2. *Process layout:* Here all similar types of operations are grouped together, e.g. in hospitals we have all equipment for emergencies in one ward, surgical patients in another, and pediatrics in another. Also, in administration where accountants work in one area, marketing in another, human resource (HR) separately, HIS in one department, etc.
3. *Service layout:* Here all similar types of services are grouped together, e.g. cardiology department offering cardiac services; similarly neurology department, gynecology department, pediatrics department, general medicine, etc.

Laboratory facilities where diagnostic services are provided with different labs like microbiology, biochemistry, clinical pathology, etc. grouped under diagnostics.

PRODUCTIVITY AND WORK MEASUREMENT

Productivity

Productivity in simple terms can be defined as the ratio of output to inputs.

| P P = O/I or Productivity = Output/Input |

Determinants of Productivity

- Technology
- Quality of labor force
- Capital resources
- Natural resources
- Social structure and attitudes
- Management
- Government policies

Classification of Productivity

1. *Labor productivity*
   - It is the ratio of output to labor input.
   - The concept of labor productivity is of matter of debate as far as hospitals are concerned as the success of hospitals depends on 'efficient patient care', for which increased input in the form of doctors, nurses, paramedical staff, etc. are required.
   - Labor productivity gained significance in West especially in manufacturing sector, because labor was scarce, and that the data on the basis of man-hours were more easily available than any other input factors.
2. *Capital productivity:* It is the ratio of output to capital input. Capital inputs in hospitals include building, capital equipment like MRI, C.T. scan, cath-lab.
3. *Particular or single factor Productivity:* When output is measured per unit of a single factor such as labor or capital, the measurement so obtained is called single factor productivity.
4. *Total factor productivity:* When all the factors of product or service are considered, it is called total factor productivity.

John Kendrick in 1950's distinguished between single factor productivity and total factor productivity.

Productivity Studies in Hospitals

Productivity study in hospitals in Taiwan was conducted by Shih Nerg Chen of Shih Hsin University, Taipei.

This study considered medical inputs in the form of
- Number of doctors
- Number of nurses
- Number of other medical personnel and
- Total number of beds

The medical outputs are comprised of
- O.P visits
- Use of ICU's
- Inpatients
- Number of surgeries performed, etc.

Techniques or Tools of Productivity

- Work-study
- Operations research
- Quality control
- Production or operations planning and control
- Industrial engineering
- Incentives and motivation
- Ergonomics

Productivity can be enhanced through the following means

- Application of scientific management
- Application of division of labor and specialization
- Implementing simplification and standardization in operations
- Improvement in the working environment
- Proper selection and training of employees
- Good industrial relations
- Philosophy and vision of management, etc.

National Productivity Council or N.P.C was formed by Government of India in 1958, on recommendations of a committee headed by Dr. Vikram Sarabhai.

NPC is a national level organization providing training, consultancy and undertaking research in the area of productivity.

Productivity Measurement in a Hospital Setup

Many hospitals, when facing periodic budget crises, embark on energetic initiatives to dramatically reduce labor, supply or purchased service costs. They adopt severe measures such as labor budget cuts, hiring freezes and layoffs, or they remove a layer of management. Such approaches are almost always short-lived, disruptive and resented, causing significant morale problems. In the long run, they are ineffective and costly. A more sustainable approach is to nurture a culture of productivity. But to effectively measure productivity, a hospital first needs to employ standards.

The Importance of Standards

Standards in this sense are mathematical constructs based on surveys of hundreds of hospitals; they represent the relationship between departmental workload and productivity. When a hospital isn't being productive, standards will help point to where staff is falling short. Standards are difficult to establish because workload measures are generally not precise, nor are they necessarily universally defined or interpreted. Specific workload measures are needed both for internal examination and external comparison with other hospitals. Productive hours include regular hours, overtime, etc.

Targets

Industry standards are defined for individual departments based on their workload. Lower values represent less staff relative to workload—in other words, greater efficiency. A given department can be expected to operate more or less favorably within the generally accepted range of standards depending on three fundamental operating characteristics:

1. *Unit configuration* or components of the department. For example, the radiology department may or may not include transportation, transcription and nursing. A broadly configured department would tend to function towards the high end of

industry standards, while a narrowly configured department could be expected to embrace lower targets.

2. *Scope of service* or daily department responsibilities. For example, the laboratory within a hospital that decentralizes phlebotomy can be expected to function near the low end of industry ranges for laboratories. A more comprehensive dietary service department that delivers patient trays, caters an abundance of meals and delivers meals on wheels would be likely to have higher targets.

3. *Intrinsic functionality* or department capability. Departments well-endowed with tools and technology should operate with greater labor efficiency, toward the lower end of standard ranges. For example, PACS technology helps pharmacy and the imaging departments to achieve labor efficiencies.

Building a culture of productivity requires that all hospital departments embrace productivity standards. It is important that the department manager view the selected standard as being objective, well-informed and achievable. The results should also be measured frequently (weekly or biweekly) against set targets.

Successful standards should be:

- *Inclusive:* Rather than being imposed, the standards should evolve from negotiation and discussion.
- *Comprehensive:* The program should include all sectors of the hospital, large and small, clinical, ancillary and support.
- *Fair and equitable:* The same approach should be used for all departments; no "sacred cow" department is exempt for organizational, political or other reasons.
- *Transparent:* The program knowledge and the ongoing productivity report should be widely disseminated. Each department's performance is the legitimate interest of every other department.
- *Well-communicated:* The expectations and results of the program should be regularly communicated and discussed.

Objectivity

There are inherent difficulties in setting productivity standards throughout the hospital, but because this task is at the foundation of a successful culture of productivity, doing it well is critical.

A crucial step is finding an individual or small team to act as an unbiased, fair and knowledgeable arbiter. Such a standard "referee," whether an employee or consultant, must know how to evaluate departmental functionality, configuration issues and scope of service implications.

THE POWER OF PRODUCTIVITY STANDARDS

Standards, when they are credible, fair and embraced by managers, can boost productivity and sustain productivity gains:

Comparison: When managers understand their current situation, they are more likely to model good ideas from other hospitals and change processes to achieve efficiency gains.

Internalization: When employees understand targets and observe their manager's acceptance of them, they are likely to help the department meet targets and contribute their own ideas.

Staffing: When a hospital has invested in a culture of productivity, each department has a precise staffing plan that is consistent with its standards. Staffing plans are openly shared, and, if a given manager is unable to meet the expectations, the organization provides assistance and training. All levels of management share staffing knowledge and capabilities in a hospital endowed with a strong culture of productivity.

Sustaining a Culture of Productivity

Hospitals that embrace a culture of productivity develop management characteristics beyond the department level, which tend to sustain and enhance productivity gains in three ways:

1. *Human resources:* Replacing vacated positions become streamlined and stress-free. Vacancies are obvious and even anticipated; there is no need to justify personnel requisitions repeatedly. The traditional employing of overstaffing for fear of bureaucratic delays is no longer necessary.
2. *Budgeting:* The budget process, as it relates to labor costs, is streamlined. The labor budget is a constantly known element of cost because labor volume changes translate directly to labor cost increases and decreases. The dreaded pressure characteristics of the annual budget cycle are minimized.
3. *Recognition:* A culture of productivity is sustained when it is aligned with recognition. When the rules and expectations are clearly understood, managers can be rewarded as they demonstrate their ability to succeed in a culture of productivity.

Building a culture of productivity based on carefully defined standards supports sustainable productivity gains and many other positive effects that permeate all areas of the hospital. Healthcare productivity levels in recent years have increased for a variety of reasons like rapidly increasing technological improvements, particularly in the areas of diagnostic and treatment equipment and procedures.

Hospitals need to analyze, develop, and implement realistic, effective productivity standards. The first step in a productivity analysis is to collect performance data for each hospital department. A workload measure should be assigned to every department. Comparing historical performance data for each department highlights problem areas. Gaining executive commitment and department manager acceptance is essential to productivity improvement initiatives. Even in departments that experience a change in function, historical data can be used to monitor performance and determine where improvement is needed.

To determine productivity levels, the hospitals should develop **"Productivity Indicators" or "Performance Indicators"**. These indicators should include all the inputs, which at best would help the hospital to judge its outcomes. In any healthcare setting, it would include the following:

1. Finance
2. Manpower
3. Technology (equipment)
4. Resource consumption

1. *Finance:* While developing the indicators for individual departments, care should be taken that nothing is left. Each and every minute detail should be noted which influences performance and utilization. To start with, if a hospital is conducting a productivity study program for the first time, they should first start with their budget variance analysis. After the variance analysis they should not stop at that point but should go further and try to find the reasons for the variance. Again, it should be noted that this exercise is a fact-finding exercise and not a fault finding one. In terms of finance one should be able to figure out the profitability aspect on per unit investment. The organization should be able to find out its rate of growth and actually how fast it can afford to grow. This can be determined by finding out exactly how much an organization invests on its inventory and how much it gets in terms of its returns, finally leading to determination of rate of growth of the organization.
2. *Manpower:* In the area of manpower, the hospital should be able to identify the ideal, actual and practical productivity levels of the workers with respect to their day to day activities. Because labor is the largest expense in healthcare organizations, hospitals that want to reduce costs need to focus on reducing labor expense. The

industry trend is to use highly sophisticated productivity measurement systems to gather, calculate, and report data to control costs. Some systems can compute cost and hourly productivity targets for every shift of everyday to help hospitals maintain cost-effective staffing levels. Although well intentioned, such systems do not achieve cost reduction; in fact, the opposite usually occurs. Because these systems are too complex to be clearly understood by most hospital department managers, the managers cannot meet the standards projected by the productivity system. A simple, logical, and rational approach is needed.

Realistic goals of productivity management include scaling back unwanted staff expansion, establishing reasonable staffing levels, and preventing unwanted staffing increases in the future. To achieve these goals, hospitals need to create achievable productivity standards and hold department managers accountable for meeting those standards. This should be a regular exercise, which will look into the total hours available for a department in a given period of time (say a year) and the total number of actual hours worked (in productive activities). Care should be taken to identify the productive and non-productive activities of the workers. Though all the activities are considered to be productive from the workers point of view, the same is not true from the managerial point of view. There should be a clear-cut line drawn between these two sets of activities. The results of this exercise would yield us the actual productivity level of the department under the study program. The next parameter to look out for would be the effective cost of manpower. The hospital should be able to determine the per hour cost (salary or wages) of the employees and effective manpower cost per unit of service rendered and how much of this is productive.

Number of productive hours X salary per hour = productive cost

This productive cost should be compared with the actual cost (per 8 hours) and this variance should be analyzed, e.g. in the case of laboratory medicine this activity will lead to number of tests per man-hour and manpower cost per test.

3. *Technology:* Technology is the other main aspect of productivity. Especially in laboratories, where we have equipment worth crores of rupees and some of which have maximum throughput of over 1200 tests per hour. This is a very sensitive area in the hospital. A constant capacity utilization monitoring system should be put into place, which would give per cent capacity utilization of the major capital equipment in the hospital. The **standard methodology to measure the utilization would be to find out the total tests performed on the equipment divided by the actual capacity**. The utilization of laboratory equipment depends highly on the workload or the number of tests performed on the equipment and if the workload is low, the utilization will also be low. Then why does hospitals go in for latest technology equipment, even when they know that there won't be optimal utilization of the equipment? This is for the simple reason that these equipment carry out tests which can be life saving in times of emergency and to deliver quality care with high accuracy and precision. It is only for the quality and precision that a hospital goes into procurement of such equipment. Moreover, this also gives the hospital a strategic advantage in the highly technology driven healthcare market.

4. *Material Consumption:* This is the most sensitive factor in terms of a department's resource consumption. The hospitals should be able to benchmark the cost of material consumption per unit of service for each department of the hospital, e.g. let

us take the example of laboratory medicine department, where in a corporate hospital, material worth crores of rupees is consumed. The kits and reagents used are imported, and highly expensive. Usually administrative or financial analysts make a mistake while benchmarking or costing of tests. Every reagent/ kit can do a number of tests, and the precise number is written on it. But, they fail to count the number of tests, which are run for quality control, calibration, and reagent testing, which in some cases have to be done simultaneously for each and every test. Each and every machine that has a backup (duplicate machine used when the active machine fails) has to be maintained and this also takes its toll on consumption. Though the tests are not run on the backup machine still, some tests are done and results are compared so that there is a little or no variance, so that when the active machine fails, the backup machine gives satisfactory results. So, in a way in some machines the tests are performed at least twice. Then there are tests, which have to be done again and again because of some reasons or the other. All these factors take their toll on the resource consumption.

Employee Related Aspects Leading to Productivity

They are learning curves, safety and health and incentive schemes.

LEARNING CURVES

The *learning curve* (Fig. 5.3) analysis is based on the premise that as an organization gains experience in manufacturing a product, the resource inputs required per unit of output diminish over the life of the product. Specifically, in the beginning of production runs, workers are unfamiliar with their tasks and the amount of time required to produce the first few units is high. But as the workers learn their tasks, their performance improves. The performance time drops off rather dramatically at first, and it continues to fall at some slower rate until a performance plateau or levelling-off is reached. This learning pattern applies to groups and organizations as well as individuals. Furthermore, it is often regular and predictable. The learning curve concepts are based on three underpinnings:

i. Where there is life, there can be learning.
ii. The more complex the life, the greater the rate of learning.
iii. The rate of learning can be sufficiently regular to be predictive.

It is, therefore, possible to estimate:
(a) The average number of labor-hours required to produce n units in a production run,
(b) The exact number of labor-hours required to produce the nth unit of production run.

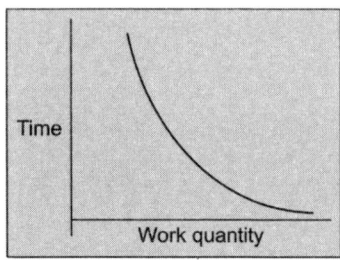

Fig. 5.3: Learning Curve

SAFETY AND HEALTH

Safety

Any accident happening in the hospital has two costs—direct and indirect or hidden costs. Direct costs can be taken care through insurance. But indirect costs like loss of morale among employees, decrease in productivity, down time of operations, loss of customers, etc. are more dangerous. *Safety has an impact on productivity, cost and loss of revenue. Thus providing safety measures for the staff are very much important, e.g. labs, operation theaters, staff in ICU's, handling bio-medical wastes, radiology department.* There are also legal complications for undertaking safety measures. Laws on occupational health, penalties on non-compliance have become severe. The safety of the community surrounding the hospital is also in the hands of the management.

Organisations evolve elaborate safety programmes to prevent accidents. A typical safety programme comprises five elements, namely

1. Development of policies, procedures and training systems.
2. Creation of an organisation to ensure safety.
3. Analysis of the causes and occurrence of accidents.
4. Implementation of the safety programme.
5. Evaluation of the effectiveness of the programme.

Health

Health is wealth for employees as well as for employers. Health of employees is affected by surroundings, job stress, noise, alcoholism, drug abuse and AIDS. Health of employees is significant as it has an impact on productivity, absenteeism and turnover. The protection of health of workers is a legal requirement too. Sections 11 to 20 of the Factories Act, 1948, deal with the health of workers. Realising the need for healthy employees, organisations take necessary steps to prevent causes which result in ill health to workers. For example, giving off for employees in a radiology department at frequent intervals, continuous free health check for those employees working in labs.

Incentive Payments

Incentives are monetary benefits paid to workmen in recognition of their outstanding performance. The primary advantage of incentives is the inducement and motivation of workers for higher efficiency and greater output. Positive response will surely come when incentives are included as a part of the total remuneration. Earnings of employees would be enhanced due to incentives. Increased earnings would enable the employees to improve their standard of living. Through incentives productivity would increase resulting in a greater number of units produced for given inputs. This would bring down the total and unit cost of production. The other advantages of incentive payments are: reduced supervision, better utilization of equipment, reduced scrap, reduced lost time, reduced absenteeism and turnover and increased output.

There is an **ethical dimension** to incentive payments as well. It is unjust to pay extra to the employees when they are already paid their usual wages and salaries. If an employee is paid for eight hours a day, he or she is expected to show better performance for the day. To show increased production, extra payments are not necessary. There are also instances where incentives lead to corruption. Supervisors and workmen join hands, false production figures are recorded and wrong time bookings are made in order to enable employees earn enhanced incentives. The amount is later shared with the supervisors who join hands with the employees in the fraud.

Incentive payments are linked to employees' performance. A standard performance is set for employees. The actual performance is then compared with the standard and depending upon the degree of efficiency, incentives are fixed. Unfortunately, these standards themselves become ceilings on the productivity of employees. Workers would be happy to attain a performance near the standards, and may not strive to cross them.

SCOPE AND TYPES OF INCENTIVE SCHEMES
Scope

Although, the incentive payments have a universal appeal, their application is confined to certain important industries. Stated differently, payment by results schemes are difficult to apply in:

a. Industries in which measurement of individual or group output is rendered difficult or impossible either by technical consideration or by psychological circumstances which might be prejudicial to output.
b. Industries in which the control of quality is necessary and is particularly difficult, or in the case of certain classes of workers, where high quality and precision of work is of prime importance.
c. Industries in which the work is especially dangerous and is particularly difficult to ensure the observance of adequate safety precautions.

As a rule, incentives must not be introduced in a newly set-up unit. Workers must be content with time-rated earnings, at least, during the first four to five years. This time period is necessary for the unit to carve a niche for itself in the market. Furthermore, as was noted earlier, incentives are likely to affect the quality of output. Any defect in quality would seriously affect fortunes of the newly set up unit, particularly in its formative years.

Types

Incentive schemes are many and varied. The International Labor Organisation (ILO) classifies all the schemes of payment by results into four categories. They are —

1. Incentives schemes where the workers' earnings vary in the same proportion as output.
2. Schemes where earnings vary proportionately less than output.
3. Schemes where earnings vary proportionately more than output.
4. Schemes where earnings differ at different levels of output.

Group Incentive Plans

A fundamental assumption common to all the individual schemes is that, the output of each worker can be accurately measured. But in some cases, the operations are performed by the group as a whole, and the contribution of each worker in the group cannot be accurately measured. In such cases, the group incentive scheme is followed. Group incentives are as common as individual plans in industrial establishments.

Any individual scheme which has already been discussed may be applied to a group of workers. But the most common is the *piece-work system*. The total earnings of a group are first determined in accordance with the incentive method which is followed, and the earnings are then distributed among the members of the group on some equitable basis. If the group consists of members with equal skill, the earnings are divided equally among them. When the members are of unequal skill, the earnings of the group may be divided among the members in proportion to their individual time-rates, or according to specified percentages, or in some cases only among a certain number of members of the group.

Some of the advantages of group incentives are
  (i) Better cooperation among workers.
  (ii) Less supervision
  (iii) Reduced incidence of absenteeism
  (iv) Reduced clerical work
  (v) Shorter training time

The disadvantages are
  (i) An efficient worker may be penalized for the inefficiency of the other members in the group
  (ii) The incentive may not be strong enough to serve its purpose and
  (iii) Rivalry among the members of the group defeats the very purpose of team work and co-operation.

Some of the group incentive plans are
1. The Rucker Plan
2. The Scanlon Plan
3. The Profit-sharing Plan

ERGONOMICS

Ergonomics is the scientific discipline concerned with designing according to the human needs and the profession that applies theory, principles, data and methods to design in order to optimize human well-being and overall system performance. The field is also called **human engineering,** and **human factors engineering.**

Ergonomics is the science of fitting the job to the worker. When there is a mismatch between the physical requirements of the job and the physical capacity of the worker, work-related musculoskeletal disorders (MSDs) can result. Ergonomics is the practice of designing equipment and work tasks to conform to the capability of the worker, it provides a means for adjusting the work environment and work practices to prevent injuries before they occur. Healthcare facilities especially nursing homes have been identified as an environment where ergonomic stressors exist.

Ergonomic research is performed to study human capabilities in relationship to their work demands. Information derived from these studies contributes to the design and evaluation of tasks, jobs, products, environments and systems in order to make them compatible with the needs, abilities and limitations of people.

Ergonomics is a science concerned with the 'fit' between people and their work. It takes into account the worker's capabilities and limitations in seeking to ensure that tasks, equipment, information and the environment suit each worker.

Ergonomics is the science of designing the job, equipment, and workplace to fit the worker. Proper ergonomic design is necessary to prevent repetitive strain injuries, which can develop over time and can lead to long-term disability. The four main contributing causes of these injuries are quick, repetitive actions, awkward position, use of force, and lack of rest. Minimization of repetitive tasks and awkward body positions can help to prevent such injuries from occurring.

To assess the fit between a person and their work, ergonomics consider:

- The job being done and the demands on the worker
- The equipment used (its size, shape, and how appropriate it is for the task)
- The information used (how it is presented, accessed, and changed).

Ergonomics draws on many disciplines in its study of humans and their environments, including **anthropometry** (the study of human body measurements. The uses of anthropometry include the creation of ergonomic furniture designs and the examination and comparison of populations.), **biomechanics** (the study of body movements and of the forces acting on the musculoskeletal system), mechanical engineering (the branch of engineering that deals with the design, production, and use of machinery and tools, as well as the generation and transmission of heat and mechanical power), **industrial engineering** (the study and practice of designing industrial operations), **industrial design** (the art of designing the shape, size, or appearance of manufactured objects), **kinesiology** (the study of the mechanics of motion with respect to human anatomy), **physiology** (the branch of biology that deals with the internal workings of living things, including functions such as metabolism, respiration, and reproduction, rather than with their shape or structure) and **psychology** (the scientific study of the human mind and mental states, and of human and animal behavior).

Five Aspects of Ergonomics

There are five aspects of ergonomics, safety, comfort, ease of use, productivity or performance, and aesthetics. Based on these aspects of ergonomics, examples are given of how products or systems could benefit from redesign based on ergonomic principles.

1. *Safety—medicine bottles*: The print on them could be larger so that a sick person who may have impaired vision (due to sinuses, etc.) can more easily see the dosages and

label. Ergonomics could design the print style, color and size for optimal viewing.
2. *Comfort—alarm clock display:* Some displays are harshly bright, drawing one's eye to the light when surroundings are dark. Ergonomic principles could redesign this based on contrast principles.
3. *Ease of use—street signs:* In a strange area, many times it is difficult to spot street signs. This could be addressed with the principles of visual detection in ergonomics.
4. *Productivity/performance—HD TV:* The sound on HD TV is much lower than regular TV. So when you switch from HD to regular, the volume increases dramatically. Ergonomics recognizes that this difference in decibel level creates a difference in loudness and hurts human ears and this could be solved by applying principles of ergonomics.
5. *Aesthetics—signs in the workplace*: Signage should be made consistent throughout the workplace not only to be aesthetically pleasing, but also that information is easily accessible for all signs.

Ergonomics in Hospitals

1. Patient handling tasks pose increased ergonomic risk to employees if they are
   - Repetitive (e.g. repeatedly doing manual adjustments for beds)
   - Done in awkward postures (e.g. reaching across beds to lift patients)
   - Done using a great deal of force (e.g. pushing wheel chairs, trolleys, stretchers, etc. across elevation changes or up ramps)
   - Lifting heavy objects (e.g. manually lifting immobile patients) or combining these factors.
   - Overexertion; trying to stop a patient from falling or picking patient up from floor or bed.
   - Multiple lifts per shift (more than 20)
   - Lifting alone, no available staff to help
   - Lifting non-cooperative, confused patients
   - Lifting patients who cannot support their own weight.
   - Expecting employees to perform work beyond their physical capabilities.
   - Awkward postures required by the activity.
   - Ineffective training of employees in body mechanics and proper lifting techniques

   Facilities should establish a safety and health program that addresses patient handling hazards and establishes patient handling criteria.

2. Many patients/residents (especially nursing home residents) are totally dependent on staff members to provide activities of daily living, such as dressing, bathing, feeding, and toileting. Each of these activities involves multiple interactions with handling or transferring of patients/residents and could result in employee injuries. Employee injuries lead to increased injury costs, higher turnover rates, increased sick/injured days, and staffing shortages.

3. Employee exposure to injury from ergonomic stressors during handling, transferring and repositioning of patients/residents. Hospital healthcare workers (especially nursing assistants, who do a majority of the lifting in many facilities) may develop musculoskeletal injuries such as muscle and ligament strain and tears, joint and tendon inflammation, pinched nerves, and others from patient/residents handling.

Good work practice includes continually identifying the most hazardous tasks and implementing engineering and work practice controls to help reduce or prevent injuries in those tasks.

Provide employees with proper assist devices and equipment to reduce excessive lifting hazards. Proper equipment selection

depends on the specific needs of the facility, patients/residents, staff, and management.
4. Trip/slips and falls from spills or environmental hazards.
   Environmental hazards such as
   - Slippery or wet floors.
   - Uneven floor surfaces.
   - Lifting in confined spaces.
   - Cluttered or obstructed work areas/passageways.
   - Poorly maintained walkway or broken equipment.
   - Inadequate staffing levels to deal with the workload, leading to single person lifts and greater chances of falls.
   - Inadequate lighting, especially during evening shifts.

Possible Solutions

Good work practice includes implementing engineering and work practices controls to help prevent slips/falls such as:
- Eliminate uneven floor surfaces.
- Create non-slip surfaces in toilet/shower areas.
- Immediate clean-up of fluids spilled on floor.
- Safely working in cramped working spaces- avoiding awkward positions, using equipment that makes lifts less awkward.
- Eliminate cluttered or obstructed work areas.
- Provide adequate staffing levels to deal with the workload.
- Keep floors clean and dry. In addition to being a slip hazard, continually wet surfaces promote the growth of mold, fungi, and bacteria that can cause infections.
- Provide warning signs for wet floor areas.
- Where wet processes are used, maintain drainage and provide false floors, platforms, mats, or other dry standing places where practicable, or provide appropriate waterproof footgear.
- Walking/working surfaces standard requires all places of employment clean and orderly and in a sanitary condition.
- Keep aisles and passageways clear and in good repair, with no obstruction across or in aisles that could create a hazard. Provide floor plugs for equipment, so power cords need not run across pathways.
- Keep exits free from obstruction. Access to exits must remain clear of obstructions at all times.

Other Recommended Good Work Practices
- Ensure spills are reported and cleaned up immediately.
- Use no-skid materials in slippery areas such as toilet and shower areas.
- Use only properly maintained ladders to reach items. Do not use stools, chairs, or boxes as substitutes for ladders.
- Aisles and passageways should be sufficiently wide for easy movement and should be kept clear at all times. Temporary electrical cords that cross aisles should be taped or anchored to the floor.
- Eliminate cluttered or obstructed work areas.
- Nurses station countertops or medication carts should be free of sharp, square corners.
- Use prudent housekeeping procedures such as cleaning only one side of a passageway at a time, and provide good lighting for all halls and stairwells, to help reduce accidents.
- Provide adequate lighting especially during night hours. You can use flashlights or low-level lighting when entering patient rooms.
- Instruct workers to use the handrail on stairs, to avoid undue speed, and to maintain an unobstructed view of the stairs ahead of them even if that means requesting help to manage a bulky load.
- Eliminate uneven floor surfaces.

- Promote safe work in cramped working spaces. Avoid awkward positions, and use equipment that makes lifts less awkward.
5. Increased potential for employee injury exists when awkward postures are used when handling or lifting patients/residents. Awkward postures include
    - Twisting while lifting.
    - Bending over to lift.
    - Lateral or side bending.
    - Back hyperextension or flexion.
    - Forces on the spine increase while lifting, lowering or handling objects with the back bent or twisted. This occurs because the muscles must handle your body weight in addition to the weight of the patient/residents being lifted.
    - More muscular force is required when awkward postures are used because muscles cannot perform efficiently.
    - Fixed awkward postures (i.e. holding the arm out straight for several minutes) contribute to muscle and tendon fatigue, and joint soreness.
    - To be considered a risk factor, awkward postures need to last more than 1 hour continuously or for several hours in the work shift.
    - Reaching forward or twisting to support a patient/resident from behind to assist them in walking.

So possible solutions include
   - Good work practice recommends avoiding awkward postures while lifting or moving patients/residents.
   - Educate and train employees about safer lifting techniques.
   - Use assist devices or other equipment whenever possible.
   - Team lifting based on assessment.
6. Employee exposure to ergonomic stressors in healthcare workplaces occurs not only during patient/resident handling tasks but also to perform other tasks in the kitchen, laundry, engineering, and housekeeping areas of facilities, for example, during transporting of equipment, moving food carts or other heavy carts, pouring liquids out of heavy pots or containers, reaching into deep sinks or containers, using hand tools, and during housekeeping tasks.

Possible Solutions

Use engineering or work practice techniques to eliminate the hazard or decrease the hazard. For example:
- *Transferring Equipment:* Strains and sprains can occur if employee is transferring equipment like IV poles, wheel chairs, oxygen cylinders, respiratory equipment, dialysis equipment, X-ray machines, or multiple items at the same time (Fig. 5.4). To reduce the hazards of transferring equipment:
    - Place equipment on a rolling device if possible to allow for easier transport, or have wheels attached to the equipment.
    - Push rather than pull equipment when possible. Keep arms close to your body and push with your whole body not just your arms.
    - Assure that passageways are unobstructed.
    - Attach handles to equipment to help with the transfer process.

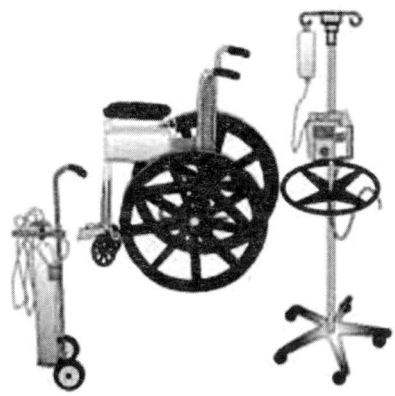

Fig. 5.4: Wheel chair

- Get help moving heavy or bulky equipment or equipment that you can't see over.
- Do not transport multiple items alone. For example, if moving a patient/resident in a wheel chair as well as an IV pole and/or other equipment get help, do not overexert yourself.

Reaching into deep sinks or containers: If washing dishes, laundry, or working in maintenance areas and using a deep sink, limit excessive reaching and back flexion by:
- Placing an object such as a plastic basin in the bottom of the sink to raise the surface up while washing items in the sink or
- Remove objects to be washed into a smaller container on the counter for scrubbing or soaking and then replace back in the sink for final rinse (Fig. 5.5).

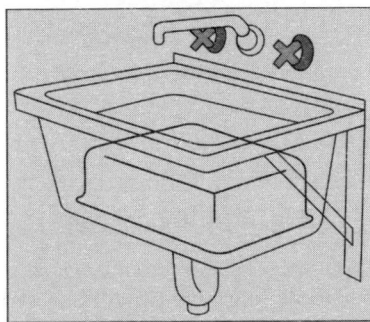

Fig. 5.5: Deep sink

Limit reaching or lifting hazards when lifting trash, laundry or other kinds of bags by
- Using handling bags for laundry, garbage, and housekeeping when possible that have side openings to allow for easy disposal without reaching into and pulling bags up and out. The bags should be able to slide off the cart without lifting (Fig. 5.6).
- Limiting the size and weight of these bags and provide handles to further decrease lifting hazards.
- Using garbage cans that have a frame *vs.* a solid can to prevent plastic bags from sticking to the inside of the can or use products that stick to the inside of the garbage, that can prevent the bag from sticking.
- Limit the size of the container to limit the weight of the load employee must lift and dump.

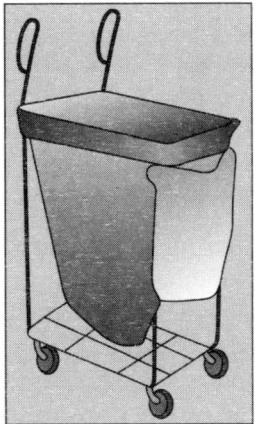

Fig. 5.6: Handling bag

- Using spring-loaded platforms to help lift items such as laundry keeping work at a comfortable uniform level (Fig. 5.7).

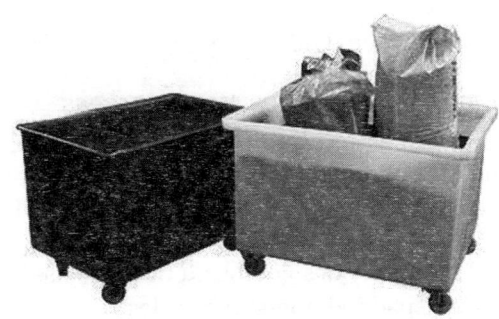

Fig. 5.7: Spring loaded platform

Limit reaching and pushing hazards from moving heavy dietary, laundry, housekeeping or other carts by:
- Keeping carts, hampers, or other carts well maintained to minimize the amount of force exerted while using these items.
- Using carts with large, low rolling resistance wheels. These can usually roll easily over

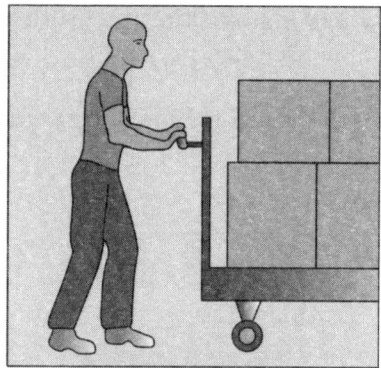

Fig. 5.8: Trolly

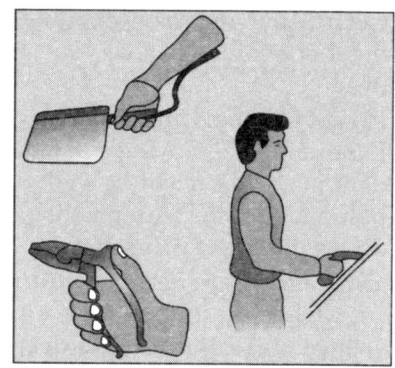

Fig. 5.9: Using hand tools

mixed flooring as well as gaps between elevators and hallways.
- Keeping handles of devices to be pushed at waist to chest height.
- Using handles to move carts rather than the side of the cart to prevent the accidental smashing of hands and fingers (Fig. 5.8).
- Keeping floors clean and well maintained.
- Pushing rather than pulling whenever possible.
- Removing from use all malfunctioning carts.
- Getting help with heavy or bulky loads.

Using hand tools in maintenance areas

Limit strains and sprains of the wrists, arms, and shoulders, of maintenance workers by choosing hand tools carefully (Fig. 5.9). Hand tools should:
- Be properly designed, and fit to the user.
- Have padded non-slip handles.
- Allow the wrist to remain straight while doing finger intensive tasks. Select ergonomic tools such as ergonomic knives or bent-handled pliers.
- Have a minimal tool weight.
- Have a minimal vibration or use vibration dampening devices and vibration-dampening gloves.
- Not be used when performing highly repetitive manual motions by hand, use

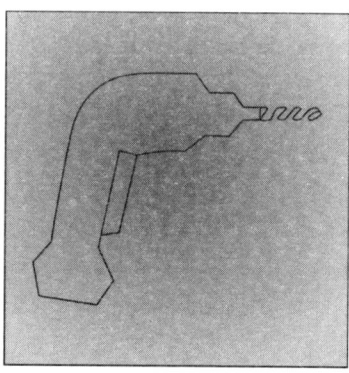

Fig. 5.10: Trigger bar

power tools (e.g. use power screwdrivers instead of manual screwdrivers) (Fig. 5.10).

Housekeeping tasks: To decrease ergonomic stressors while performing cleaning tasks, employees should (Fig. 5.11):
- Alternate leading hand.
- Avoid tight and static grip and use padded non-slip handles.
- Clean objects at waist level if possible, rather than bending over them (e.g. push wheel chairs up a ramped platform to perform cleaning work, or raise beds to waist level before cleaning).
- Use knee pads when kneeling.
- Use tools with extended handles, or use step stools or ladders to avoid or limit overhead reaching.

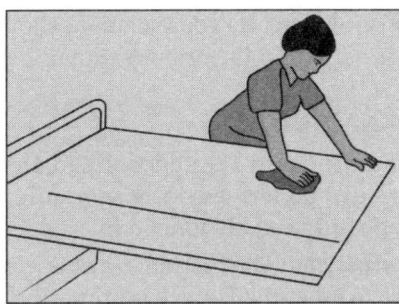

Fig. 5.11: Housekeeping

- When sweeping or dusting use flat head dusters and push with the leading edge; sweep all areas into one pile and pick up with a vacuum (Fig. 5.12).
- Use chemical cleaners and soaks to minimize force needed for scrubbing.
- Frequently change mopping styles while mopping (e.g. push/pull, and rocking side to side) to alternate stress on muscles.
- Be sure buckets, vacuums, and other cleaning tools have wheels or are on wheeled containers with functional brakes.
- Alternate tasks or rotate employees through stressful tasks.
- Avoid awkward postures while cleaning (e.g. twisting and bending).
- Use carts to transport supplies rather than carrying.
- Use buffers and vacuums that have lightweight construction and adjustable handle heights.

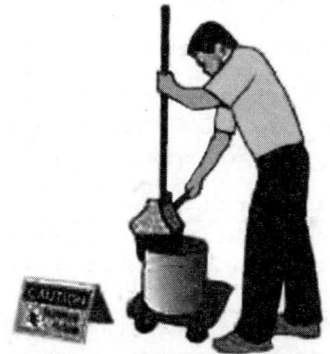

Fig. 5.12: Housekeeping work

- Use spray bottles and equipment that have trigger bars rather than single finger triggers.
7. *Recordkeeping:* Without proper recordkeeping, illness and injury trends would go unreported and unstudied and valuable information about causes and possible prevention of injuries would be lost.

Possible Solutions

- Follow the recordkeeping standard.
- Employers must record each fatality, injury or illness that:
  - Is work related
  - Is a new case
- Exposure to ergonomic stressors in healthcare workplaces can result in a variety of disorders in affected workers referred to as musculoskeletal disorders (MSDs). MSDs may develop gradually over time or may result from instantaneous events such as a single heavy lift. These conditions will be classified in recordkeeping forms as either injuries or illnesses. It is critical for recording keeping data to be kept accurately and that employers do not under report these events.

WORK STUDY

Work study is a generic term used for those techniques particularly **method study and work measurement** which are used in the examination of human work in all its context, and which lead systematically to the investigations of all facts which affect the efficiency and economy of the situation being reviewed in order to effect improvement.

Method study: The systematic recording and critical examination of existing and proposed ways of doing work as a means of developing and applying easier and more effective methods and reducing cost.

Work measurement: The application of techniques designed to establish the time for a qualified worker to carry out a specified job at a defined level of performance.

The main objective of work study is to improve the effectiveness of important parameters of production such as men, machines and methods.

Method study and work measurement are closely linked. Method study is concerned with the reduction of the work content and operation, while work measurement is concerned with the investigation and reduction of ineffective time and the subsequent establishment of time standards for the operation on the basis of the work content as established by methods study. Usually a method study should precede work measurement.

Basic Work Study Procedure

There are eight basic steps, some of which are common to both Method Study (MS) and Work Measurement (WM)
1. Select (MS and WM)
2. Record (MS and WM)
3. Examine (MS and WM)
4. Develop (MS)
5. Measure (WM)
6. Define (WM)
7. Install (MS)
8. Maintain (MS)

Before work study good relations should be developed within the organization.

METHOD STUDY

Method study in its generalized field of activity can be termed work simplification. Method study can be done in five stages:

Identifiction: The first stage is the selection of work to be studied which is primarily based on
- Economic consideration
- Technical consideration
- Human consideration

For example, nursing procedures, diagnostic procedures such as X-rays, lab work, etc.

Recording: After identifying the job, a record is to be made of all relevant facts relating to the present method. For recording several symbols are used.

CHRONOLOGICAL SEQUENCE ANALYSIS

In this analysis, breakdown the process under study into events or activities chronologically. There could be product/material-oriented process charts or person-oriented process chart. Usually in hospitals person-oriented process charts are drawn.

Symbol	Name of activity	Definition
◯	Operation	Whenever something is produced or task accomplished
→	Transportation	A transportation occurs when an object is moved from one operation to another
▭	Inspection	When a qualitative or quantitative appraisal or verification is made
D	Delay	State of inactivity or delay
▽	Storage	Storage occurs when a material is kept and protected against unauthorized removal
▭→	Combined activity	A combined activity occurs when two activities occur simultaneously

Using these symbols some charts are used for work study

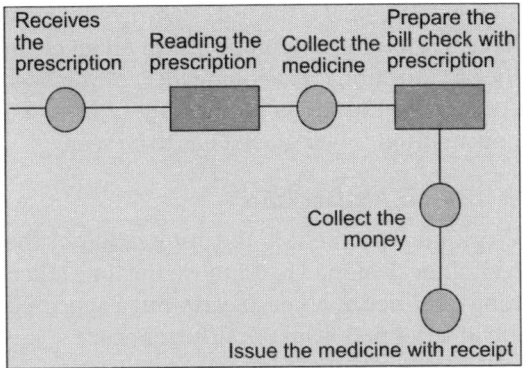

Fig. 5.13: Housekeeping

For chronological sequence analysis various charts are used:

1. *An outline/operation process chart* is the one which gives an overall picture by recording only the main operations and inspections, e.g. pharmacist in the O.P pharmacy.
2. A more detailed type is the **flow process chart** which is a graphic representation of the chronological sequence of all operations, transportation, inspection, delays, storage occurring during a process or procedure and includes information considered desirable for analysis such as time required, distance moved, etc.

Following are the different types of flow charts

i. *Material or product type*—Which records what happens to a material or product, e.g. recording the activities of a portable X-ray machine.
ii. *Form process chart*—It is a graphic symbolic representation of process flow of paper work form. This is useful in organization and method studies, e.g. hospital stores.
iii. *Two-hand process chart*—In which activities of the employees' hands (limbs) are recorded chronologically to one another, e.g. while studying activities of E.C.G technician or a cook in the dietary.
iv. *Multiple activity chart*—When more than one subject (worker, machine or equipment) is recorded.

Example of Flow Process Chart in Pharmacy

Movement and flow of activities: For this we will be using certain diagrams to indicate visually the path of movement. There are various types of charts or diagrams for movement and flow of activities charting (Fig. 5.14).

i. *Flow diagram*—Which shows rough view of space, machines with

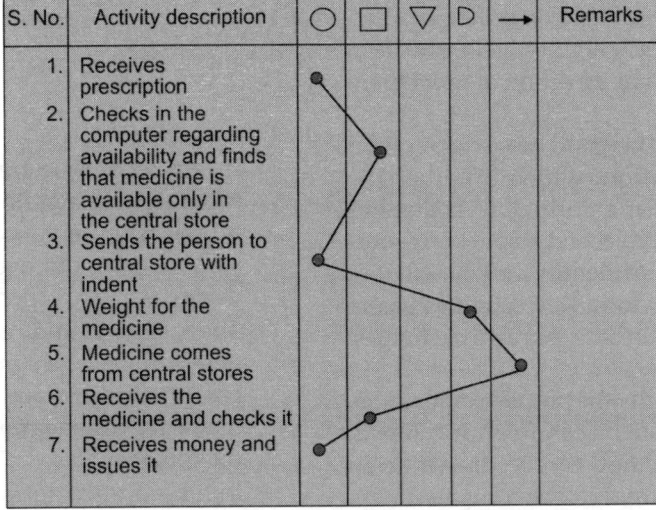

Fig. 5.14: Flow process chart in pharmacy

connecting set of arrows to indicate the route of travel followed by workers,

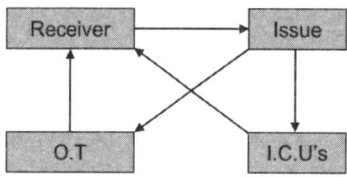

Fig. 5.15: Flow diagram on sterile supplies

materials or equipment, e.g. flow diagram on sterile supplies (Fig. 5.15).
ii. *String diagram*—It is a model on which a thread or string is used to trace and measure the path of workers, materials or

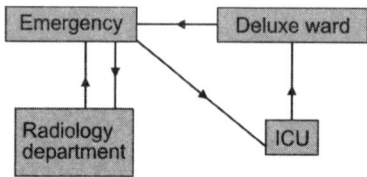

Fig. 5.16: Movement of mobile X-ray

equipments during a specified sequence of events, e.g. movement of mobile X-ray (Fig. 5.16).
iii. *SIMO or Simultaneous motion chart*—developed by Gilbreth.
iv. *Cycle graph*—It is a record of the path of the movement, usually traced by a continuous source of light on a photograph
v. *Chronological graph*—Cycle graph in which speed or direction of movement is recorded.

Examination: The third stage of method study is examination, which involves the critical and systematic study of facts that has been collected in the second stage, i.e. recording. We will be able to identify the key activities and put away activities. Key activities has to be retained, whereas some 'put away activities' can be deleted.

Development: After the proper examination, the new method can be carefully developed. This approved method can be drawn up in process-flow chart and can be compared with the existing method.

Installation: It is the final stage in which we have to gain the acceptance from all levels in the organization for installing the new method. After this continuous monitoring of how the new method is being used has to be seen.

WORK MEASUREMENT

Work measurement is the application of the technique designed to establish the time taken for a qualified worker to carry out a specified job at a defined level of performance.

Work Measurement Procedure

The basis steps followed sequentially are
1. Select
2. Record
3. Measure
4. Examine
5. Compile
6. Define

The above steps of work measurement are essentially three-stage procedure of analysis measurement and synthesis.

Techniques of Work Measurement

The principal technique used to measure work are
1. Time study
2. Work sampling
3. Pre-determined motion time system (PMTS)
4. Analytical estimating
5. Synthesis from standard data
6. MOST

1. **Time Study**
   - It is a technique for determining as accurately as possible from a limited number of observations, the time necessary to carry out a given activity at a defined standard of performance (Fig. 5.17).
   - The basic time study equipment consists of a stopwatch, a study board, pencils, pocket calculator, and measuring instruments for distance and time (like ruler, micrometer, etc.).
   - In time study a normal performance is estimated and the actual performance

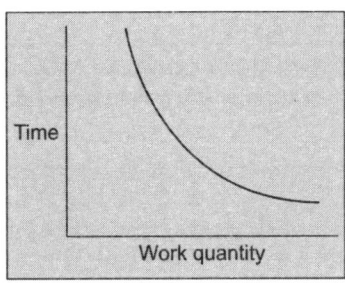

Fig. 5.17: Time study

is compared with the normal performance and rating is done.

2. *Work Sampling*
   - It is a technique developed by L.H.C. Tippet, in 1935 while working for British Cotton Industry Research Institute.
   - It is useful in obtaining information about certain long cycle work or non-repetitive type of jobs for which it is clearly impractical to use continuous observation method.
   - Work sampling is a method of randomly observing work, noting state or condition of the object being studied.
   - From the proportion of observations in each category, inferences are drawn concerning the total work activity under study.

3. *Pre-determined Motion Time System (PMTS)*
   - Every element of work is composed of some combinations of human motions.
   - All work can be broken down into elements that are usually a fundamental movement of the body or organs.
   - After this analysis, the basic motions that have been isolated have a time allotted to them on the basis of predetermined motion times. This is the measurement stage.
   - The synthesis stage involves combining the basic motions in specific combinations and frequencies to form basic elements, which would go to complete the total work operation.

4. *Analytical Estimating:* In this case, the job will be broken down into its constituent elements in certain type of non-repetitive work, and analysis is done. In this analysis, we can find that there will be certain basic elements or factors, which are critical in that particular work.

5. *Synthesis From Standard Data:* Here the standard data from previous research will be available in the organization.

6. *'Most' Measurement System*
   - MOST stands for Maynard Operation Sequence Technique, was conceptualized in 1967 and formalized in 1975.
   - The basic assumption here is that for an overwhelming majority of work, there is a common denominator from which work can be studied: the displacement of objects.
   - MOST is a system to measure work by concentrating on the movement of objects.
   - Most technique is composed of following basic sequence models:
     1. General move sequence—For the spatial movement of object through air.
     2. The controlled move sequence—For the movement of an object when it remains in contact with a surface or is attached to another object during movement.
     3. The tool sequence—For the use of common hand tools.

Work study can be used in hospitals setting for nursing patterns and staffing, ward-design and hospital layout, improvement in services like catering, laundry work, domestic cleaning, documentation, etc.

As per this analysis, total time required for performing one X-ray is 25 minutes. This exercise has to be repeated at least three times by three separate technicians. After this, time spent by each technician is to be analyzed and among that the least time can be considered as the standard time.

Travel ft.	Symbol and minutes	Descripiton	Explanation
			X-ray technician reaches his department, signs his attendance and started his work.
	☐ 5	Inspecting	Examining the X-ray machines, materials, etc.
10 ft	→ 2	Transportation	Visit to dark room and coming back to X-ray table.
	☐ 2	Inspection	Meeting a patient and examining a prescription.
	● 3	Operation	Prepare new film positioning machine and patient.
8 ft	→ 1	Transportation	Repositioning patient, correcting and positioning exactly.
	● 2	Operation	Completing X-ray and sending for processing.
8 ft	→ 1	Transportation	Reaching to dark room.
	● 2	Operation	Fixed the film for processing.
	D (5)	Delay	Waiting some time for X-ray.
	☐ 2	Inspection	Examine whether the film has come properly or not.

Time spend for completing one X-ray

●	Operation	=	7 minutes
→	Transportation	=	4 minutes
■	Inspection	=	9 minutes
D	Delay	=	5 minutes
	Total time	=	25 minutes

Time motion study can be used for productivity analysis and can be used in hospitals to achieve greater output with required quality.

VALUE ENGINEERING

- Value engineering (VE) or Value analysis (VA) is an important and powerful approach for improvement in the performance of the products, services, systems or procedures and reduction in costs without jeopardizing their function.
- L.D. Miles defined value analysis as an organized creative approach, which has for its purpose the efficient identification of unnecessary cost, i.e. cost which provides neither quality, use, life, appearance, nor customer features.
- The basic objective of VA/VE is to achieve equivalent or better performance at a lower

cost maintaining all functional and quality requirements.
- It does this largely by identifying and eliminating hidden, invisible and unnecessary costs.
- VE should not be treated as a mere cost reduction technique of the product or service. It is more comprehensive and the improvement in value is attained without any sacrifice in quality, reliability, maintainability, and aesthetics, etc.

Historical Perspective
- Value Engineering had its origin at General Electric Company under the leadership of L.D. Miles. L.D. Miles wrote the book "Techniques of Value Analysis and Engineering" and is considered as father of VE.
- VE/VA can be applied in hospitals also. Tata Main Hospital, Jamshedpur is the first Indian hospital to apply VE.

Value and Functions
Value is usually confused with the monitory price or cost of the item. However, value is not synonymous with the cost. Value may be perceived as the ratio of sum of positive and negative aspects of an object. Thus value can be considered as a composite of quality and cost. It is more in terms of worth and utility. Thus a ratio of quality to cost can be treated as value of the product. If costs can be reduced for same quality or quality can be improved with the same cost, then value improvement can be said to occur. The term value can be divided into:
a. *Use value:* The properties and qualities, which accomplish a useful purpose or service.
b. *Esteem value:* The properties, features or attractiveness that causes us to want or own it.
c. *Cost value:* The sum of labor, material and various other costs required to produce it.
d *Exchange value:* The properties or qualities, which enable us to exchange it for something else we want.

Identification of functions constitutes an important aspect of value of VE. The term function is used to mean the purpose or use of a product/service. Functions can be of two types:
a. *Basic functions:* The primary purpose of a product or service.
b. *Secondary functions:* Other purpose not directly accomplishing the primary purpose but supporting it.

VALUE ENGINEERING PROCESS
The formal procedural model of VE process is called **VE job plan**. Three different approaches to conduct VE programme are:
1. Job plan due to mudge
2. DARSIRI method
3. FAST (Function Analysis System Technique).

1. *Job plan due to mudge* is a well-recognized approach and it has seven phases:
    I. *General phase:* This phase is aimed at creating right environment for VE to be effective. This includes
    - Good human relations
    - Inspire teamwork
    - Work on specifics
    - Overcome roadblocks
    - Apply good business judgment
    II. *Information phase:* The objective of this phase is to gain an understanding of the project being studied and to obtain all essential facts relating to the project as also to estimate the potential of value improvement.
    - Secure facts
    - Determine costs
    - Fix cost on specifications and requirements
    III. *Function phase:* The objectives of this phase is to define the functions that a product/service actually performs and is required to perform as well as to

relate these functions to the cost and worth of providing them. Two techniques of this function are

1. *Define function:* The method of functional analysis requires functions to be described with only two words, i.e. verb and noun. By restricting the functional specification, clear description of the functions is possible. The rules of function description are as follows:
   - Determine the users need for the product or service
   - Use only one verb and one noun
   - Avoid goal-like words or phrases such as improve, maximize, etc.
   - List a large number of two word pairs and then select the best pair.
2. *Evaluate Functional Relationship:* The technique attempts to determine relative importance of various functions. Paired comparison technique will be used at this stage.
   I. *Creation phase:* The objective of this phase is to create ideas for value alternatives to accomplish the functions defined in the previous phase. This phase requires creativity to be the focal point. In brainstorming free-wheeling is permitted. Two powerful techniques to promote creativity are
      - Establish positive thinking
      - Develop creative ideas
   II. *Evaluation phase:* The objective of this phase is to select for further analysis the most promising of the ideas generated during the creative phase. The four techniques associated with this phase are:
      - Refine and combine ideas
      - Establish cost on all ideas
      - Develop function alternatives
      - Evaluate by comparison— Decision matrix approach can be effective here.
   III. *Investigation phase:* In this phase selected ideas are refined into workable and acceptable solutions providing lower cost methods for performing the desired function.
   IV. *Recommendation phase:* This is final phase in which finally selected value alternative is recommended for acceptance and implementation. Two techniques associated with this phase are
      - Present facts
      - Motivate positive action

2. **Darsiri method:** Similar to job plan of mudge, the seven steps are
   1. D – Data collection
   2. A – Analysis
   3. R – Record of ideas
   4. S – Speculation
   5. I – Investigation
   6. R – Recommendation and
   7. I – Implementation

3. **FAST diagram:** Functional analysis system technique was developed in 1965 by charles. W. Bythway. It gives an understanding of the interaction of function and cost. FAST diagram can also be used in the function phase of VE job plan due to mudge.

Accountancy for Hospital Managers

Ghousia

AN INTRODUCTION TO ACCOUNTANCY

Accountancy has rightly been termed the language of business. The basic function of the language is to serve as the means of communication. It communicates the results of business operation to various holders and parties who have some stake in the business, viz. the proprietor, creditors, investors, government, other agencies, though accounting is generally associated with business, it has been used by persons like housewives, government and other individuals. For example, housewife has to keep the record of the money received and spent by her during a particular period of time as she can record receipts of money on one page of her household dairy while payments for different items such as milk, food, clothing, education, etc. on some other page in a chronological order. Such a record will help her in knowing about the sources from which she received cash and the purposes it utilized and also whether the receipt is more than the payments or vice versa.

The balance of cash in hand or deficit, if any at the end of a period. In this case a housewife records her transactions regularly; she can collect valuable information about the nature of her receipts and payments. For example, she can find out the total amount spend by her during a period on different items, say milk, food, education, entertainment, etc. Similarly, she can find the sources of her receipts such as salary of her husband, rent from property, cash gift, etc. thus, at the end of the period she can see for herself about her financial position, i.e. what she owns and what she owes. This will help her in planning her future income and expenses.

The need for accountancy is all the greater for a person who is running a business. He knows:

What he owns?

What he owes?

Whether has earned profit or suffered a loss on account of running a business.

What is his financial position, i.e. whether he will be in the position to meet all the commitments in the near future or he is in the process of becoming a bankrupt?

History of Accounting

Accounting is as old as money itself. In India, Chanakya in his book, Arthashastra has emphasized the existence and need of proper accounting and auditing. Modern system of accounting owes its origin to pacoili, who lived in Italy in the 18th century. In those days business were not so complex due to their being small and easily manageably by the proprietor himself but the things has changed very fastly during last fifty years. The advent of industrial revolution has resulted in large scale production, cut-throat competition and widening of markets. This has also reduced the effectiveness of personnel supervision resulting in decentralization of authority and responsibility. Today there is greater need for coordination and control. Old technique of management by the intuition is no longer considered dependable in the situation in which the modern firm operates. Accountancy has grown in importance and changed in its structure with the evolution of complex and giant industrial organizations. In the recent past changes in the technology have also brought a remarkable change in the field of accounting. It has been recognized as a tool for mastering the various economic problems which a business organization has to face.

Classification of Accountancy

The word accountancy can be classified into three categories (Fig. 6.1):
a. Financial accounting
b. Management accounting
c. Cost accounting

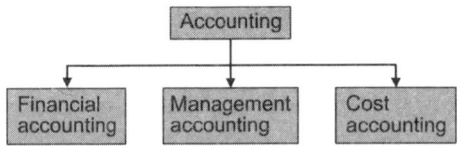

Fig. 6.1: Classification of accountancy

Financial Accounting

Financial accounting has come to existence with the development of large scale business in the form of joint stock companies. As public money in share capital, Companies Act of 1956 has provided a legal framework to present the operating result and financial position of the company. Financial accounting is concerned with preparation of profit and loss account and balance sheet to disclose information to the shareholders. It is oriented towards the preparation of financial statements, which summaries the results of operation for the select period of time and show the financial position of the business on a particular date. Financial accounting is concerned with providing information to the external users preparation of financial statement is a statutory obligation. It is required to be prepared in accordance with generally accepted accounting principles (GAAP) and practices. In fact, the corporate laws that govern the enterprises not only make it mandatory to prepare such accounts, but also lay down the format and information to be provided in such accounts. In sharp contrast, management accounting is entirely optional and there is no standard format for preparation and presentation of the reports. Financial accounts relate to the business as a whole, while management accounts focuses on parts or segment of the business.

Management Accounting

Management accounting is the new approach to accounting. The term management accounting is composed of two words —*management* and *accounting*. It refers to a accounting for the management. It is the modern tool and provides the technique to management for interpretation of accounting data which serves the need of management for decision making.

Managers in all types of organization need information about business to plan accurately for future and make decision for achieving goals of the organization.

As uncertainty is the characteristic of decision-making process, it cannot be eliminated but it can be reduced, hence the function of management accounting is to reduce uncertainty and help management in decision making.

Management accounting is that field of accounting which deals with providing information including financial accounting information to managers for their use in planning, decision making, performance evaluation, control, management of cost and cost determination for financial reporting.

Cost Accounting

Cost accounting is the formal system of recording cost. It may be defined as "the process of accounting for cost which begins with recording of income and expenditure and ends with preparation of periodical statement and reports for ascertaining and controlling cost".

The main objectives of cost accounting are
  i. To ascertain cost of a product or a service
  ii. To determine selling price
  iii. To control cost and

iv. To provide guidance to management for decision-making and policy formulation.

Definition and Role of Accounting

From the above discussion it is clear that the period of time, the concept of accounting and the role of accountant has undergone a revolutionary change. Earlier accounting was considered simply as a process of recording business transactions and the role of accountant as that of record-keeper but now accounting is considered to be a tool of management which provides vital information concerning the organization's future. Accounting today is thus more of an information system rather than a mere recording system.

It would be useful to give in a chronological order the definitions given by some of the well established accounting bodies which show how the concept of accounting has changed over the period of times.

In 1941, the American Institute of Certified Public Accounting (AICPA) defined accounting as follows:

"Accounting is the art of recording, classifying and summarizing in the significant manner and in terms of money, transactions and events which are in parts at least of a financial character and interpreting the results thereof".

In 1966, the American Accounting Association (AAA) defined accounting as follows:

"Accounting is the process of identifying, measuring and communication economic information to permit informed judgment and decision by users of the information"

In 1970, Accounting Principles Board (APB) of American Institute certified public accounting enumerated the functions of accounting as follows:

"The role of accounting is to provide quantitative information, primarily of financial nature, about economic entities, that is needed to be useful in making economic decisions".

Thus accounting may be defined as the process of recording, classifying, summarizing, analyzing and interpreting the financial transactions and communicating the result to the person interested in such information.

An analysis of the definition bring out the following functions of accounting:

1. *Recording:* This is the basic function of accounting. It is concerned not only with ensuring that all business transactions of financial character are in fact recorded but also that they are recorded in an orderly manner. Thus recording is done in the book called "journal". This book may be further sub-divided into various subsidiary books like cash journal (for recording cash transactions), purchase journal (for recording purchase of goods), sales journal (for recording credit sales of goods), etc. The number of subsidiary books to be maintained depends on the nature and size of the business.

2. *Classifying:* Classification is concerned with the systematic analysis of the recorded data, with a view to group transactions of one nature at one place. This work is done in the book called "ledger". This book contains individuals account heads under which all financial transactions of similar nature are collected. For example, there may be separate account head for traveling expenses, printing and stationery, advertising, etc. All expenses under these heads after being recorded in the journal will be classified under separate heads in the ledger. This will help in finding out the total expenditure incurred under each of the above heads.

3. Summarizing: This involves presenting the classified data in a manner which is

understandable and useful to the internal as well as external end-users of accounting statements.

This process leads to the presentation of the following statements:
   i. Trial balance
   ii. Income and expenditure statement
   iii. Balance sheet.

4. *Dealing with financial transactions*: Accounting records only those transactions and events in terms of money which are of a financial character.

   Transactions which are not of a financial character are not recorded in the books of accounts. For example, if a company has a team of dedicated and trusted employees, it is of great use to the business but since it is not of financial character and capable of being expressed in terms of money, it will not be recorded in the books of the business.

5. Analyzing and interpreting: The recorded financial data is analyzed and interpreted in the manner that the end-users can make a meaningful judgment about the financial condition and profitability of the business operations. The data is also used for preparing the future plan and framing of policies for executing such plans.

6. Communication: The accounting information after being meaningfully analyzed and interpreted has to be communicated in a proper form and manner to the right person. This is done through preparation distribution of accounting records, which include besides the usual income statement and the balance sheet, additional information in the form of accounting ratios, graphs, diagrams, funds flow statement, cash flow statement, etc. the initiative, imagination and innovative ability of accountant are put to test in this process.

Accounting Cycle

As accounting has been defined as recording, classifying and summarizing the financial transactions and interpreting the results, therefore accounting cycle involves the following stages.

Recording of transactions: This is done in the book called 'journal'.

Classifying of transactions: This is done in the book called 'ledger'.

Summarizing of transactions: This includes preparation of the trial balance, profit and loss account and balance sheet of the business.

Interpreting the results: This involves computation of various accounting ratios to know about the liquidity, solvency and profitability of business and various statements which help management in decision making (Fig. 6.2).

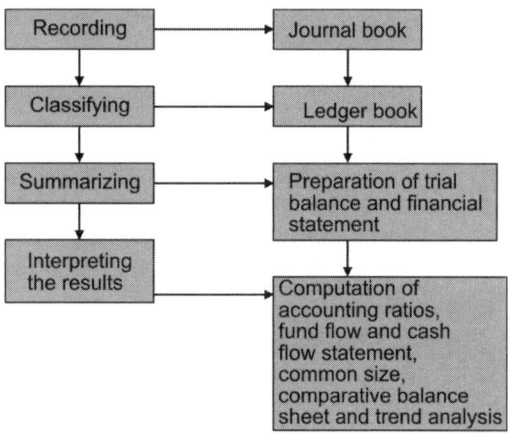

Fig. 6.2: Accounting cycle

Principles of Accounting

Accounting principles may be defined as those rules adopted by the accountants universally while recording accounting transactions.

   "They are a body of doctrines commonly associated with the theory and procedures of accounting, serving as an explanation of current practices and as a guide for selection or procedures where alternatives exist."

These principles can be classified into two categories

1. Accounting concepts
2. Accounting conventions.

Accounting Concepts

The term "concept" includes those basic assumptions or conditions upon which the science of accounting is based. The following are the important accounting concepts.
- Separate entity concept
- Going concern concept
- Money measurement concept
- Cost concept
- Dual aspect concept
- Accounting period concept
- Periodic matching concept
- Realization concept

Accounting Conventions

The term convention includes those customs or traditions which guide the accountant while preparing the accounting statement. The following are the important accounting conventions.
- Convention of conservatism.
- Convention of full disclosure.
- Convention of consistency.
- Convention of materiality.

Each of the above concepts and conventions are explained below

Accounting Concepts

Separate Entity Concept

In accounting, business is considered to be a separate entity from the proprietor. It may appear to be ludicrous that one person can sell goods to himself but this concept is extremely helpful in keeping business affairs strictly free from the effect of private affairs of the proprietor. Thus when a person invest, say ₹ 10,000 in the business, it will be deemed that the proprietor has given that much of money to the business, it will be shown as a 'liability' in the books of the business. In case the proprietor withdraws ₹ 3000 from the business for his personnel use, then it will be charged to him and the net amount payable by the business will be shown as 7000 only.

Going Concern Concept

According to this concept it is assumed that the business will continue for a fairly long time to come. There is neither the intention nor the necessity to liquidate the particular business venture in the foreseeable future. On account of this concept, the accountant while valuing the assets does not take into account forced sale value of assets. Moreover, he charges depreciation on fixed assets on the basis of their expected lives rather than on their market value. This concept does not imply permanent continuance of the enterprise, it rather presumes that the enterprise will continue its operation for a long enough to charge against income.

Money Measurement Concept

Accounting records only monetary transactions. Those transactions which cannot be expressed in terms of money do not find its place in the books of accounts. For example, if a business has a team of loyal and dedicated employees, which is an asset to the business but since they are not measurable in terms of money, they are not shown in the books of accounts.

Measurement of business transactions in terms of money will help in understanding the position of business in much better form. For example, if business owns ₹ 15000 cash, 1000 kg of raw material, 3 trucks, furniture, 20 machinery, 10000 sq ft building space, etc., these items cannot be added together, it gives a meaningful total of what business owns. But however, if these items are expressed in terms of money such as ₹ 15000 cash, ₹ 20000 worth raw material, ₹ 800000 trucks, ₹ 50000 furniture, ₹ 10,0000 machinery, ₹ 500000 building, all such items can be added for much more intelligible and precise estimate about the assets of the business will be available.

Cost Concept

This concept is closely related to going concern concepts. According to this concept:

An asset is ordinarily entered in the books of accounts at the price paid to acquire it, and this cost is the basis of all subsequent accounting for assets.

For example, if the business buys a building for ₹ 1,00,000, this would be recorded in the books at ₹ 100,000, even if the market value at that time happens to be ₹ 150,000 and in case a year later the market value of this building comes down to ₹ 1,20,000 ,it will be ordinarily continue to be shown at ₹ 1,00,000 and not at ₹ 1,20,000.

Dual Aspect Concept

This is the basic concept of accounting. According to this concept every business transaction has a dual effect. For example, a person starts a business with the capital (initial investment), say of ₹ 10,000. This transaction has two aspects. On the one hand, business has an asset of ₹ 10000 and on the other hand, business has to pay to the proprietor a sum of ₹ 10000, which is taken from the proprietor as capital.

This can be shown in the form of equation:

Capital (equities) = cash (assets)

₹ 10,000 = ₹ 10,000

The term assets denote the resources owned by the business, while the term equities denote the claim by various parties against the assets of the business. Equities are of two types:

Owner's equity (fund) or capital

Outsider's equity (fund) or liability

Owner's equity or capital is the claim of owners against the assets of the business while the outsiders equity or the liability is the claim of outside parties, such as the creditors, debenture-holders, etc. against the assets of the business. As the assets of the business are claimed by someone, i.e. either by owners or outsiders, the total asset will be equal to the total of liabilities. Thus,

Equities = asset

Liabilities + capital = asset

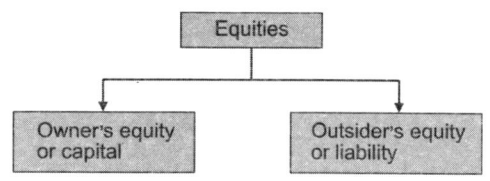

The above equation is also used to denote the relationship of equities to assets, it can well be stated as "for every debit, there is an equivalent credit".

The entire system of double entry bookkeeping is based on this concept.

Accounting Period Concept

According to this concept, the life of the business is divided into appropriate segments for studying the results shown by the business after each segment. As the life of the business is considered to be indefinite, according to the going concern concept, measuring the income and studying the financial position after a long period would not be helpful in taking proper corrective measures in appropriate time, thus it is necessary that this long period is divided into small segments where business will stop and see back, how things are going. In accounting, such segment is called "accounting period" and it is usually one year.

At the end of each accounting period in income statement, a balance sheet or financial statement is prepared. The income statement discloses the profit or loss made by the business during the accounting period, while the balance sheet shows the financial position of the business as on the last day of the accounting period.

Periodic Matching of Cost and Revenue Concept

This concept is based on the accounting period concept. In order to ascertain the profit made by the business during the period of time, it is necessary that the 'revenue' of the period should be matched with the cost or expenses of the period.

In other words, income made by the business during the period can be measured only when the revenue earned during the period is compared with the expenditure incurred for earning that revenue.

For example, if a salesman is paid commission in January 2001, for the sales made by him in December 2000, the commission paid to him in January 2001 should be taken as the cost for sales made by him in December 2000. This means that revenue of December 2000 should be matched with cost incurred for earning that revenue in December 2000, though paid in January 2001. On account of this concept, adjustments are made for all outstanding expenses, accrued income, prepaid expenses and unearned income, etc. while preparing the final accounts at the end of the accounting period.

Realization Concept

According to this concept revenue is recognized when a sale is made. Sale is considered to take place at the point when the property in goods transferred to the buyer and he become legally liable to pay.

For example: If Mr. 'x' places an order with Mr. 'y' for supply of a certain good yet to be manufactured. On receipt of a order, Mr.'s' purchases raw material, employs workers, produces the goods and delivers to them to Mr. 'x'. He makes payment on receipt of goods. In this case the sale will be presumed to have been made not at the time of receipt of order but at the time when the goods are delivered to Mr. 'a' with certain exceptions to this concept in case of hire purchase and contract account.

Accounting Conventions

Convention of Conservatism

In the early stages of accounting, certain anticipated profits which were recorded, did not materialized. In those days profits were assumed for the future the period and recorded but when actual profit was realized, there was a difference between the assumed profit and the actual profit which resulted in less acceptability or loss of faith in accounting figures by the end users. On account of these reasons, accountant follows the rule 'anticipate no profit but provide for losses' while recording business transactions. Due to this conventions inventory is valued 'at cost or market price whichever is less'. Similarly, a provision is made for possible bad and doubtful debts out of current year's profit.

Convention of Full Disclosure

According to this convention accounting reports should disclose fully and fairly the information they purport to represent. They should be honestly prepared and sufficiently disclose information which is material interest to the end users such as proprietor, creditors customers and investors.

Convention of Consistency

According to this convention accounting practices should remain unchanged from one period to another. For example, if the business follows the practice of valuing the stock at "cost or market price", whichever is less, it should be continued year after year. Similarly, if depreciation is charged on fixed assets according to straight line method, then business should consistently follow this practice year after year.

Convention of Materiality

According to this convention the accountant should attach importance to material details and ignore insignificant details, otherwise accounting will be unnecessarily overburden with minute details. The question what constitutes a material detail, is left to the accountant and it varies from business to business.

For example: While sending the each debtor a statement of his account, a complete detail has to be given but when the statement of outstanding debtors is prepared for the top management, figures may be round up to the nearest value, in other words, the ignoring of 'Paisa' is permitted for preparing financial statement as well as by the Companies Act of 1956.

System of Bookkeeping

Bookkeeping is the art of recording business transactions systematically and in summarized form in a separate set of books. This recording of transaction may be done according to any of the following two systems:

Single entry system: According to Kohler, "It is the system bookkeeping in which as a rule only records of cash and personal accounts are maintained, it is always incomplete double entry, varying with circumstances".

This system is developed by some business houses for their convenience and maintained only some essential records. As all records are not maintained, the system is not reliable and can be used by small firms.

Double entry system: This system of bookkeeping was originated by venetian merchant of fifteenth century. It is the only system of recording the twofold aspect of the transition.

As every business transaction involves transfer of money or money's worth and as such consists of two aspects:
a. The receiving aspect
b. The giving aspect

These two aspects go together, because receiving necessarily implies giving and vice versa. The record of any business transaction will be complete only when both these aspects are recorded. This recording of two aspects of the transaction is called double entry system of bookkeeping.

To understand the double entry system of bookkeeping, one need to remember the fundamental rule of bookkeeping while recording the transactions in the books. They are as follows:

a. Debit the account which receives the benefit.
b. Credit the account which gives the benefit.

Type of accounts

All those transactions that take place in every business deals with
a. Number of people, firms, or companies,
b. Possesses assets such as cash, goods, machinery, building, etc.
c. Pays expenses such as salaries, rent commission, discount, etc.

All these transactions are divided into three types of accounts. They are:
a. Personal account
b. Real account
c. Nominal account

Personal Account

This account deals with all those transactions with
a. Natural persons in various capacities such as suppliers, buyers, lenders and borrowers of loan, investors of capital, etc. Ram account, Raheem account, Krishna account, etc.
b. Legal or notional persons such as incorporated companies assuming the status of a banker, insurance, etc. Government and semi-government institutions, clubs, associations unions, etc. e.g. A.B.C. Co Ltd, Canara Bank, Indian Railways, Hyderabad Municipal Corporation, etc.

The proprietor brings money into the business and draws money from the business for the personal expenses. Hence two separate accounts are maintained in his books of accounts.
1. Capital account shows the amount invested in the business and
2. Drawing account shows the amount withdrawn for the personal use.

Therefore, capital account and drawing account are personal accounts.

Real Account

Account relating to properties or assets is known as 'real account' as every business needs assets such as machinery, furniture, vehicle building, etc. for running the activities separate account is maintained for every assets a business owns. Real account can be classified into two categories. They are:

Assets: Assets are meant for the use in the business for a long period of time.

Goods: These are meant for resale, the trader buys goods and sells goods, return defective goods to his suppliers and also receives defective goods from his customers.

Real account can further be classified as 'tangible' and 'intangible'.

Tangible properties are sub-divided into physical resources such as land building, machinery, furniture, etc. and non-physical resources such as securities, account receivables.

Intangible items may be valuable such as goodwill, trademarks, patents which had exchange value or fictitious (worthless) like registration cost of a partnership firm.

Nominal Account

Nominal account relate to such items which are meant for name sake only, these items pertain to expenses and gains such as interest, rent, salary, commission, discount, etc. A separate account is opened for each head of expense or income.

Rules of Debit and Credit

An account has two sides, the left-hand side is known as 'debit side' or 'dr' and the right-hand side is known as 'credit side' or 'cr' (Table 6.1).

The benefits received by the account are recorded on the left-hand side or debit side and the benefit imparted by the account are recorded on the right-hand side or credit side.

As every transaction affects two accounts, this effect will have to be entered in both of them, on debit side in one account and on credit side in another account. Therefore, it is necessary to find out which account is to be debited and which is to be credited, for this purpose one has to identify the class to which these two accounts belong, i.e. personal, real or nominal account and then a certain rule of debit and credit is to be applied.

Personal Account

The account of the person receiving the benefit or receiver of the transaction is debited and the account of the person giving to the benefit or giver of the transaction is credited.

Rule: "Debit the receiver and
Credit the giver"

Real Account

When an asset is coming into the business the account of that asset is debited. When an asset is going out of the business, the account of that asset is credited.

Rule: "Debit what comes in and
Credit what goes out"

Nominal Account

When an expense is incurred or loss is suffered, the account will represent the

Table 6.1: Rules of debit and credit

Date	Particulars	LF	Amount	Date	Particulars	LF	Amount
	Particulars of benefit received				Particulars of benefit given		

expense or the loss is debited. When any income is earned or gain is made, the account will represent this income or gain is credited.

Rule: "Debit all expenses and losses.

Credit all income and gains".

These rules of accounts are followed while preparing journal and ledger accounts (Fig. 6.5).

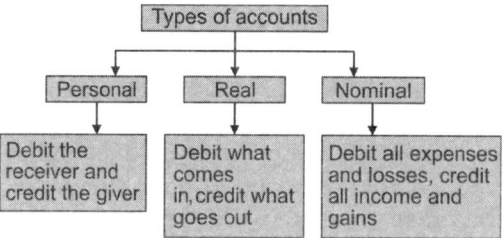

Fig. 6.5: Different types of accounts

Books of Accounts

Business houses maintain several books of accounts for recording business transactions. The proprietor or manager of the business house decides the number and kinds of books of accounts that has to be maintained. This is based on different factors like:

a. The legal forms of business
b. The nature and size of the business
c. The volume of the business transactions.

Every business has to maintain two books of account which is mandatory, i.e.

a. Journal book
b. Ledger book

Journal

The transactions are recorded in the books called journal. A journal, therefore, may be defined as a book containing a chronological record of transactions. It is the book in which the transactions are recorded under double entry system. Thus journal is the book of the original record. A journal does not replace but precedes the ledger.

In the journal, entries are made datewise and shown in each case which account is to be debited and which is to be credited and it also includes brief particulars of each transaction. This process of recording the transactions in the journal is termed journalizing. Entries from the journal are recorded in the book called ledger. Hence the journal is called the 'book of original entry'.

Advantages of Journal

The transactions are recorded in the chronological order. This reduces the chance of omitting any transaction.

The transactions are accompanied by narration. Thus, the entry is supplemented with basic information regarding the transaction. This narration is very useful in understanding the nature of compounding entries.

Debit and credit amount are written side by side. It minimizes the chance of wrong amount.

The journal is a complete and chronological record of business transactions. Therefore, it facilitates easy and quick reference.

The journal helps in posting the entries in the ledger.

The journal helps accountants and auditors in finding out the mistakes committed in ledger and trial balance.

Date (1)	Particulars (2)	LF (3)	Debit (₹) (4)	Credit (₹) (5)
Year/ month and day	Name of the account debited ...dr to name of the account credited (narration)		Amount	Amount

The proforma of journal is given below:

It is noticed from the above that journal has five columns.

Column 1 is meant for recording date on which the transaction takes place.

Column 2 gives the brief details of each transaction.

Column 3 entered the page number of the ledger on which the account concerned has been correspondingly debited and credited.

Column 4 records the amount with which the account is debited.

Column 5 records the amount with which the account is credited.

Narration

A narration is the reason or explanation of an entry. A journal entry is incomplete without a narration. This should be given with details, calculations, reference to documents, period, etc. whereever necessary. The narration should start with the word 'being'.

Transactions are of different types

i. *Transactions relating to purchase and sale of good for cash.*

Illustration 6.1:

Journalize the following transactions:

Date	Particulars	Amount
2002/Jan. 5	Bought goods for cash	30,000
6	Sold goods for cash	25,000
8	Bought goods for cash from Ramu	26,000
10	Sold goods to Ravi for cash	45,000

ii. *Transaction relating to purchased or sale of goods on credit:* In case of credit transaction cash is not immediately paid. The settlement of account is postponed. Therefore while recording such transactions, it is necessary to involve the personal account of the parties concerned.

Illustration 6.2:

Journalize the following transactions

Date	Particulars	Amount
2004/Jan 10	Sold goods to Aryan on credit	25,000
16	Bought goods from Suman	15,000
18	Purchase goods from Ramana	10,000
20	Sold goods on credit to Kapil	5,000

Sometimes the name of the parties or the word cash or on creditor on account is not mentioned, for example, transactions give as 'bought goods' or 'sold goods', these transactions shall be treated as cash transactions.

iii *Transactions relating to purchase or sale of assets:* Assets such as plant and machinery, building, furniture, vehicle, etc. are bought for use in the business and not for resale, therefore, the particular asset account is debited when it is bought, similarly when the asset is sold, the particular asset account is credited.

Solution: Journal entries

Date	Particulars	LF	Debit (₹)	Credit (₹)
2002/Jan. 5	Purchase a/c…………….…dr to cash a/c (being goods purchased for cash)		30,000	30,000
6	Cash a/c……………….dr to sales a/c (being goods purchased for cash)		25,000	25,000
8	Purchase a/c……………….dr to cash a/c (being goods purchased for cash)		26,000	26,000
	Cash a/c……………….dr to sales a/c (being goods sold for cash)		45,000	45,000

Note: While recording cash purchase or cash sale, it is not necessary to involve the personal account of the parties concerned, though the name of the parties are clearly given, it is not recorded in the journal entries.

Solution (Illustration 6.2): Journal entries

Date	Particulars	LF	Debit (₹)	Credit (₹)
2004/Jan. 10	Aryan a/c .... dr to sales a/c (being goods sold on credit)		25,000	25,00
16	Purchases a/c................dr to Suman a/c (being goods purchased on credit)		15,000	15,00
18	Purchases a/c................dr to Ramana a/c (being goods purchased on credit)		10,000	10,000
20	Kapil a/c ....dr to sales a/c (being goods sold on credit)		5,000	5,000

Note: The term on credit or on account indicates that it is a credit transaction but sometimes when the name of the persons concerned is given without using the word on credit or on account, these are also credit transactions.

Illustration 6.3:

Journalize the following transactions:

Date	Particulars	Amount
2004/Feb. 12	Purchased building	5,00,000
13	Brought furniture from Godrej and Co.	15,000
15	Sold machinery	25,000
18	Sold old computer to Gupta	1,000

Solution: Journal entries

Date	Particulars	LF	Debit (₹)	Credit (₹)
2004/Feb. 12	Building a/c..................dr to cash a/c (being building purchased)		5,00,000	5,00,000
13	Furniture a/c...................dr to Godrej and Co a/c (being furniture purchased on credit)		15,000	15,000
15	Cash a/c....................dr to machinery a/c (being machinery purchased)		25,000	25,000
18	Gupta a/c ....dr to computer a/c (being computer sold to Gupta on credit)		1,000	1,000

iv. Transaction relating to return of goods: When goods are found to be defective, they are returned to the seller by the customers.

Illustration 6.4:

Journalize the following transactions:

Date	Particulars	Amount
2004/Jan. 14	Aryan returned goods	2,500
18	Returned good to Suman	1,000
20	Returned good to Ramana	1,500
24	Kapil returned goods	500

Solution: Journal entries

Date	Particulars	LF	Debit (₹)	Credit (₹)
2004/Jan 4	Sales returned a/c.............dr to Aryan a/c		2,500	2,500
	(being goods recurred by Aryan for being defective)			
18	Suman a/c ....dr to purchase return a/c		1,000	1,000
	(being goods returned to Suman)			
20	Ramana a/c ....dr to purchase return a/c		1,500	1,500
	(being goods returned to Ramana)			
24	Sales returned a/c.............dr to Kapil a/c		500	500
	(being goods recurred by Kapil for being defective)			

v. Transactions relating to expenses and income:
Illustration 6.5:

Journalize the following transactions:

Date	Particulars	Amount
2004/Jan. 4	Paid salaries	25,000
5	Paid rent	4,000
18	Received dividend on shares	5,500
23	Received commission Suresh	4,000

Solution: Journal entries

Date	Particulars	LF	Debit (₹)	Credit (₹)
2004/Jan. 4	Salaries a/c.....................dr to cash a/c		25,000	25,000
	(being salaries paid)			
5	Rent a/c.........................dr to cash a/c		4,000	4,000
	(being rent paid)			
18	Cash a/c.........................dr to dividend a/c		5.500	5,500
23	Cash a/c ....dr to commission received a/c		4,000	4,000
	(being commission received)			

vi. Transactions relating to receipts and payments of cash
Illustration 6.6:

Journalize the following transactions:

Date	Particulars	Amount
2004/Jan. 4	Received cash from Arun on account	5,000
5	Paid to Ramana on account	2,000
18	Took loan from Venkat	25,000
23	Gave loan to Sohan	30,000

Solution: Journal entries

Date	Particulars	LF	Debit (₹)	Credit (₹)
2004/Jan. 4	Cash a/c.....................dr Arun a/c		5,000	5,000
	(being cash received on account)			
5	Ramana a/c ....dr to cash a/c		2,000	2,000
	(being cash paid on account)			
18	Cash a/c......................dr to loan from Venkat a/c		25,000	25,000
	(being loan taken)			
23	Loan to Sohan a/c............dr to cash a/c		30,000	30,000
	(being loan given to Sohan)			

vii. Transactions relating to receipt and payment by cheque: When the payment is received by cheque, the amount will be debited to bank account because the cheque is deposited in the bank, this increases the bank balance, when payment is made by cheque, bank account will be credited because the bank balance will be reduced.

Illustration 6.7:

Journalize the following transactions:

Date	Particulars	Amount
2005/Jan. 4	Received cheque from Hari	10,000
5	Paid to Giri on account by cheque	5,500

Solution: Journal entries

Date	Particulars	LF	Debit (₹)	Credit (₹)
2005/Jan. 4	Bank a/c ....dr to Hari a/c		10,000	10,000
	(being cheque received from Hari)			
5	Giri a/c ....dr to bank a/c		5,500	5,500
	(being cheque issued to Giri)			

viii. Transaction relating to proprietor: Business and its proprietor are treated as separate entities. Whatever he brings to the business is treated as capital and is credited to his capital account. Similarly when he withdraws cash from the business for his personal use, his drawing account is debited.

Illustration 6.8:

Journalize the following transactions in the books of Srikanth.

Date	Particulars	Amount
2004/Jan. 4	Commenced business	2,50,000
5	He withdrew cash for personal use	15,000
18	He took goods for domestic use	5,000
23	He withdrew from bank for personal use	5,000

Solution: Journal entries in the books of Mr. Srikanth

Date	Particulars	LF	Debit (₹)	Credit (₹)
2004/Jan. 4	Cash a/c...............dr to capital a/c (being capital bought into the business)		2,50,000	2,50,000
5	Drawings a/c..............dr to cash a/c (being cash withdraw for personal use)		15,000	15,000
18	Drawings a/c..............dr to purchases a/c (being goods withdraw for personal use)		5,000	5,000
23	Drawings a/c..............dr to bank a/c (being cash withdraw from bank for personal use)		5,000	5,000

ix. Transactions relating to discount

Discount is the concession allowed by the seller to the buyer in the price to be paid by him. There are two types of discount: i. trade discount and ii. cash discount.

i. *Trade discount:* This discount is allowed by the seller to a buyer who deals in the same goods as that of the seller. Trade discount is not recorded in the books of accounts because it is shown as the deduction in the invoice. The amount which remains after deduction of trade discount is recorded in the books of accounts

ii. *Cash discount:* This discount is allowed to those buyers who make payment during a prescribed period. At the time of sale the buyer is debited with the net amount of the invoice. Later if cash discount is allowed at the time of payment, it must be adjusted in the personal account of the debtor, this would show that his account stands cleared and nothing remains due. Thus, this discount is always recorded in the books of accounts.

Illustration 6.9:

Journalize the following transactions in the books of Kamalakar.

Date	Particulars
2006/Jan. 1	Purchased goods from Mahesh at 20% trade discount. The list price of these goods were ₹ 8000.
2	Returned goods to Mahesh as these were defective. The list price of these goods were ₹ 700.
3	Sold goods to Dinesh for cash. The list price of these goods were ₹ 2000. Trade discount of 5% and a cash discount of 1 % were allowed to him.
4	Received ₹ 9850 from Krishna and allowed him a discount of ₹ 150.
6	Paid to Amala ₹ 2950 and she allowed us a discount of ₹ 50.

Solution: Journal entries in the books of Kamalakar.

Date	Particulars	LF	Amount	Amount
2006/Jan. 1	Purchases a/c...............dr to Mahesh a/c (being goods purchases at 20% trade discount)		6,400	6,400
2	Mahesh a/c...............dr to purchase return a/c (being goods returned to Mahesh after deducting 20% trade discount)		560	560

(Contd...)

(Contd...)

Date	Particulars	LF	Amount	Amount
3	Cash a/c......................dr discount a/c ....dr to sales a/c (being goods sold for cash at 5% trade discount and 1% cash discount)		1881 19	1900
4	Cash a/c dr discount a/c.................dr to Krishna a/c (being cash received from Krishna and allowed him a discount)		9850 150	10,000
6	Amala a/c.....................dr to cash a/c to discount a/c (being cash paid to Amala and discount received from her)		3,000	2,950 50

Working notes

1. 8000*20/100 = ₹ 1600, ₹ 8000 – ₹ 1600 = ₹ 6,400
2. 700*20/100 = ₹ 140, ₹ 700 – ₹ 140 = ₹ 560
3. 2000 *5/100 = ₹ 100, ₹ 2000 – ₹ 100 = ₹ 1900.
4. 1900*1/100 = ₹ 19, ₹ 199 – 19 = ₹ 1,881.

x. Transactions relating to bad debts: When debtors (customers) become insolvent or bankrupt, the trader will not be able to realize full amount due from him. A part of it will remain unrealized. The unrealized amount is called 'bad debts'. It is a loss to the business. Hence it is debited to bad debts and credited to the concern 'debtor a/c'. If in case bad debts is realized later, the amount recovered shall be treated as a business income. It will be credited to 'bad debts recovered a/c and credited to cash a/c.

Illustration 6.10:

Journalize the following transactions:

Date	Particulars
2002/Sep. 1	Subba Rao, a debtor become insolvent, he owed ₹ 5000. A final dividend of 50 paise in a rupee was received.
Sep. 25	Received ₹ 1000 from Subba Rao whose account was written off previously as bad.
Oct. 15	Raheem was declared insolvent and he owed ₹ 1000 and only 50 paise in a rupee was realised.
Nov. 10	Received ₹ 500 from Raheem.

Solution: Journal entries

Date	Particulars	LF	Amount	Amount
2002/Sep. 1	Cash a/c ....dr bad debts a/c................ dr to Subba Rao a/c (being cash received from him in full and final settlement of his account)		2,500 2,500	5,000
Sep. 25	Cash a/c......................dr to bad debt recovered a/c (being bad debt recovered from Subba Rao)		1000	1000
Oct. 15	Cash a/c ....dr to bad debt a/c .... dr to Raheem a/c (being cash received in full settlement from Raheem)		500 500	1000
Nov. 10	Cash a/c ....dr to bad debt recovered a/c (being bad debts recovered from Raheem)		500	500

Compound or Combined Entry

So far we have seen transactions which involve only two accounts. Sometimes a transaction may involve more than two accounts, sometimes there may be more transactions of the same nature taking place on the same date, in such a situation, such transactions may be recorded by means of a single journal entry, instead of passing separate entries. Such an entry is called 'combine' or 'compound' or 'composite journal entry'. It may be recorded in the following three ways:
1. By debiting one account and crediting two or more accounts.
2. By debiting two or more accounts and crediting one account.
3. By debiting two or more accounts and crediting two or more accounts.

Illustration 6.11:

Journalize the following transactions:

Date	Particulars
2001/Sep. 1	Goods worth ₹ 2000 are purchased for cash and worth ₹ 3000 are purchased from Sohan
5	Paid cash to Girish ₹ 980, and he allowed a discount of ₹ 20
10	Goods sold for cash ₹ 4000, goods sold to Surender ₹ 6000
15	Sold to Arvind ₹ 2000, sold to Sawanth ₹ 4000, sold to David ₹ 6000
20	Ramana started business by investing ₹ 50,000 in cash, ₹ 40,000 in goods and ₹ 10,000 in furniture
25	A running business with the following assets and liabilities was purchased from Tarun for ₹ 1,28,000, buildings ₹ 80,000; furniture ₹ 24,000; stock ₹ 40,000; creditors ₹ 16,000

Solution: Journal entries

Date	Particulars	LF	Amount	Amount
2001/Sep. 1	Purchases a/c ………….dr to cash a/c to Sohan a/c (being goods purchased for cash and on credit from Sohan)		5,000	2,000 3,000
5	Girish a/c ………………dr to cash a/c to discount received a/c (being cash paid to Girish and discount received)		1,000	98020
10	Cash a/c……………………..dr Surender a/c ……………….dr to sales a/c (being goods sold for cash and on credit)		4,000 6,000	10,000
15	Arvind a/c…………….dr Sawanth a/c……………. dr David a/c……………….. dr to sales a/c (being goods sold on credit)		2,000 4,000 6,000	12,000
20	Cash a/c………………….dr purchases a/c…… ……….dr furniture a/c…………….dr to capital a/c (being assets introduced in the business)		50,000 40,000 10,000	1,00,000
25	Building a/c…………….dr furniture a/c…… ………..dr stock a/c………………..dr to creditors a/c to Tarun a/c (being assets and liabilities taken from Tarun)		80,000 24,000 40,000	16,000 1,28,000

Opening Entry

When a new accounting year begins, the previous year's balance in different account is brought forward into the new books of accounts. This is done by means of a journal entry called 'opening entry'. In this entry all assets accounts are debit and liabilities are credited.

Illustration 6.12:

Mr. Srikanth has the following assets and liabilities on December 31, 2006
Cash ₹ 5,000, stock of goods ₹ 45,000, furniture ₹ 10,000,
Bank loan ₹ 20,000,
Pass opening entry on January 1, 2007.

Solution: Journal entries

Date	Particulars	LF	Amount	Amount
2007/Jan. 1	Cash a/c......................dr stock a/c		5,000	
	....................dr furniture a/c...............dr		45,000	
	to bank loan a/c		10,000	
	to capital a/c (being balances brought forward			20,000
	from the previous year)			40,000

Illustration 6.13:

Journalize the following transactions in the books of Mr. Ram and Co Ltd.

Date	Particulars	Amount
2001/Jan. 4	Business commenced	5,00,000
6	Bought goods for cash	2,000
8	Sold goods for cash	3,000
10	Hired goods for cash	2,500
12	Sold goods to Kishore	1,500
14	Sold good to Ramesh	3,500
16	Purchased goods on account from Subba Rao	5,500
17	Ramesh returned goods	500
19	Returned good to Subba Rao	800
21	Brought furniture Godrej Co	10,000
23	Sold old computer	2,000
25	Paid salary	2,500
25	Paid rent	4,200
27	Received dividend from Suresh	300
28	Paid commission to Ravi	150
29	Cash deposited in bank	5,000
30	Cash withdrawn for personal use from bank	4,000
31	Withdraw cash for office use from bank	2,200
31	Received cheque from Ramesh	3000

Solution

Date	Particulars	LF	Amount	Amount
4/1/01	Cash a/c...................dr to capital a/c (being business commenced)		500000	500000
6/1/01	Purchase a/c..............dr to cash a/c (being goods purchased for cash)		2000	2000
8/1/01	Cash a/c.......................dr to sales ....a/c (being goods sold for cash)		3,000	3,000
10-/1/01	Purchases a/c ....dr to cash a/c (being goods purchased)		2,500	2,500
12/1/01	Kishore a/c....................dr to sales a/c (being goods sold on credit)		1500	1500
14/1/01	Ramesh a/c....................dr to sales a/c (being goods sold to credit)		3,500	3,500
16/1/01	Purchases a/c...............dr to Subba Rao a/c (being goods purchased on credit		5500	5500
17/1/07	Sales returned a/c............dr to Ramesh a/c (being goods returned by Ramesh)		500	500
19/1/01	Subba Rao a/c...............dr to purchase return a/c (being goods returned to Subba Rao)		800	800
21/1/01	Furniture a/c...................dr to Godrej and Co. a/c (being furniture purchased on credit)		10,000	10,000
23/1/01	Cash a/c........................dr to computer a/c (being old computer sold)		2,000	2,000
25/1/01	Salary a/c.......................dr rent a/c.........................dr to cash a/c (being salary and rent paid)		2,5004,200	6,700
27/1/01	Cash a/c..........................dr to dividend a/c (being dividend received from Suresh)		300	300
28/1/01	Commission a/c..................dr to Ravi a/c (being commission paid)		150	150
29/1/01	Bank a/c.........................dr to cash a/c (being cash deposited into bank)		5,000	5,000
30/1/01	Drawing a/c....................dr to bank a/c (being cash withdrawn from bank for personal use)		4,000	4,000
31/1/01	Cash a/c.........................dr to bank a/c (being cash withdrawn from bank for office use)		2,200	2,200
31/1/01	Bank a/c ....dr to Ramesh a/c (being cheque received from Ramesh)		3,000	3,000

Illustration 6.14:

Journalize the following transactions in the books of Mr Nigam.

Date	Particulars
2001/Jan. 1	Assets: cash in hand ₹ 1000, cash at bank ₹ 5,000, machinery ₹ 10,000, Furniture ₹ 2,000; stock of goods ₹ 3,000, due from Suresh ₹ 1,000, due from Mahesh ₹ 1,500, due from Raheem ₹ 2000 liabilities, loan ₹ 5,000, amount due to Kamlesh ₹ 2,000.
4	Received from Mahesh by cheque ₹ 1,500
5	Cash deposited with bank ₹ 1,500
6	Withdrew from bank for business ₹ 1,000
8	Withdrew from bank for personal use ₹ 500
10	Loan repaid ₹ 5,000
12	Suresh account was settled with a discount of ₹ 100
14	Paid to Kamalesh in full settlement of his account and he allowed us a discount of ₹ 100
15	An amount written off as bad debts in the year 1999 was received ₹ 500
16	Raheem become insolvent and only 50 paise in a rupee could be received
18	Purchase good from Kavitha ₹ 5,100
19	Sold goods to Anil ₹ 3,550
20	Paid to Kavitha by cheque ₹ 5,000 and she allowed a discount of ₹ 100
25	Anil returned defective goods worth of ₹ 550
27	Received commission from Kapil ₹ 1000, received dividend on shares ₹ 1500,
28	Sold goods to Sunil for cash, the list price of these goods were ₹ 2500, trade discount of 5% and a cash discount of 1% were allowed to him.
29	Paid rent: ₹ 5,000; salary ₹ 20,000, commission ₹ 1200
30	Withdrew from bank for office use ₹ 25,000
31	Received cheque from Anil in full settlement of his account ₹ 3,000

Solution: Journal entries in the books of Mr. Nigam.

Date	Particulars	LF	Amount (dr)	Amount (cr)
2001/Jan. 1	Cash a/c................dr bank a/c................dr machinery a/c............. dr furniture a/c ....dr stock a/c ....dr debtors a/c................dr to loan a/c to creditors a/c to capital a/c (being assets and liabilities brought into the new books) capital = assets – liabilities		1,000 5,000 10,000 2,000 3000 4,500	5,000 2,000 18,500
4	Bank a/c................dr to Mahesh a/c (being cheque received from Mahesh)		1,500	1,500
5	Bank a/c................dr to cash a/c (being cash received and deposited into the bank)		1,500	!,500

(Contd...)

(Contd...)

Date	Particulars	LF	Amount (dr)	Amount (cr)
6	cash a/c.....................dr to bank a/c (being cash withdrew for office use)		1,000	1,000
8	drawings a/c...............dr to bank a/c (being cash withdrew for personal use)		500	500
10	loan a/c.....................dr to cash a/c (being loan repaid)	5,000	5,000	
12	cash a/c.....................dr discount a/c................dr to Suresh a/c (being cash received and discount allowed to him)		900 100	1,000
14	Kamalesh a/c ....dr to cash a/c to discount a/c (being cash paid and discount received)		2,000	1,900 100
15	Cash a/c.....................dr to bad debts recovery a/c (being bad debts recovered)		500	500
16	cash a/c.....................dr bad debts a/c ....dr to Raheem a/c (being cash received and bad debts recorded)		1,000 1,000	2,000
18	purchases a/c ....dr to Kavitha a/c (being goods purchased)		5,100	5,100
19	Anil a/c.....................dr to sales a/c (being goods sold on credit)		3,550	3,550
20	Kavitha a/c...................dr to bank a/c to discount a/c (being cheque paid and discount received)		5,100	5,000 100
25	Sales retune a/c...........dr to Anil a/c (being goods returned)		5,50	5,50
27	cash a/c.....................dr to commission a/c to dividend a/c (being commission and dividend received)		2,500	1,000 1,500
28	Cash a/c.....................dr discount a/c................dr to sales a/c (being goods sold for cash at a trade discount of 5% and a cash discount of 1% allowed)		2351* 24	2375

(Contd...)

(Contd...)

Date	Particulars	LF	Amount (dr)	Amount (cr)
29	Rent a/c............................dr salaries a/c .... dr commission a/c...........dr to cash a/c (being rent, salary and commission paid)		5,000 20,000	1,200 26,200
30	Cash a/c........................dr to bank a/c (being cash withdrawn for office use)		25,000	25,000
31	Bank a/c.......................dr to Anil a/c (being cheque received from Anil in full settlement of his account)		3,000	3,000

Working notes*

Trade discount

₹ 2500*5/100 = ₹ 125

₹ 2,500 – ₹ 125 = 2375

Cash discount

₹ 2375 *1/100 = 23.74 or 24 ₹

₹ 2375 – ₹ 24 = ₹ 2351

Ledger Account

Recording every transaction in the accounts involved is the main work of the book-keeping. From the above sections we have seen how the transactions are recorded in the journal with the view to know which account to be debited and which to be credited. Thus journal entry simply functions as guidelines to record transactions on debit and credit side of the concerned account. These guidelines to be followed and accounts must be entered in the ledger.

The ledger is the chief book of accounts. All business transactions are recorded in the first instance in the journal but they must find their place ultimately in the ledger account in a duly classified form. Ledger is also called the book of final entry because all the transactions that are entered in the journal must be transferred to ledger.

Therefore, ledger is the book which contains various accounts. In other words, ledger is the set of accounts of the business enterprise whether real, nominal or personal. Ledger is the register having a number of pages which are serially numbered. One account is usually assigned on one page of the ledger, it may be carried in the form of a bound ledger or a loose leaf ledger.

The process of transferring accounts from journal to ledger is called "posting".

Posting

The term 'posting' means transferring the debit and credit items from the journal to their respective account in the ledger. It should be noted that the exact name of the account used in the journal should be carried to ledger. Posting can be done any time but it should be completed before the financial statements are prepared.

Rules Regarding Posting

The following rules must be observed while posting transactions in the ledger from the journal.

1. The pages of the ledger consecutively numbered and one page is allotted to one account. This means that there should be a separate account for every account that is mentioned in the journal. For example, salaries account, sales account, sale return account, purchase account, purchase return account, cash account, etc.

2. The title of the account or the name of the account should be prominently written on the top of the page assigned to it.

The word 'dr' should be written on the left side of the account and the word 'cr' should be written on the right side of the account and the headings of the columns should be filled.

On the debit side (left side) every entry in the 'particulars' column must begin with the word 'to'. On the credit side (right side), every entry in the 'particulars', column must begin with the word 'by'.

The first line in the journal entry must be posted on the debit side of the ledger account and the second line on the credit side. However, a reference should be made of the other account which has been credited in the journal. For example, for salaries paid, the salaries account should be debited in the ledger, but at the same time a reference should be given of the cash account which has been credited in the journal.

Write the amount in the debit column of the journal in the 'amount' column on the debit side of the ledger account and the amount in the credit column of the journal in the 'amount' column on the credit side of the account.

Sub-division of Ledger

In the small business houses, it is possible to keep all the account in one ledger. But as the business grows, the ledger can be divided into various sub-division from the viewpoint of convenience and simplicity. The usual division of ledger is shown below.

General ledger: This contains all the accounts other than debtors and creditors. That is, the ledger which contains all the real and nominal accounts. It includes assets account, goods account, liabilities other than the creditors and debtors. It is also called impersonal ledger or main ledger or principal ledger.

Books of accounts

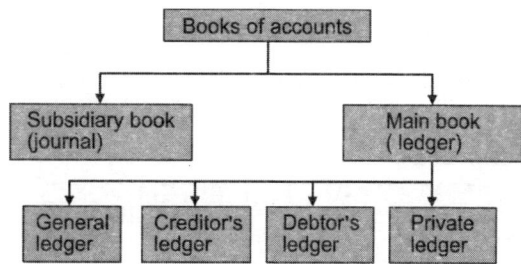

Creditor's ledger: This ledger contains personal accounts of suppliers or creditors from whom the goods were purchased on credit. This ledger is known as purchase ledger or bought ledger.

Debtor's ledger: This ledger contains the personal accounts of the customers or debtors to whom the goods are sold on credit. This ledger is also known as sales ledger or sold ledger.

Private ledger: This ledger contains the personal account of the proprietor, i.e. the capital account, current account, drawings account, etc. and final accounts (trading, profit and loss account and balance sheet).

Proforma of ledger

Particulars	JF	Date	Particulars	JF	Amount

Illustration 6.13: From the above, the following has been taken to explain ledger postings'

Date	Particulars	JF	Amount	Date	Particulars	JF	Amount
04/01/2001	to capital a/c		5,00,000	06/01/2001	by purchases a/c		2,000
08/01/2001	" sales a/c		3,000	10/01/2010	" purchases a/c		2,500
23/01/2001	" computer a/c		2,000	25/01/2001	" rent a/c		4,200

(Contd...)

(Contd...)

Date	Particulars	JF	Amount	Date	Particulars	JF	Amount
27/01/2001	dividend a/c		300		salary a/c		2,500
31/01/2001	bank a/c		2,200		bank a/c		5,000
				31/01/2001	by balance c/d		4,91,300
							5,07,500
			5,07,500				
01/02/2001	to balance b/d		4,91,300				

Capital a/c

Date	Particulars	JF	Amount	Date	Particulars	JF	Amount
31/01/2001	to bal c/d		5,00,000	04/01/2001	by cash a/c		5,00,000
			5,00,000				5,00,000
				01/02/2001	by bal b/d		5,00,000

Purchase a/c

Date	Particulars	JF	Amount	Date	Particulars	JF	Amount
06/01/2001	to cash a/c		2,000	31/01/2001	by bal c/d		10,000
10/1/2001	to cash a/c		2,500				
16/1/2001	to Subba Rao a/c		5,500				
	to bal b/d		10,000				10,000
01/02/2001			10,000				

Sales a/c

Date	Particulars	JF	Amount	Date	Particulars	JF	Amount
31/01/2001	to bal c/d		8,000	08/01/2001	by cash a/c		3,000
				12/01/2001	by Kishore a/c		1,500
				14/01/2001	by Ramesh a/c		3,500
			8,000				8,000
				01/02/2001	by bal b/d		8,000

Kishore a/c

Date	Particulars	JF	Amount	Date	Particulars	JF	Amount
12/01/2001	to sales a/c		1,500	31/01/2001	by bal c/d		1,500
			1,500				1,500
01/02/2001	to bal b/d		1,500				

Ramesh a/c

Date	Particulars	JF	Amount	Date	Particulars	JF	Amount
14/01/2001	to sales a/c		3,500	17/01/2001	by sales return a/c		500
				31/01/2001	by bank a/c		3,000
			3,500				3,500

Subba Rao a/c

Date	Particulars	JF	Amount	Date	Particulars	JF	Amount
19/01/2001	to purchase return a/c		800	16/01/2001	by purchases a/c		5,500
31/01/2001	to bal c/d		4,700				
			5,500				5,500
				01/02/2001	by bal b/d		4,700

Sales return a/c

Date	Particulars	JF	Amount	Date	Particulars	JF	Amount
17/01/2001	to Ramesh a/c		500	31/01/2001	by bal c/d		500
			500				500
01/02/2001	to bal b/d		500				

Purchase return a/c

Date	Particulars	JF	Amount	Date	Particulars	JF	Amount
31/01/2001	to bal c./d		800	19/01/2001	by Subba Rao a/c		800
			800				800
				01/02/2001	by bal b/d		800

Furniture a/c

Date	Particulars	JF	Amount	Date	Particulars	JF	Amount
21/01/2001	to Godrej and Co a/c		10,000	31/01/2001	by bal c/d		10,000
	to bal b/d		10,000				
01/02/2001			10,000				10,000

Godrej and Co a/c

Date	Particulars	JF	Amount	Date	Particulars	JF	Amount
1/01/2001	to bal c/d		10,000	21/01/2001	by furniture a/c		10,000
							10,000
			10,000	01/02/2001	by bal b/d		10,000

Computer a/c

Date	Particulars	JF	Amount	Date	Particulars	JF	Amount
31/01/2001	to bal c/d		2,000	23/01/2001	by cash a/c		2,000
			2,000				2,000
				01/02/2001	by bal. b/d		2,000

Rent a/c

Date	Particulars	JF	Amount	Date	Particulars	JF	Amount
25/01/2001	to cash a/c		4,200	31/01/2001	by bal c/d		4,200
			4,200				4,200
01/02/2001	to bal b/d		4,200				

Salary a/c

Date	Particulars	JF	Amount	Date	Particulars	JF	Amount
25/01/2001	to cash a/c		2,500	31/01/2001	by bal c/d		2,500
							2,500
			2,500				
01/02/2001	to bal b/d		2,500				

Dividend a/c

Date	Particulars	JF	Amount	Date	Particulars	JF	Amount
31/01/2001	to bal c/d		300	27/01/2001	by cash a/c		300
			300				300
				01/02/2001	to bal b/d		300

Commission a/c

Date	Particulars	JF	Amount	Date	Particulars	JF	Amount
28/01/2001	to ravi a/c		150	31/01/2001	by bal c/d		150
			150				150
01/02/2001	to bal b/d		150				

Bank a/c

Date	Particulars	JF	Amount	Date	Particulars	JF	Amount
29/01/2001	to cash a/c		5,000	30/01/2001	by drawing a/c		4,000
31/01/2001	to ramesh a/c		3,000	31/01/2001	by cash a/c		2,200
				31/01/2001	by bal c/d		1,800
			8000				8000
01/02/2001	to bal b/d		1,800				

Ravi a/c

Date	Particulars	JF	Amount	Date	Particulars	JF	Amount
31/01/2001	to bal c/d		150	28/01/2001 s	by commission a/c		150
			150		by bal b/d		150
				01/02/2001			150

Drawing a/c

Date	Particulars	JF	Amount	Date	Particulars	JF	Amount
30/01/2001	to bank a/c		4,000	31/01/2001	by bal c/d		4,000
			4,000				
01/02/2001	to bal b/d		4,000				4,000

References

Ashok Narkar, *Bookkeeping and Accountancy*, Reliable publications, Mumbai.

C.C. Rama Gopal, *Accounting for Managers*, New Age Publications, pp. 335–337.

Dr. Jawahar Lal, *Accounting for Management*, Himalaya Publications.

Dr. S.N. Maheswari, *An Introduction to Accountancy*, Vikas Publishing House, New Delhi, 9th edition, pp. 1.3–1.6, 1.18–1.22.

Elements of Commerce and Bookkeeping, Vikram Series.

7

Information Technology in Healthcare

GVRK Acharynlu

INTRODUCTION

Information technology (IT) has the potential to improve the quality, safety, and efficiency of healthcare. Diffusion of IT in healthcare is generally low (varying, however, with the application and setting) but surveys indicate that providers plan to increase their investments. Drivers of investment in IT include the promise of quality and efficiency gains. Barriers include the cost and complexity of IT implementation, which often necessitates significant work process and cultural changes. Certain characteristics of the healthcare market including payment policies that reward volume rather than quality, and a fragmented delivery system can also pose barriers to IT adoption. Given IT's potential, both the private and public sectors have engaged in numerous efforts to promote its use within and across healthcare settings. Additional steps could include financial incentives (e.g. payment policy or loans) and expanded efforts to standardize records formats, nomenclature, and communication protocols to enhance interoperability. However, any policy to stimulate further investment must be carefully considered because of the possibility of unintended consequences.

By providing new ways for providers and their patients to readily access and use health information, information technology (IT) has the potential to improve the quality, safety, and efficiency of healthcare. However, relatively a few healthcare providers have fully adopted IT. Low diffusion is due partly to the complexity of IT investment, which goes beyond acquiring technology to changing work processes and cultures, and ensuring that physicians, nurses, and other staff use it. In addition, certain aspects of the market such as payment policies that reward volume rather than quality and the fragmentation of care delivery do not promote IT investment, and may hinder it. Because of its potential, policy makers need to better understand how information technology is diffusing across providers, whether action to spur further adoption is needed, and if so, what steps might be taken. Any policy to stimulate further investment must be carefully considered because of possible unintended consequences such as implementation failures due to organizations' inability to make the necessary cultural changes. This chapter is a first step in increasing our understanding of the current state of IT in the healthcare industry.

Despite considerable attention to the topic, much remains unknown about the role of IT in the healthcare setting. What types of IT are being used? What is the link between use of IT and quality improvements? How much investment have hospitals and physicians already made in information technology, and in what kinds? What factors drive IT investments (e.g. financial returns, quality improvement goals, other factors)? What factors hinder IT investments and implementation (e.g. work flow changes, lack of compatibility with other IT, costs)? What current steps are being taken by public and private entities to encourage further diffusion of IT? What additional actions might make sense?

Delivering quality healthcare requires providers and patients to integrate complex information from many different sources. Thus, increasing the ability of physicians, nurses, clinical technicians, and others to readily access and use the right information about their patients should improve care. The ability for patients to obtain information to better manage their condition and to communicate with the health system could also improve the efficiency and quality of care. This potential to improve care makes broader diffusion of IT desirable.

The larger healthcare market poses additional barriers to investment in IT. Payment systems that tie reimbursement to the volume of services delivered, for example, may penalize providers who improve quality in ways that result in fewer units of service. To the extent that IT investments lead to reduced volume, many who make the investment will not reap all of the benefits. Systems that integrate care across settings tend to be more advanced users of IT because they are able to capture some of these efficiencies. In addition to barriers posed by payment systems, a fragmented delivery system leads to redundant investments by multiple providers who lose the benefit of economies of scale. Although this aspect of our delivery system is a barrier to adoption, widespread use of IT could help providers coordinate care across settings, overcoming some of the problems of fragmentation.

Both the private and public sectors have engaged in numerous efforts to promote use of IT within healthcare institutions and across care delivery settings.

Information systems for all intents and purposes brought automation of various processes to the healthcare industry. Now doctors have the ability to do sonograms to determine the sex of a baby or to insert a heart in a patient using a computer. Thirty years ago this was not even a consideration. The health-care field used to be a safe, cozy profession with hospitals and clinics living on their own little island. With the advancement of IT, com-munication has been enhanced threefold. Clinics have the ability to share patient infor-mation with a hospital at the push of a button and vice versa. Instead of walking across a large hospital to talk to another doctor, nurses can email, instant messaging (IM), or send patient information to a doctor's PDA without having to leave a workstation or the patient's rooms (Table 7.1).

Table 7.1: Examples of health information technology for hospitals and physicians

Type of information technology	Applications
Hospitals	
Administrative and financial	Billing
	General ledger
	Cost accounting systems
	Patient registration
	Personnel and payroll
	Electronic materials management
Clinical	Computerized provider order entry for drugs, lab tests, procedures
	Electronic health record
	Picture archiving and communication systems for filmless imaging
	Results reporting of laboratory and other tests
	Clinical decision support systems
	Prescription drug fulfillment, error-alert, transcriptions

(Contd...)

Table 7.1: Examples of health information technology for hospitals and physicians (Contd...)

Type of information technology	Applications
Infrastructure	Electronic monitoring of patients in intensive care units
	Desktop, laptop, cart-based, and tablet computers
	Servers and networks
	Wireless networks
	Voice recognition systems for transcription, physician orders, and medical records
	Bar-coding technology for drugs, medical devices, and inventory control
	Information security systems
Physicians	
Administrative and financial	Billing
	Accounting
	Scheduling
	Personnel and payroll
Clinical	Online references (drug compendia and clinical guidelines)
	Receiving lab results and other clinical information online
	Electronic prescribing computerized provider order entry clinical decision support systems electronic health record
	E-mail communication with patients
Infrastructure	Desktop and laptop computers
	Handheld technology
Servers and network	

HEALTHCARE INFORMATION TECHNOLOGY (HIT)

Healthcare information technology (HIT) is a new discipline that promotes comprehensive management of medical information and its secure exchange between healthcare consumers and providers. In general, healthcare IT is expected to enhance healthcare quality by improving individual patient care, preventing medical errors, reducing healthcare costs through administrative efficiencies and decreased paperwork and expanding access to affordable care. Also, public health officials are counting on healthcare IT workers to assist in early detection of infectious disease outbreaks around the country, improve tracking of chronic diseases and decrease patient care costs.

Health information technology (HIT) consists of an enormously diverse set of technologies for transmitting and managing health information for use by consumers, providers, payers, insurers, and other groups with an interest in health and healthcare. In general it includes the capture, storage, use and/or transmission of health information through electronic processes.

Health information technology (HIT) provides the umbrella framework to describe the comprehensive management of health information and its secure exchange between consumers, providers, government and quality entities, and insurers. Health information technology (HIT) is in general increasingly viewed as the most promising tool for improving the overall quality, safety and efficiency of the health delivery system. Broad and consistent utilization of HIT will:
- Improve healthcare quality
- Prevent medical errors

- Reduce healthcare costs
- Increase administrative efficiencies
- Decrease paperwork
- Expand access to affordable care

Health information technology (HIT) is "the application of information processing involving both computer hardware and software that deals with the storage, retrieval, sharing, and use of healthcare information, data, and knowledge for communication and decision making". Technology is a broad concept that deals with a species' usage and knowledge of tools and crafts, and how it affects a species' ability to control and adapt to its environment. However, a strict definition is elusive; "technology" can refer to material objects of use to humanity, such as machines, hardware or utensils, but can also encompass broader themes, including systems, methods of organization, and techniques. For HIT, technology represents computers and communications attributes that can be networked to build systems for moving health information. Informatics is yet another integral aspect of HIT.

COMPONENTS OF HIT

There are many components of HIT which include:

Applications: These are the "programs" that are used to perform HIT functions. These applications include but are not limited to: Patient Registries, Accounting/Practice Management Systems (PMS), CPOE/CDS (Computerized Physician Order Entry with Clinical Decision Support), Prescribing, Electronic Medical Records (EMRs), Electronic Health Records (EHRs), Patient Health Records (PHRs), Results Reporting, Electronic Documentation, Appointment Scheduling, Patient Kiosks, Telemedicine, Interface Engines.

Electronic Medical Record: "An electronic record of health-related information on an individual that can be created, gathered, managed, and consulted by authorized clinicians and staff within one healthcare organization."

Electronic Health Record: "An electronic record of health-related information on an individual that conforms to nationally recognized interoperability standards and that can be created, managed, and consulted by authorized clinicians and staff across more than one healthcare organization.

Personal Health Record: "An electronic record of health-related information on an individual that conforms to nationally recognized interoperability standards and that can be drawn from multiple sources while being managed, shared, and controlled by the individual."

Health Information Exchange: "The electronic movement of health-related information among organizations according to nationally recognized standards."

Health Information Organization: "An organization that oversees and governs the exchange of health-related information among organizations according to nationally recognized standards."

Regional Health Information Organization: "A health information organization that brings together healthcare stakeholders within a defined geographic area and governs health information exchange among them for the purpose of improving health and care in that community."

Communications Standards: These are the various sets of standards that are necessary in order for HIT systems to communicate with each other in a uniform manner. These standards encompass

Messaging Standards

HL7, ADT, NCPDP, X12, DICOM, UB92, HCFA, ASTM, EDIFACT, etc.

Messaging standards are the form and structure that is required for the information to move and be tracked from one system to another; and

Coding Standards

LOINC, ICD-9, CPT, NDC, RxNorm, Snomed CT, etc.

Coding standards are the form and structure of the procedure codes that are necessary to communicate what procedure was performed for a particular patient during a visit.

It is important to note that a "user" does not need to know what all of these codes and structures are, however, it is important to realize that these codes and structures are necessary in order for systems to work together towards the goal of being "interoperable".

Interoperability is an important concept in HIT. Without interoperability the healthcare system will not be able to benefit to the fullest extent possible from the implementation of HIT. Interoperability is the *ability of a system to work with or use the parts or equipment of another system*. In order for the healthcare system to reap the benefits of widely used HIT systems it will be important for those systems to communicate with each other and share vital information.

HIPAA Security/Privacy: This plays an important role in all exchange of health information using HIT. Healthcare providers, institutions and vendors must comply with HIPAA in any and all exchange of personal health information (PHI). There is also much debate at the present time with regard to HIPAA being or not being stringent enough to protect privacy in an all HIT world. A balance will need to be developed that allows for healthcare information to be exchanged in order to provide improved quality of care for the patient and still maintain his/her confidentiality.

Devices: these are the various hardware components that make HIT work and include such things as: desktops, laptops, tablet PCs, servers, mice, pens, bar coding devices and more. As HIT continues to develop and we continue to exchange information with our providers we will see in-home devices such as blood pressure monitors and scales have the ability to transmit data directly to our provider for him/her to review and monitor our care. This is available and is occurring now.

USE OF HIT

HIT is useful in a number of areas, the foremost being quality of care. It is utilized to improve quality care to the patients that health centers serve. Being able to monitor groups of patients with chronic conditions, receive alerts automatically and in a timely manner when lab values are abnormal, having clinical decision support reminders pop up to inform a provider of a recommended treatment or intervention when the patient is in front of the provider, providers being informed of possible adverse reactions or drug interactions when they are prescribing, and pharmacists not having to decipher a physician's hand-writing are only some of the advantages of HIT that will assist to improve quality care. On a broader scale when provider offices, hospitals, clinics and all healthcare providers are able to share information about a patients care a truly team approach to care is made possible with elimination of many of the repeat procedures that are now required because basic patient care information is not available.

ELECTRONIC HEALTH RECORD (EHR)

An electronic health record (EHR) is a real-time, point-of-care, patient-centric information resource for clinicians that represents a major domain of health information technology (HIT). More recently, an EHR has been defined as "a longitudinal electronic record of patient health information, produced by encounters in one or more care settings".

It includes patient information such as a problem list, orders, medications, vital signs, past medical history, notes, laboratory results, and radiology reports, among other things. The EHR generates a complete record of a clinical patient encounter or episode of care and underpins care-related activities such as decision-making, quality management, and clinical reporting. Some distinguish between the terms EHR and electronic medical record (EMR), with EMR focusing on ambulatory care systems. However, in practice, the terms are interchangeable. The term EHR relates to computerized patient health records stored within and among institutions.

Health IT encompasses a broad array of new technologies designed to manage and share health-related information. The most basic type of health information technology is a system that electronically collects, stores and organizes health information about patients. When properly implemented, such a system can help coordinate patient care, reduce medical errors and improve administrative efficiency.

Some call the information collected an electronic health record (EHR); others call it an electronic medical record (EMR). Though some health informatics experts make a distinction between EHRs and EMRs, these terms are often used interchangeably in the media. Efforts are underway to develop consensus definitions for these terms and others. For convenience, we will use the term "electronic health record," or "EHR" to refer broadly to systems that collect and store patients' medical information in digital form. An EHR differs from a personal health record (PHR), which is a health record that is "owned" and maintained by an individual patient, rather than by payers or providers.

Electronic record systems come in a variety of shapes and sizes. Some collect and share patient information only within a certain institution or within a certain provider group, while others are integrated into larger information networks. The capabilities of EHR systems and the extent to which they are integrated into provider practices also vary. "Fully functional" EHR systems collect and store patient data, supply patient data to providers on request, permit physicians to enter patient care orders, and assist providers in making evidence-based clinical decisions.

Another technology is known as computerized physician order entry (CPOE), an important part of a fully functional EHR system. This allows physicians to order prescription drugs and laboratory tests digitally, thereby eliminating errors associated with illegible handwritten prescriptions. CPOE systems check for the accuracy of prescription orders, flagging any orders that appear extreme. One study concluded that CPOE systems for prescriptions could reduce preventable medication errors by 55 percent because they ensure, at a minimum, that orders are complete and legible.

The process of automating healthcare records includes six major stages: creating infrastructure, transferring scheduling, transferring billing, automating medical records, putting it all together and implementing software that can analyze a patient's health issues and identify trends. A discussion of each of these stages is as follows

- *Stage 1: IT infrastructure:* Healthcare is an industry unlike any other. A physician's office needs to interact with and be connected to patients, their employers, insurance companies, state agencies, federal agencies and pharmacies. For decades, phones and fax machines facilitated those connections. Although automating this process further will save time and money for the patients and insurance companies, it will create additional costs for medical professionals. Exchanging information using specialized software backed by massive computers, servers and high-speed internet connections costs money. Medical professionals also must contend with new federal laws forcing them to save more patient information and, at the same time, protect the security of that information. This puts additional pressure on medical professionals to invest in their computer networks and the people who run them. The tasks associated with this first step focus on the installation of computers, servers and medical software. Workers hired to perform these tasks will have varying education levels along with specialized computer and software training.

- *Stage 2: Scheduling:* Along with appointment scheduling automation, this step includes automation of general office management. Most hospitals and physicians' offices now use computers and basic software packages to record and store some patient and scheduling information. The workers hired for this step need basic computer literacy training.
- *Stage 3: Billing:* Hospitals, clinics and physicians' offices tend to have billing specialists who understand the medical codes needed to exchange information with insurance companies, medicare, medicaid and employers.
- *Stage 4: Medical records:* Converting the medical histories of millions of patients from old mainframe computers or paper records to modern electronic files is a daunting task with multiple legal constraints regarding privacy and data backups. Billing records include basic coding, whereas medical records contain a more complex list to track patient histories and disease trends. Such complexity requires workers with high-level training in both medical practice and information technology.
- *Stage 5: Putting it all together:* This step pulls together the infrastructure, patient scheduling, billing, medical records, prescriptions and business processes. Physicians can buy and install a software program to move from paper records to electronic records, but the move changes the processes of a doctor's office.
- *Stage 6: Analytics:* A key benefit of moving to electronic medical records is the ability to install and run software programs that analyze patient health problems, identify trends and more accurately track billing problems.

TECHNOLOGY IN HEALTHCARE

Technology in healthcare is going to shape the health delivery process globally. Technology in healthcare can start as simply as taking a phone call to a doctor, up to building a seamlessly integrated healthcare workflow. On the one hand, IT functions as an enabler in delivering faster and more accurate medical information to end users and at the same time reducing the manual labor-intensive process. Technology will probably never be able to replace a doctor's judgment or a nurse's touch. But it can help tip the balance by improving workflow and making manual and routine tasks more efficient. The automation of tasks such as temperature taking will free up time for other nursing tasks. Also, with a rapid decrease in hardware size and increase in mobility and connectivity, doctors will always know the technological change.

Technology will increasingly be deployed right next to the clinical care and the patient in a number of ways. Using biometrics, RFID, and barcode to establish patient identity before treatment administration. Bedside clinical information displays to keep patients engaged in their own care. Computer navigation via integration of a multitude of medical imaging datasets through the real-time display of anatomy during surgery. This will be taken further via telemedicine, head up displays and hepatics feedback technologies. Knowledge bases will increasingly be deployed to bring about best evidence healthcare. Evidence-based driven guidelines will bring about rule-based diagnosis and treatment. Algorithm-driven diagnosis is already well tried and tested and will be implemented in EMR to bring about cost-effective diagnosis and increasingly, the same will apply to the treatment of chronic diseases.

With the increasing use of electronic medical records, there are many advantages to their use in patient care. When looking at electronic medical records and patient safety, using this technology can reduce the amount of medication errors and better organize patient information. The use of remote health monitoring through telemedicine has changed the way in which healthcare professionals are able to provide care to people living in rural locations. The professional will use a variety of telemedicine remote monitoring tools to monitor the person's health.

With affordable wireless communications technology and availability of inexpensive wireless-based laptops, portables and CD-ROM based problem resolution and diagnostic technology, the value of wireless technology is clearly seen in improving service productivity, efficiency and profitability. Though healthcare organizations have been slow to embrace wireless technology, more and more organisations are finding that they can save money and improve care with this technology, and as it eliminates the need for wired connections, it increases mobility of the patients and healthcare professionals, invariably improving treatment outcomes.

The benefits of wireless technology in healthcare could be far reaching if used in an appropriate manner. Doctors could store information in real-time, access patient records and medical reference materials from the internet, send e-mails through handheld devices that are connected to a server.

Wireless networks would allow doctors in a hospital, with their hand held devices, to stay in touch with each other at all times, arrange their schedules instantaneously and receive results of procedures and investigations not just at any time but also almost anywhere within the hospital's vicinity.

This would lead to better and more efficient care. Doctors in remote areas can be equipped with a hand held device and be able to send details of their patients from their homes to a hospital's database, receive the results of any investigations or procedures done and access the Internet for any medical reference no matter where he is and what time it is. This could be especially useful when applied in medical disaster response where communications is frequently inadequate and medical responders need access to adequate, effective and reliable communication.

The following technologies and terms are often included in discussions of information technology in healthcare.

- *Electronic health record (EHR):* EHRs were originally envisioned as an electronic file cabinet for patient data from various sources (eventually integrating text, voice, images, handwritten notes, etc.). Now they are generally viewed as part of an automated order-entry and patient-tracking system providing real-time access to patient data, as well as a continuous longitudinal record of their care.

- *Computerized provider order entry (CPOE):* CPOE in its basic form is typically a medication ordering and fulfillment system. More advanced CPOE will also include lab orders, radiology studies, procedures, discharges, transfers, and referrals.

- *Clinical decision support system (CDSS):* CDSS provides physicians and nurses with real-time diagnostic and treatment recommendations. The term covers a variety of technologies ranging from simple alerts and prescription drug interaction warnings to full clinical pathways and protocols. CDSS may be used as part of CPOE and EHR.

- *Picture archiving and communications system (PACS):* This technology captures and integrates diagnostic and radiological

images from various devices (e.g. X-ray, MRI, computed tomography scan), stores them, and disseminates them to a medical record, a clinical data repository, or other points of care.
- *Barcoding:* Barcoding in a healthcare environment is similar to brocade scanning in other environments: An optical scanner is used to electronically capture information encoded on a product. Initially, it will be used for medication (for example, matching drugs to patients by using bar codes on both the medications and patients' arm bracelets), but other applications may be pursued, such as medical devices, lab, and radiology.
- *Radio frequency identification (RFID):* This technology tracks patients throughout the hospital, and links lab and medication tracking through a wireless communications system. It is neither mature nor widely available, but may be an alternative to bar coding.
- *Automated dispensing machines (ADMs):* This technology distributes medication doses.
- *Electronic materials management (EMM):* Healthcare organizations use EMM to track and manage inventory of medical supplies, pharmaceuticals, and other materials. This technology is similar to enterprise resource planning systems used outside of healthcare.
- *Interoperability:* This concept refers to electronic communication among organizational so that the data in one IT system can be incorporated into another. Discussions of interoperability focus on development of standards for content and messaging, among other areas, and development of adequate security and privacy safeguards

QUALITY AND HEALTH INFORMATION TECHNOLOGY

One of the primary motivators for adopting many clinical health IT applications is the belief that they improve the quality of patient care. Yet, further research is needed to better document and understand the link between IT and quality, including the types of quality problems, information technology can be used to solve and implementation strategies to ensure that quality objectives are met.

Quality healthcare relies on physicians, nurses, patients and their families, and others having the right information at the right time and using it to make the right decisions.
Yet the health information needed to make these decisions changes frequently, the guidelines and clinical evidence continually evolve, as does knowledge about the condition of the patient. IT may provide a tool to store, integrate, and update this information base.

Beyond improving care in individual settings, health IT also has the potential to address the problems presented by a fragmented delivery system. Most patients receive care from many desperate providers. The primary means of coordination is often through discussion with the patients about what other services they have received and what the other providers thought about their conditions. Information technology used across settings could create a "virtual" integrated delivery system without requiring formal mergers or affiliations.

Information Technology Priorities for Hospitals

- Upgrading security protocols
- Reducing medical errors, promoting patient safety
- Replacing, upgrading inpatient clinical systems
- Implementing wireless systems
- Implementing electronic health records
- Upgrading network infrastructure
- Designing process, workflow
- Improving the IT department
- Bar-coded medication management
- Electronic health records

- Clinical information systems
- CPOE
- PACS
- Enterprise-wide clinical information sharing
- Point-of-care decision support

Information Technology in Physicians' Practices

Like hospitals, physicians are more likely to use IT for administrative functions (such as billing, claims submission, and scheduling) than for clinical functions (such as electronic health records, clinical decision support, access to formularies or other references, or computerized provider order entry). Physicians must also invest in infrastructure to support their IT applications.

- Billing and claims submission
- Scheduling and patient appointment reminders
- Lab orders and results
- Communication with hospital
- Claims status
- Patient records
- Patient eligibility
- Diagnostic imaging and radiology
- Referrals
- Procurement of supplies
- Charge capture
- Clinical protocols and pathways
- Prescribing
- Telemedicine

Linking Healthcare Providers Through Information Technology

For information technology to become widespread, individual providers must adopt it. Once that happens, connecting them electronically could bring additional benefits. Healthcare today involves considerable sharing of information among providers such as physicians' offices, hospitals, imaging centers, and clinical laboratories, as well as among providers and payers. A healthcare information infrastructure would provide the networks and standards to allow providers within a community to share information electronically. In addition, patients could use it to access their medical records or other healthcare information from all providers. A primary focus of those advocating a healthcare information infrastructure is development of standards for messaging so that one IT system can communicate with another.

TELEMEDICINE

Telemedicine is the use of telecommunications technology for medical diagnosis and patient care when the provider and client are separated by distance. Telemedicine includes pathology, radiology, and patient consultation from the distance.

The term an umbrella encompasses various technologies as part of a coherent health service information resource management program. Telemedicine is the capture, display, storage and retrieval of medical images and data towards the creation of a computerized patient record and managed care. Advantages include move information, not patients or providers; enter data once in a healthcare network; network quality specialty healthcare to isolated locations; and build from hands-on experience.

Different Tasks Doctor can do with Telemedicine

- Consult with patients from a distance; means that specialists do not have to travel to all regions to provide care
- Can perform robotic surgery
- Sending of digital X-rays; blood test results by e-mail
- Online 24-hour health consultant centre using website and e-mail
- Questions and answers using e-mail
- Use of forums and discussion groups

Different Hardware and Software Requirements for Successful Telemedicine

- Good Internet connection with high broadband width

- Video conferencing equipment, e.g. webcam, speakers and microphone; video conferencing software (for consultations)
- E-mail accounts and websites hosted on web servers
- Digital X-ray machines
- Robotic surgery equipment
- Electronic medical records which are compatible or central record system.

Telemedicine is the transfer of electronic medical data (i.e. high resolution images, sounds, sometimes video briefings and records of specific operations and patient record) from the remote areas to a center where the experts or well-equipped hospitals are available. Taking advantage of telecommunication, medical electronics, and Information technologies, telemedicine acts as a potential source to reduce healthcare expense, to improve healthcare service in remote areas, and to support modern home healthcare, etc. Telemedicine can deliver healthcare services, where distance is the critical factor. Recent works in communication technologies have inspired the development of telemedicine to a large extent. There are many different disciplines in telemedicine, such as teleradiology, telemonitoring, teleconsultation, teleconference, and telepsychiatry . The common problem met during the development of a telemedicine system is how to integrate the existing techniques to meet the requirements for telemedicine applications.

The people in India, particularly in rural and remote areas are found struggling to access timely medical treatment. The region of the country is characterized by densely populated communities spread over vast distances; there is a lack of qualified personnel in certain sectors of the health service. Telemedicine has come originally to serve rural populations, or any people who are geographically dispersed—where time and the cost of travel make access to the best medical care difficult. Nowadays, telemedicine is forming a new architecture in healthcare services. By using information and communication technologies, the healthcare professionals in the specialized fields such as cardiology, urology, oncology, psychiatry, surgery and many others, can access or exchange information for diagnosis, treatment and prevention of disease. This new age concept also provides solutions for the continuing education and research among healthcare providers for improving the health of individuals and their communities. Thus, the telemedicine ensures delivery of right medical advice at the right place at the right time using new computer-based communication technologies for medical purposes.

HOSPITAL INFORMATION SYSTEM (HIS)

Hospital is an institution suitably located, constructed, organized, managed and personnel led to supply scientifically, economically efficiently and unhindered, all or any recognized part of the complex retirements for the prevention, diagnosis and treatment of physical, mental and the medical aspect of social illness; with functioning facilities for training new workers in the many special professional, technical and economic fields essential to the discharge of its proper functions and with adequate contacts with physicians, other hospitals, medical schools and all accredited health agencies engaged in the better health program. Hospital is an institution for the medical, surgical, obstetrics, or psychiatric care and treatment of patients. It is an institution for healthcare providing treatment by specialized staff and equipment, and often but not always providing for longer-term patient stays. In a typical hospital the following people actively work to deliver medical services, medical (Physicians, surgeons, anesthetist, pathologist, microbiologist, radiologist), nursing (education, quality assurance, infection, administration), paramedical (physiotherapist, occupation, lab-technicians, radiographers, etc.), pharmacy department staff; dietary department staff; support services (CSSD, housekeeping, laundry, biomedical, maintenance), admin (HR), finance, and HID. All the work is done by using the hospital infrastructure (OP, ER, IP), building and medical equipment, expertise (doctors, surgeons, nursing staff and other staff), support services, etc.

Information is an arrangement of information (data), processes, people, and information technology that interacts to collect, process, store, and provide an output to the information needed to support organization. Hospital Information System (HIS) is an area of medical informatics, the aim of an HIS is to achieve the best possible support of patient care and administration by electronic data processing. The information that is readily accessible, timely, complete, accurate, legible, and relevant is critical to healthcare providers for efficient patient care. In order to provide quality care cost containment, and ensure adequate access, the need for comprehensive information is much greater than today. The demand for information has increased due to unprecedented advances in information technology. Main function of the hospital information system is to establish administrative control over functional activities, preparing operating budget, report gene-ration for government and other agencies. Distribution of expenses while computing the cost of operations, planning of additional facilities, staff, equipment, training programs and quality of patient care. If a person is sick/injured admitted to the hospital, depending on the condition of the patient, the necessary treatment is provided by the physician in order to get the patient condition stable, i.e. in the OP, ER or IP. The following are the various activities taking place in a hospital in the outpatient clinics, ER, inpatient wards, ICU, CCU, and NICU. A patient is admitted in the hospital for any treatment; the following information is collected and documented in the record to provide effective and efficient care:

- Care of sick/injured
- Conduct medical education
- Medical research and other functions
- Demographic information
- Patient history
- Physical examination
- Progress notes
- Problem list
- Investigation
- Diagnosis
- Consultation
- Treatment—Medical and Surgical
- Results

A hospital information system (HIS) takes on the tasks of collecting, storing, manipulating, and presenting the data, helping to generate the information needed to make the decisions in a hospital. We partition the presentation of the issues into five sections.

A hospital information system is a computerized system designed to meet the information needs of the hospital. This includes many diverse types of data, such as patient information, clinical laboratory, radiology and patient monitoring, patient census and billing, staffing and scheduling, outcome assessment and quality control, pharmacy ordering, decision support, finance and accounting, supplies, inventory, maintenance and orders management, etc.

Over the last few decades, medical sciences have made great strides leading to radical improvements in the modes of investigations, therapeutic activities and surgical procedures. This has enhanced the imperative need to have authentic and accurate information system.

Information Versus Data

Selecting the right data for processing and performing data analysis require knowledge. Knowledge is acquired by people through training and experience, and may be encoded in expert or knowledge-based systems.

Current HISs are not knowledge based, so that personnel must supply the knowledge needed to control the functions of an HIS.

When the data are used to initiate actions and perform actions with a higher degree of confidence than would otherwise be possible, we have created and used information. Information and the actions affected by information are the end objective of our medical information systems. There are many paths to obtain information, but a system designer must keep objectives at this level in view.

In order to generate an action, there has to be a decision-maker with the authority to carry out the activity. Providing information to a person who cannot effect change is only frustrating. In information system design, it is necessary to identify the person who will benefit from the information.

The actions initiated by the decision-maker will change the state of the world. These changes will be observed, recorded, and entered as data into the systems. Subsequent requests for information will reflect those changes, and cause new decisions to be made. There is also a knowledge loop. As the decision-maker learns from the effect of the actions, the actions may change as well. If the knowledge is transmitted to others, by memos, papers, books, or perhaps by encoding in knowledge-based systems, the new knowledge can be applied to instances outside of the local system.

Administrative and Management Information

The hospital information system also has to provide administrative and management information. Having a complete profile of the patient makes it easier to predict utilization of services, length of stay, and potential for complications. This information can in turn be used to predict resource consumption in the hospital. For reimbursement it can also be important that services provided are documented so that healthcare costs can be properly allocated.

ORGANIZATION AND INFORMATION

To permit information to be exploited, it must reach the individuals in the hospital who can act on it. At times, it is necessary to change the organization and the level of authority of individuals in the system so that the HIS can be effective. A good hospital system that provides reliable information will allow delegation of decision-making tasks to people for whom that responsibility would previously have been troublesome. Without some delegation, it may happen that as a computer system increases productivity, the load on individuals who were previously responsible for certain types of decisions becomes excessive, while lower-level personnel are underutilized.

Data Sources for Information

When information needs are identified, the sources for the data and the transformation functions required to provide that information have to be determined. The traditional sources for data have been discussed in the first section; they are the physicians, nurses, and admission personnel who interact with the patient. There are other potential sources of data that are underutilized. A detailed history may be obtained from the patients themselves. For long-term chronic diseases, the family may provide important data and help in obtaining a complete picture of the patient. Previous medical records contain another component of the patient's picture and can contain data that are easily forgotten or not considered relevant by a patient who is concerned only about a current problem.

Health Information Systems

Health Information Management System, health informatics or medical informatics is the intersection of information science, computer science, and healthcare. It deals with the resources, devices, and methods required to optimizing the acquisition, storage, retrieval, and use of information in health and biomedicine. Thus, it is seen as a computerized system providing standardized data and recordkeeping procedures to support medical, environmental health and industrial hygiene activities. Health informatics tools include not only computers but also clinical guidelines, formal medical terminologies, and information and communication systems.

On the other hand, a *hospital information system* (HIS), variously also called clinical information system (CIS) is a comprehensive, integrated information system designed to manage the administrative, financial and clinical aspects of a hospital. This encompasses paper-based information processing as well as data processing machines.

It can be composed of one or a few software components with specialty-specific extensions as well as of a large variety of sub-systems in medical specialties (e.g. Laboratory Information System, Radiology Information System).

CISs are sometimes separated from HISs in that the former concentrate on patient-related and clinical-state-related data (electronic patient record), whereas the latter keeps track of administrative issues. The distinction is not always clear and there is contradictory evidence against a consistent use of both terms.

It is important to talk briefly and differentiate e-Health from the other types of health related systems. E-Health (also written e-health) is a relatively recent term for healthcare practice which is supported by electronic processes and communication. The term is inconsistently used: some would argue it is interchangeable with healthcare informatics and a subset of health informatics, while others use it in the narrower sense of healthcare practice using the Internet.

The term can encompass a range of services that are at the edge of medicine/healthcare and information technology:

Electronic medical records: Enable easy communication of patient data between different healthcare professionals (GPs, specialists, care team, pharmacy).

Telemedicine: It includes all types of physical and psychological measurements that do not require a patient to travel to a specialist. When this service works, patients need to travel less to a specialist or conversely the specialist has a larger catchment area.

Consumer health informatics (or citizen-oriented information provision): Both healthy individuals and patients want to be informed on medical topics.

Health knowledge management (or specialist-oriented information provision): For example, in an overview of latest medical journals, best practice guidelines or epidemiological tracking.

Virtual healthcare teams: These consist of healthcare professionals who collaborate and share information on patients through digital equipment (for transmural care).

mHealth or m-Health: It includes the use of mobile devices in collecting aggregate and patient level health data, providing healthcare information to practitioners, researchers, and patients, real-time monitoring of patient vitals, and direct provision of care (via mobile telemedicine).

Medical research uses e-health Grids that provide powerful computing and data management capabilities to handle large amounts of heterogeneous data.

Sub-domains of healthcare informatics: These include clinical informatics, nursing informatics, imaging informatics, consumer health informatics, public health informatics, dental informatics, clinical research informatics, bioinformatics, veterinary informatics, and pharmacy informatics.

Benefits of Health Information System

In order to realize the full potential of information systems, healthcare organizations must plan for and implement strategies that are designed to maximize benefits of such system. Some of the benefits include:

- Information systems can improve cost control.
- Increase the timeliness and accuracy of patient care and administration information.
- Increase service capacity, reduce personnel costs and inventory levels, and improve the quality of patient care.
- Hospital Information System (HIS) is vital to decision making and plays a crucial role in the success of the organization
- Managers, clinicians and other healthcare workers can now access the information with the help of HIS without delay or errors.
- Improved quality of documentation
- Improved quality of patient care
- Reduced error
- Enhanced ability to track patient record
- Improved Hospital image
- Ensures flawless integration within the various departments of the hospital.

It is no doubt that a carefully planned hospital information system and intelligently used information will be a great asset to any healthcare industry.

The hospital information managers must have the necessary skills to facilitate and manage this transition and bridge the gap in the changing patterns switch over to 21st century.

Definitions of Hospital Management Information Systems and Its Components

A system which acquires, stores, processes, and delivers patient related information in a hospital with required details in response to a query or routinely or periodically as per predetermined format to those who need it is called a "Hospital Information System".

Such a system may also integrate information pertaining to areas not directly related to patient care such as personnel and financial information.

A hospital information system which deals with only patient related information is termed patient information system or medical information system. Occasionally, use of the terminology is not so rigorous and often used interchangeably.

A hospital, by virtue of the nature of job it performs, generates a vast amount of data in all its activity centers (clinical, non-clinical and administrative activities). The information processed from this data has action imp-lication for the recipient for management functions like planning, organizing, staffing, directing and controlling. Such information is called management information. When several sub-systems pertaining to various activity centers are integrated together into an interacting and inter-related bigger system, then it may be termed management information system.

Table 7.2 will give some of the major HIS implementations at some corporate hospitals. Other corporate hospitals imple-ment HIS to a few independent modules only.

Table 7.2: Major HIS implementations

Hospital	HIS Modules	Implementers
Wockhardt	ADT (Admission Transfer Discharge), emergency, wards, laboratory, billing, help desk, purchase, pharmacy, blood bank, HR, physicians and specialties	Wipro and Wockhardt IT team
Hinduja	Pharmacy, laboratory, OPD, HR, billing, analytical modules for tracking drug stock	Internal IT team

(Contd...)

Table 7.2: Major HIS implementations (Contd...)

Fortis	Backend pharmacy systems, medical use, medical care equipment, front-office billing, smart card and access control, HR and payroll	Internal IT team
Apollo	Pharmacy, laboratory, OPD, HR, billing, analytical modules for tracking drug stock	Wipro and Internal team

NEED FOR HOSPITAL INFORMATION SYSTEM (HIS)

The two primary processes in hospitals are the specialist cure process and the care and support process. The patients and the information about patients are exchanged between the two primary processes.

A hospital can be considered as a microcosm. A variety of functions are performed by a large number of functionaries to produce a product, which may be termed patient care.

With ever increasing expectations and demands of the patients, medical professionals, fast changing medical technology and with the inclusion of healthcare in consumer protection act and many other factors such as the changing economic conditions, which include long term high inflation, high interest rates and low real growth, structural changes in economy caused by global competition and new information technology economics such as telecommunications cost performance and cost performance of circuitry and mass storage, the healthcare institutions are reengineering their core processes to the challenges faced by them.

So information is increasingly being recognized as an indispensable, valuable commodity required by management to plan and control business operations effectively. Moreover, higher level managers need information for strategic and tactical planning. As hospitals attempt to develop innovative programs and make strategic decisions about their future direction, the quality and availability of information for decision making has continued to gain greater importance.

The competitive pressures that pervade the healthcare industry have further heightened the need to use hospital information system (HIS) as a competitive weapon. The increasingly competitive pressures have fostered new incentives for the development of organizational strategies that reach far beyond the traditional mission statement that hospitals have long relied upon.

Information systems are only as good as the quality of their data. Most materials management information systems contain obsolete, duplicate, and inaccurate data. As tools for procurement become more automated and efficient, it becomes more important that the data is up to date and correct. Cleansing and managing thousands of lines of data—which are often created by multiple users at different points in time is a huge task. A hospital can greatly improve its cost savings by integrating, verifying, standardizing, and monitoring the data going into and out of their materials information systems.

FUNCTIONAL MODEL OF A HOSPITAL INFORMATION SYSTEM

Healthcare industry is one of the most information intensive and technologically advanced in our society. Thus, the information should be accessible easily, timely, complete, accurate, reliable and relevant information in making important strategic or patient care decisions. The end objective of medical informatics is the integration of data, knowledge, and tools necessary to apply that data and knowledge in the decision-making process associated with patient care. The focus on the structures and algorithms necessary to manipulate the information separates medical informatics from other medical disciplines where information content is the focus. To be more precise, the entire hospital system that is being practiced with the manual system has to be completely transformed into electronic by using the latest information technology, for example, HIS which contains the domain functionality, flow charts, screens, database that are developed, tested and produced as application software for implementation in order to convert a hospital into a computerized format.

From admission to diagnostic and medical support services, the modern healthcare centers rely on wide range of software applications. Some of the distinctive advantages of HIS include improved quality of patient care, improved communications within the hospital, increased productivity, reduced costs and reduced chances of errors and the enhanced ability to track patient records. Today HIS and electronic medical records (EMR) have become the minimum prerequisites for delivering quality healthcare.

Information requirements can be grouped as

- Operational requirements, which include up-to-date factual information that are necessary for day-to-day tasks.
- Planning requirements that comprise short- and long-term decisions about patient care and decisions about hospital management.
- Documentation requirements such as maintenance of records, accreditation and legal records.

Application domain: The application layer includes: patient management, medical care, nursing, medical support, administrative, ancillary services. The information bus deals with services. The middleware layer should include authorization component, patient component, activity component, resource component, and healthcare record and knowledge component. The persistent layer related to images, bio-signals, alphanumeric data, web pages. While developing the electronic hospital information system, in order to achieve inter-operability, portability and data exchange healthcare information system must apply standards. Some of the standards are as follows: ISO, HL7, HIPAA, ICD, PACS, DICOM, ASTM, SNOMED,CPT, etc.

Passive storage: Electronic medical record (EMR): Up to this point the medical record has served as a passive storage devise, while the EMR as an active tool that can provide the clinician with decision-support capabilities and access to knowledge resources, reminders, and alerts.

Signal processing (EEG, EMG, ECG): Computers are useful devices for processing electrical signals from various sources, such as ECG for detection of heart dysrhythmias and EEG for analysis and detection of spike and sharp waves that can sometimes be missed by the neurologist.

Image processing: Image processing includes radiography, US, CT scanning, MRI/MRA, SPECT/PET scanning, cerebral angiography. Image processing and pattern recognition are important fields in medical informatics, specifically in neuroinformatics as an emerging domain for CT scanning, MRI of the brain, and other new techniques such as SPECT and PET scanning and functional MRI (fMRI). For example, processing of spatially distributed patterns of brain activation in fMRI data sets using computerized analysis helps determine pathophysiology of many neurologic disorders and define functional structures of the brain. For example, EMG expert systems such as EMG Assistant can help electromyographers through a sophisticated analysis of the input data and provide them with the most likely diagnosis that objectively best explains the findings.

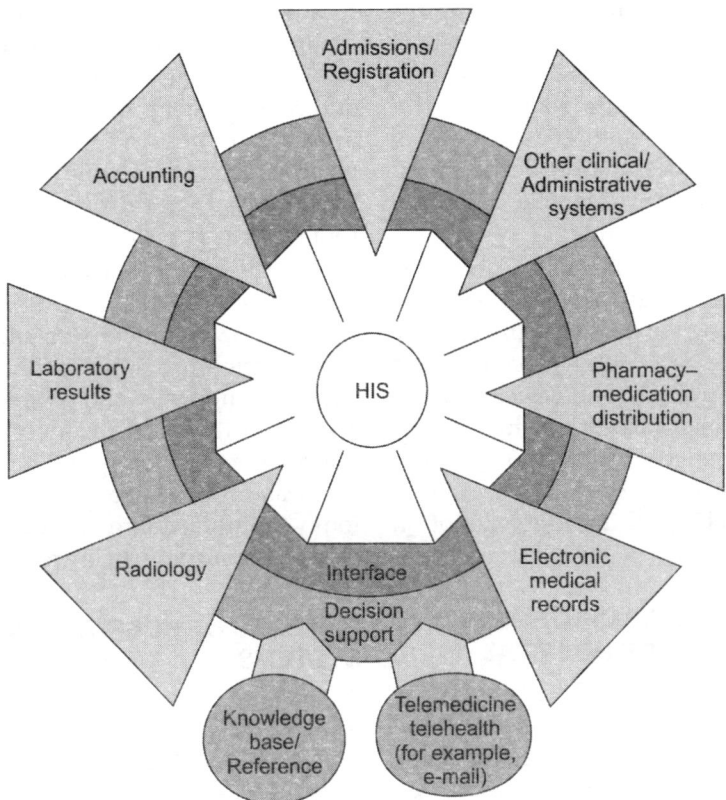

These programs can help doctors understand the readings as they develop the field experience to analyze the data themselves.

Core Functions

The eight core functions that an EMR software system should have:
- Health information and patient data
- Computerized order management
- Laboratory results management
- Decision support system
- Electronic communication and connectivity
- Patient support and education
- Administrative processes
- Reporting

Additionally, the following functionalities help better adoption of the EMR by physicians:
- Transition or flexibility in moving from desktop to handheld computing devices
- Structured data entry to accommodate the diversity of specialized care
- Options to express findings and conclusions in free text or definition of normal
- Graphical data entry for body maps and radiology images
- Automatization and improvement of transcription and upload process
- Enhancement of faxback service and upgrade to electronic file transfer or Web access service
- Enhancement of decision support systems and implementation of artificial intelligence such as drug interaction service and various clinical guidelines.

Decision support system: Decision support systems are real-time computerized algorithms that help physicians in their clinical practice. For example, when clinicians perform a task (e.g. order entry) using the EHR, they are warned if the task appears to be inappropriate on the basis of patient data. The system presents this warning automatically using consensus-based clinical decision support "rules" that are derived from medical knowledge (or financial data) and patient-specific information.

Provider order entry systems: Computer-based provider order entry (CPOE) systems helps in improving the quality of patient care and reducing the costs. Studies have shown that CPOE system lead to better accuracy and completeness of medical orders, which in turn lead to reduced lengths of stay and costs and allow fast transmission of orders, legibility, and on-line tracking of the life cycle of an order.

APPLICABILITY OF COMPUTERS IN DIFFERENT AREAS OF HOSPITAL

Application of computers effects directly or indirectly the efficiency of all the areas of the hospital functions. Some of the areas of prime importance for gainful computerization are :

- Medical Records Department.
- Laboratory records and reports.
- Imaging records and reports.
- Admission, discharge and billing procedures.
- Stores.
- Dietary department.
- Housekeeping.
- Human resource department (personnel functions)
- Management information system.

Hospitals in India, unlike hospitals in other countries, irrespective of their size and location can maintain adequate records. What is needed is the standardization of forms, procedures and methods of analysis and evaluation.

Computers have long offered the promise of putting clinicians closer to the information they use in making patient care decisions. Up to now the real effects of computers in this realm have been small. As demonstrated and discussed at the recent Health information and Management Systems Society (HIMSS) annual meeting in Orlando, the medical record is slated to become the key component in the medical information system of tomorrow.

What is being envisioned and tested is a medical record in computerized form (a Computerized Patient Record, or CPR) that will be the clinicians' primary means of accessing not only the patients healthcare record, but also reference and research information, including such decision-support tools as clinical practice guidelines and today's standard fare of bibliographic databases and journal article archives.

BENEFITS OF HOSPITAL INFORMATION SYSTEMS

Benefits of computer based medical information system : Although the impact of HIS will be seen differently among the various departments, there are generic benefits that affect all users. The relative importance of these benefits will vary, of course, depending on the mission of a given department. Some of these benefits are:

- *Requisitions:* Service requests are more timely, accurate and complete. Departments can elect to receive requisitions in a convenient fashion.
- *Reports:* Reports from the service department to the requestor are more timely and accurate and are better organised from the viewpoint of the user.
- *Status:* Visibility into the status of a service request or resulting report is improved. Status can usually be determined from any terminal, eliminating the need to telephone or visit the performing department.
- *Workload:* Departments can look ahead at their workload (e.g. scheduled admissions on a particular day or investigative

procedures ordered) and also look back (e.g. procedures done last month).
- *Clerical effort:* Most routine clerical work (e.g. patient lists, appointment lists, charge tickets, etc.) is eliminated.
- *Audit trails:* Service requisitions can be traced to reports and charges without error or ambiguity (e.g. matching microbiology reports to specimens).
- *Location independence:* The relationship between location and information is largely eliminated. Information is now available to authorized personnel at any terminal in the hospital.

A Hospital Information System (HIS) is a computerized system designed to meet the information needs of all (or most) of a hospital. This includes many diverse types of data, such as:
- Patient information
- Clinical laboratory, radiology, and patient monitoring
- Patient census and billing
- Staffing and scheduling
- Outcomes assessment and quality control
- Pharmacy ordering, prescription handling, and pharmacopoeia information
- Decision support
- Finance and accounting
- Supplies, inventory, maintenance, and orders management

Advantages of Hospital Information Systems

- Increased time nurses spend with patients
- Access to information
- Improved quality of documentation
- Improved quality of patient care
- Increased nursing productivity
- Improved communications
- Reduced errors of omission
- Reduced medication errors
- Reduced hospital costs
- Development of a common clinical database
- Improved patient's perception of care
- Enhanced ability to track patient's record
- Enhanced ability to recruit and retain staff

Improve Patient Care

1. Make patient information from other hospitals available where the patient is currently being treated.
2. Improve the accessibility of patient related information to healthcare professionals through improved handling of medical records and getting results of investigations more quickly.
3. Improve patient administration procedures, resulting in shorter waiting times and better service.

Form an Integral Part of a Larger Quality Improvement Programme

1. Standardization of patient administration and management procedures across hospitals.
2. Provision of information to evaluate performance and audit healthcare.

Improve management efficiency of hospitals

1. Allow hospitals to manage their own finances
2. Improve revenue collection
3. Improve management decision making through the availability of integrated management information
4. Save costs through the identification of primary cost drivers at hospital level and the monitoring of mechanisms introduced to lower costs

Planned Functions for Hospital Information System

- Master patient index
- Admission, discharges, and transfers
- Patient recordtracking
- Appointments
- Order entry and reporting of results

- Departmental systems for laboratory, radiology, operating theatre, other clinical services, dietary services, laundry
- Financial management
- Management information and hospital performance indicators.

APPLICATION OF HIS

Decision support system: This is required to allow retrieval of pertinent information to assess operational effectiveness. It allows the investigation of physician utilization, revenue analysis, census comparison, etc.

Laboratory information system: The LIS is required to be fully integrated with the hospital information system and to include control on laboratory workflow from requisition and specimen collection and processing to results reporting. This includes the services, chemistry, microbiology, blood bank etc.

Order entry/results reporting: It includes online communication of physician orders, and patient information between nursing and ancillary departments.

Pharmacy information system: Pharmacy information system includes medication administration record, patient profiles, medication charges, inventory control, etc.

Human resources: This is required for managing entire functions of human resources.

Materials management (purchasing): Materials management module helps in procurement control and manages inventory, supplies and equipment throughout the hospital.

Nursing care and management: This handles all the processes involved in the daily transactions that occur in a ward, these transactions involve test requisitions placed for the patient, medicines consumed by the patient, bedside procedures performed, medical equipment connected to the patient, and recording of all visits by the doctor. Furthermore, it allows for the capturing of nursing assessment data, nursing plans and checklists, nursing charting/progress notes, nurse management and nursing quality assurance.

Physicians' access and notes: The purpose of using this is to provide physicians associated with the hospital, an easy means of communicating with the 'Hospital Information System'. Simultaneously the system should provide a facility for the doctors to organize their notes and activities within the hospital.

Accident and emergency management: The Accident and Emergency (A and E) module allows the hospital to record data accurately and quickly for patient treatment. It also allows users to record casualty details, and 'discharge status'.

Inpatient management (ADT): It supports two main functions: the administration of wards (nursing units) and the handling of admissions, discharge and transfer of patients in those wards.

Medical records: It is required, to be fully, integrated with, inpatient management and patient accounting. It supports the operational needs of a modern medical records department including transcription, case indexing, abstracting, statistical reporting, and charge location, with complete integration with patient billing function.

Outpatient management: The outpatients management supports the setting up and maintenance of clinics and the administration and scheduling of outpatient appointments.

Patient registration system: The hospital needs a registration system, which will utilize a central patient registration database that contains basic information on each patient. The patient registration database will serve as a master patient index supports all other systems in patient identification. The system allows the search of a patient record by using any combination of fields.

Housekeeping and laundry: A submodule is needed to help the hospital schedule housekeeping activities and follow-up on incurred cost and progress of work.

RADIO FREQUENCY IDENTIFICATION (RFID)

Radio frequency identification (RFID) is revolutionizing the way organizations around the world track the location and movement of goods and assets. RFID technology utilizes inexpensive wireless RFID chips or tags that report their location to nearby scanners. Items with RFID tags can be tracked from a supplier's factory floor to the retailer's store shelves.

The technology is already helping major retailers better control their inventory. Soon other organizations are expected to find innovative uses for RFID.

Hospitals will be able to instantaneously pinpoint the exact location of expensive equipment through RFID systems. Not only will the technology help hospitals maximize the use of equipment, but it will also help them provide better care. In the pharmaceutical industry, companies may soon use RFID to help monitor the distribution of drugs around the world. This will help them reduce product counterfeiting while helping them better control inventory and monitor product quality.

The Basics of RFID

Automatic identification (auto ID) technologies help machines or computers identify objects by using automatic data capture. RFID is one type of auto ID technology that uses radio waves to identify, monitor, and manage individual objects as they move between physical locations. Although there are a variety of methods for identifying objects with RFID, the most common method is by storing a serial number that identifies a product and its related information. RFID devices and software must be supported by an advanced software architecture that enables the collection and distribution of location-based information in real time.

Tags and Readers

An RFID system consists of tags and readers. RFID tags are small devices containing a chip and an antenna that store the information for object identification. Tags can be applied to containers, pallets, cases, or individual items. With no line-of-sight requirement, the tag transmits information to the reader, and the reader converts the incoming radio waves into a form that can be read by a computer system. An RFID tag can be active (with a battery) or passive (powered by the signal strength emitted by the reader).

Active Tags

These can be read from a long-range distance of more than 100 feet.

These are ideal for tracking high-value items over long ranges, such as tracking, shipping containers in transit.

Active tags have high power and battery requirements, so they are heavier and can be costly.

Passive Tags

These can only be read from a short-range distance of approximately 5–10 ft.

These can be applied in high quantities to individual items and reused.

Passive tags are smaller, lighter, and less expensive (and therefore more prevalent) than active tags.

RFID, smart cards, and other form factors RFID technology is currently being used in conjunction with smart card technology in the financial industry, primarily in Europe. Financial institutions are issuing smart cards to record personal finance information such as account balances. RFID technology is also being used in other form factors such as key fobs, bulk metal tags, garment disks, and even metal nails that can be driven into pallets.

RFID and Barcodes

Although it is often thought that RFID and barcodes are competitive technologies, they are in fact complementary. The primary element of differentiation between the two is that RFID does not require line-of-sight technology. Barcodes must be scanned at specific orientations to establish line-of-sight, such as an item in a grocery store, and RFID tags need only be within range of a reader to be read or scanned. Although RFID and barcode technologies offer similar solutions, there are significant advantages to using RFID.

Tags can be read rapidly in bulk to provide a nearly simultaneous reading of contents, such as items in a stockroom or in a container.

Tags are more durable than barcodes and can withstand chemical and heat environments that would destroy traditional barcode labels. Barcode technology does not work if the label is damaged.

Tags have read and write capabilities and can be updated. Barcodes contain static information that cannot be updated unless the user reprints the code.

Tags can potentially contain a greater amount of data compared to barcodes, which commonly contain only static information such as the manufacturer and product identification.

Tags do not require any human intervention for data transmission, whereas barcodes do.

It is easy to see how RFID has become indispensable for a wide range of automated data collection and identification applications. With the distinct advantages of RFID technology, however, comes an inevitably higher cost. RFID and barcode technologies will continue to coexist in response to diverse market needs. RFID, however, will continue to expand in markets for which barcode or similar optical technologies are not as efficient.

Healthcare and Pharmaceutical

The benefits of RFID for the healthcare and Pharmaceutical industry will far exceed the supply chain level in the near future. In addition to ensuring safer pharmaceuticals, RFID will improve the drug manufacturing processes and inventory control, increase patient safety, streamline business processes, reduce costs, protect brand values, and reduce counterfeiting.

In the United States, illicit counterfeiting organizations are successfully introducing potentially unsafe diverted and counterfeit drugs into the drug distribution system. Anti-counterfeiting techniques, such as authentication and track-and-trace technologies, facilitate the identification of counterfeit drugs and minimize consumer exposure. Perhaps most importantly, the technologies reduce the financial impact that counterfeit drugs have on the existing prescription drug distribution system. For any drug distribution shipment in the United States, there is a significant danger of drug counterfeiters intercepting the shipment, altering the drugs, and then distributing them to pharmacies or directly to consumers.

The following fictional scenario shows how RFID, a track-and-trace technology, is used by one pharmaceutical company for inventory control, anti-counterfeiting efforts, and more.

Providing inventory management, validating, tracking shipments and processing recalls.

RFID Solutions for Healthcare Industry

RFID has made its way into almost all the day to day operations of a healthcare facility. Let's take a look at these areas and see how the different RFID technologies are being used and why.

Patient tracking

RFID is being used to track and authenticate patients, from new born babies to seniors suffering from dementia and everything in between. The technologies that are being used for patient tracking include almost all the RFID technologies. LF and HF are used for applications such as bedside care and mother and baby matching. UHF is being used to monitor patient movement and establish geo-fencing as required. Active technology is a more robust form of movement and motion tracking.

Wait Time Monitoring

RFID technology is being deployed to monitor patient wait times in real time. Reusable active technology, for example, an ER sees exactly the number of patients in the queue and length of wait time by patient.

Medication Authentication and Control

Bedside care has leap frogged the use of bar codes and embraced RFID to ensure the right medication is given to the right patient. Nursing staff find RFID easier to work with than bar codes and realize the additional privacy that RFID brings to the process. For example, when the nurse is away from the computer on wheels (COW) administering medication to a patient the computer can be programmed to go into screen save mode thus maintaining patient information confidentiality. Bedside care RFID typically employs contact like HF technology. Nurses or meds administrators can be virtually adhered to a the COW using UHF technology.

Surgery Asset Management

The use of RFID is reducing the chance of overlooking things such as sponges or other surgical kit components after an OR procedure. Many ORs are using LF technology to tag everything used in a surgery. Once the procedure has been completed, the patient is scanned to make nothing has been left behind.

Handwashing

Monitoring the hand cleaning stations at touch points has been a way of improving compliance to hand washing protocols. Healthcare workers simply wear an RFID badge. Hand wash stations at every touch point are equipped with an RFID reader. Every time a hand wash station is used the reader records the user's identity and length of stay in front of the reader. The accumulated data allows an organization to see how well hand washing protocol is being followed.

By using RFID to tag high demand items like pumps many institutions have reported fewer shortages of these critical items when required and less time lost searching for these items. By using UHF technology any critical piece of equipment can be tagged and tracked throughout a facility making them easy to locate when required. Asset tracking saves valuable people time as well as valuable capital funds.

Inventory Management

RFID can help an institution manage its entire supply inventory. RFID provides the real-time visibility that barcode just can't deliver. RFID is also being used to manage shared storage areas such as locked pharma cabinets. Access to these cabinets can be restricted, controlled and audited using HF RFID. Inventories inside these cabinets can be seen real-time and from remote locations such as a supplier DC. Most back room inventory systems are using UHF technology. HF is commonly used in smart storage cabinets.

Parking

RFID is being used for **parking control** by many establishments. Parking falls into two categories: Public and Reserved. Public parking is usually metered parking or pay as you go. RFID can be used to record the entry and exit time of each visit. The billing is based on the length of stay and the time of day. HF (High Frequency) RFID is most commonly used for cash transaction applications such as public pay as you go parking. Reserved parking using RFID can use a wider variety of technologies varying from HF to UHF (Ultra High Frequency) to active technologies. UHF or Active technologies are used for the convenience of the reserved parking client. Both RFID parking solutions, public and reserved, can be implemented as an automated, unmanned, stand alone system.

RFID is used by many establishments to control access to restricted entry and exit points as well as restricted areas within a facility. The most commonly used technologies are LF (Low Frequency) or HF because they are contact like and allow facilities to maintain a high degree selective security. Unmanned, controlled access security provides the audit trail information required for restricted access areas.

RFID is being used to track and locate critical files such as patient charts and records. The most commonly use technology is UHF. Searching for misplaced files consumes 100's of man hours each year.

A healthcare facility is like a small city. There is a complete army of engineers that keep things running and maintained. RFID is being used to tag key service points that need regular maintenance. The RFID tag when read tells the service technician what and how to perform the service. An RFID driven maintenance program ensures all equipment is serviced on time and according to specification.

Laundry Management

Whether the laundry service is outsourced or in-house, RFID is being used to manage this massive and essential service. Healthcare facilities use 100s of thousands of garments. The logistics of cleaning, ironing, folding, shipping and storing laundered items would be unmanageable without RFID. Early RFID laundry applications used HF technology which is slowly being replaced by UHF technology because of read distance being greater and tag costs being lower.

Waste Management

RFID has completely changed the waste management game. By using RFID waste disposal, companies can co-ordinate and identify all types of waste including hazardous waste. RFID helps identify and monitor all waste generated within a facility as well as track all waste removal. UHF is the most commonly used technology in waste management.

E-HEALTH

Everybody talks about e-health these days, but a few people have come up with a clear definition of this comparatively new term. Barely in use before 1999, this term now seems to serve as a general "buzzword," used to characterize not only "Internet medicine", but also virtually everything related to computers and medicine. The term was apparently first used by industry leaders and marketing people rather than academics. They created and used this term in line with other "e-words" such as e-commerce, e-business, e-solutions, and so on, in an attempt to convey the promises, principles, excitement (and hype) around e-commerce (electronic commerce) to the health arena, and to give an account of the new possibilities. The internet is opening up to the area of healthcare. Intel, for example, referred to e-health as "a concerted effort undertaken by leaders in healthcare and hi-tech industries to fully harness the benefits available through convergence of the Internet and healthcare." Because the internet created new opportunities and challenges to the traditional healthcare information technology industry, the use of a new term to address these issues seemed appropriate. These "new" challenges for the healthcare information technology industry were mainly (1) the capability of consumers to interact with their systems online (B2C = "business to consumer"); (2) improved possibilities for institution-to-institution transmissions of data (B2B = "business to business"); (3) new possibilities for peer-to-peer communication of consumers (C2C = "consumer to consumer").

So, how can we define e-health in the academic environment? One JMIR Editorial Board member feels that the term should remain in the realm of the business and marketing sector and should be avoided in scientific medical literature and discourse. However, the term has already entered the scientific literature (today, 76 Medline-indexed articles contain the term "e-health" in the title or abstract). What remains to be done is, in good scholarly tradition, to define as clearly as possible what we are talking about. However, as another member of the Editorial Board noted, "stamping a definition on something like e-health is somewhat like stamping a definition on 'the Internet': It is defined how it is used—the definition cannot be pinned down, as it is a dynamic environment, constantly moving."

It seems quite clear that e-health encompasses more than a mere technological development. The term and concept of e-health can be described as follows:

e-health is an emerging field in the intersection of medical informatics, public health and business, referring to health services and information delivered or enhanced through the Internet and related technologies. In a broader sense, the term characterizes not only a technical development, but also a state of mind, a way of thinking, an attitude, and a commitment for networked, global thinking, to improve healthcare locally, regionally, and worldwide by using information and communication technology.

This definition hopefully is broad enough to apply to a dynamic environment such as the Internet and at the same time acknowledges that e-health encompasses more than just "Internet and Medicine".

As such, the "e" in e-health does not only stand for "electronic," but implies a number of other "e's," which together perhaps best characterize what e-health is all about (or what it *should* be). Last, but not the least, all of these have been (or will be) issues addressed in articles published in the Journal of Medical Internet Research.

The 10 e's in "e-health"

1. *Efficiency:* One of the promises of e-health is to increase efficiency in healthcare, thereby decreasing costs. One possible way of decreasing costs would be by avoiding duplicative or unnecessary diagnostic or therapeutic interventions, through enhanced communication possibilities between healthcare establishments, and through patient involvement.

2. *Enhancing quality of care:* Increasing efficiency involves not only reducing costs, but also at the same time improving quality. E-health may enhance the quality of healthcare, for example, by allowing comparisons between different providers, involving consumers as additional power for quality assurance, and directing patient streams to the best quality providers.

3. *Evidence based:* E-health interventions should be evidence-based in a sense that their effectiveness and efficiency should not be assumed but proven by rigorous scientific evaluation. Much work still has to be done in this area.

4. *Empowerment of consumers and patients:* By making the knowledge bases of medicine and personal electronic records accessible to consumers over the Internet, e-health opens new avenues for patient-centered medicine, and enables evidence-based patient choice.

5. Encouragement of a new relationship between the patient and health professional, towards a true partnership, where decisions are made in a shared manner.

6. Education of physicians through online sources (continuing medical education) and consumers (health education, tailored preventive information for consumers).

7. Enabling information exchange and communication in a standardized way between healthcare establishments.

8. Extending the scope of healthcare beyond its conventional boundaries. This is meant in both geographical sense as well as in a conceptual sense. E-health enables consumers to easily obtain health services online from global providers. These services can range from simple advice to more complex interventions or products such as pharmaceuticals.
9. *Ethics:* E-health involves new forms of patient-physician interaction and poses new challenges and threats to ethical issues such as online professional practice, informed consent, privacy and equity issues.
10. *Equity:* To make healthcare more equitable is one of the promises of e-health, but at the same time there is a considerable threat that e-health may deepen the gap between the "haves" and "have-nots". People, who do not have the money, skills, and access to computers and networks, cannot use computers effectively. As a result, these patient populations (which would actually benefit the most from health information) are those who are the least likely to benefit from advances in information technology, unless political measures ensure equitable access for all. The digital divide currently runs between rural vs. urban populations, rich vs. poor, young vs. old, male vs. female people, and between neglected/ rare vs. common diseases.

LATEST TRENDS IN HEALTHCARE IT

E-prescribing: It involves prescription orders that clinicians input electronically, which are then transmitted to the pharmacy. It provides decision support to the clinician, such as drug interaction flags and allergy-related information is usually included. E-prescribing eliminates hard-to-read handwritten prescriptions, as well as errors in dispensing (such as wrong drug or contraindicated drug).

Electronic clinical notes systems: It includes information on a patient's demographics, medical history, physician/nurse notes, and/ or follow-up orders.

Electronic lab orders: This computerizes ordering of lab tests.

Electronic lab results: It may allow quicker receipt and review of results by clinicians; this process usually includes decision support, such as highlighting results out of the normal range.

Electronic images available throughout a hospital: It helps in electronically storing of images (CT, MRI, PET scans) available to the medical team beyond the doors of the radiology department.

Electronic reminders for guideline-based interventions: It assists physicians by proactively suggesting care on evidence-based knowledge and patient-specific data.

THE LEGAL ASPECT OF HEALTH INFORMATICS

Health informatics law deals with evolving and sometimes complex legal principles as they apply to information technology in health-related fields. It addresses the privacy, ethical and operational issues that invariably arise when electronic tools, information and media are used in healthcare delivery.

Health informatics law also applies to all matters that involve information technology, healthcare and the interaction of information. It deals with the circumstances under which data and records are shared with other fields or areas that support and enhance patient care.

THE FUTURE HEALTH INFORMATION SYSTEMS

The global hospital information systems (HIS) market was valued at $7.4 billion in 2010, and is forecast to grow at a compound annual growth rate (CAGR) of 10% to reach about $14.7 billion by 2017. The high growth forecast for the period of 2010–2017 is significantly influenced by accelerated efforts from the public and private sectors around the world to contain rising healthcare costs and enhance quality of care. The inflow of key Information Technology (IT) technologies such as dictation and speech recognition solutions, and mobile healthcare solutions into the healthcare market space will also contribute substantially to growth prospects in this market. These technological advancements attempt to offset major deterrents to IT adoption in healthcare settings, such as significant upfront investments and ineptitude of medical professionals, with large electronic data entry and handling. Rapid adoption in emerging economies due to enhanced focus of key healthcare IT players will also accelerate growth of the HIS market. With the concept of interconnected healthcare systems seeming to materialize, starting with the US healthcare IT market; vendors have accelerated their efforts in assimilating necessary capabilities to tap the significant market potential. Intense market consolidation activity has resurfaced in the last two years.

Health systems of the future will be influenced by a variety of factors that directly and indirectly affect health. These include the interactive effects of changing disease patterns, population distribution, and environmental factors. Health systems of the future must be prepared to deal with an increasing number of behaviourally determined health problems while maintaining capabilities to control emerging and re-emerging infectious diseases.

Ageing populations that are increasingly concentrated in urban centres will reduce the need for fully equipped and staffed peripheral facilities while increasing the need for home and community level services. Even though the long-term economic outlook for the Western Pacific Region continues to be optimistic, affordability of health services will be a major issue in the organization of health systems in the next 50 years.

Improved access brought about by concentrations of population as well as improvements in transport and communications will bring about more demands on health systems. At the same time these health systems will be supported by smaller working populations. This situation will be compounded by the added healthcare costs resulting from the availability of services of substantially improved quality but which require ever higher levels of sophisticated technological support. The major technological developments in-fluencing health systems of the future are in the areas of biogenetics, body imaging, computerized information handling and communications.

Advances in biological research will lead to the development of new and better antimicrobial drugs and vaccines to deal with infectious diseases; increasingly accurate means of diagnosing and predicting hereditary, degenerative and neo-plasmic disorders, and production of more effective pharmaceutical remedies to alleviate and cure a wide range of human afflictions. Radiological, ultrasonographic, and nuclear magnetic resonance techniques will combine with immunology, other biological methods, and fibre-optic endoscopy to extend non-invasive body imaging not only for diagnosis but also for the delivery of therapeutic materials to diseased and damaged sites.

BIBLIOGRAPHY

Buckly A, Edwards C, Ward J & Bztheway A, 'The Essence Of Information System', Prentice Hall, England, 1996.

Brigl B, Ammenwerth E, Dujat C, Gräber S, Grosse A, Häber A, et al. Preparing strategic information management plans for hospitals: a practical guideline. *Int J Med Inform.* 2005;**74**:51–65. doi: 10.1016/j.ijmedinf.2004.09.002.

Borzekowski, R., "Healthcare Finance and the Early Adoption of Hospital Information Systems," Washington, D.C.: Discussion Paper No. 2002-41, Finance and Economics Discussion Services from the Board of Governors of the Federal Reserve System (U.S.), 2002.

Davis BG & Olsen MH, 'Management Information System', McGraw-Hill, New York, 1984.

Dolin RH, Alschuler L, Boyer S, Beebe C, Behlen FM, Biron PV, Shabo Shvo A. HL7 Clinical Document Architecture, Release 2. *J Am Med Inform Assoc.* 2006;**13**:30–39. doi: 10.1197/jamia.M1888.

Degoulet, P. and Fieschi, M. Introduction to Clinical Informatics, Springer Verlag, New York, NY, 1997.

De Lone, W.H. and McLean, E.R., "Information systems success: the quest for the dependent variable", Information Systems Research, Vol. 3 No. 1, pp. 60–95, 1992.

Healthcare Information and Management Systems Society. Electronic health record attributes and essential requirements. 2003. Available at: http://www.himss.org/content/files/ehrattributes070703.pdf. Accessed September 22, 2006.

Hasmann A, Haux R, van der Lei J, De Clercq E, Roger-France F., editor. II. Ubiquity: Technologies for Better Health in Aging Societies. European Notes in Medical Informatics; 2006. pp. 328–332.

Hersh, W.R. Medical Informatics: Improving Healthcare through Information. JAMA. 2002; 288(16):1955–1958.

Joint Commission for accreditation of healthcare organizations. http://www.jointcommission.org/

J.H. Van Bemmel, M.A. Musen (Eds.), Handbook of Medical Informatics, Springer, Heidelberg, Germany, 1997.

Kaihara S. Realization of the Computerized Patient Record: Relevance and Unsolved Problems. International Journal of Medical Informatics. 1998; 49(1):1–8.

Kuhn KA, Giuse DA. From Hospital Information Systems to Health Information Systems. Methods of Medical Informatics. 2001; 40(4): 275–287.

Lucas, H.C., "The evolution of an information system: from key-man to every person", Sloan Management Review, Vol. 19, No. 2, pp. 39–53, 1978.

Miller, R.H., Sim, I., and Jewman, J. (2003). *Electronic Medical Records: Lessons from Small Physician Practices.* California Healthcare Foundation.

Niland JC, Rouse L, Stahl DC. An informatics blueprint for healthcare quality information systems. *J Am Med Inform Assoc.* 2006;**13**:402–417. doi: 10.1197/jamia.M2050.

Van der Loo, R.P., van Gennip, E.M.S.J. and Baker, A.R. (1995), "Evaluation of automated information systems in healthcare: an approach to classifying evaluative studies", Computer Methods and Programs in Biomedicine, Vol. 48 No. 1, pp. 45–52.

Index

A
Accident and emergency department 103
Accountancy 146
Accounting conventions 150–152
Accounting cycle 111
Administration 2
Air flow 111
Architectural brief 90
Architectural drawings 91

B
Benchmarking 56–57
Benefits of hospital information system 23–27
Blood bank 117
Bookkeeping 153
Books of account 155
BPR 54, 55

C
CAMF 113
Cardiac catheterization laboratory 136
Catering unit 119
Capitation 30
Central sterile supply department 130
Commissioning 94
Compound or combined entry 162
Construction 94
Control chart 52–54
Controlling 1, 6, 12, 14–16
Cost
 accounting 148
 leadership 116
CPR 113

D
Darsiri method 144
Day care services 114
Decision making 1
 Dialysis unit
Differentation 116
Directing 1, 14, 16
Doctor manager 27

E
E-health 31–34
Electrical drawings
Electronic health record (EHR) 7, 8
Ergonomics 130–137
Evidence-based care 24

F
Facility location 117
Fast diagram 144
Financial accounting 147
Functional brief 90
Future of health information system 34–35

G
Generic strategy 115
Green
 building 79
 hospital 80

H
Healthcare information technology 3–5
Health
 information system 14–15, 17–18
 maintainance organizations 23
Heating, ventilation and air conditioning
HEPA filters
HIPAA security/privacy 6
HIS 114
Histogram 49
Hospital 1–4, 16
 adminstration 3–4, 14
 management information system 19
 organization 1, 4, 9, 16
 planning 82
Housekeeping and waste management 120
Human resources 2–3

I
Incentive payments 129
Indices relating to the hospital
Information technology 1–2
Inpatient unit
Intensive care unit
IT priorities for hospitals 12

J
Job plan due to mudge 143

K
KBS 112

L
Laboratory services 115
Labor and delivery suites 103
Laminar air flow
Learning curve 128
Licensee drawings
Linen and laundry services 123
Ledger account 167

M
Managed healthcare 22
Management 1–3, 7–10, 12
 accounting 147
Managing
 care in hospitals 38–43
 doctors 33–38

Market wide strategy 115–116
Master plan 86
Mechanical drawings
Medical
   gases 137
   imaging services 125, 128
Medicine 20
Method study 138
Modular grids 91

N

NABH 46
Negotiating 28
Nominal account 154
Nursing unit 99

O

Objectives goals 10–13, 15
Opening entry 163
Operations 110
   management 110–112
   strategy 114, 115
Operation unit 106
Organizing 1, 6, 12–13, 16
Outpatient services 97

P

PACS 112
Pareto 51

Personal
   account 154
   administration 1
Process 47
Production management 110
Productivity 123

Q

Quality and health information technology 1

R

Radio frequency identification (RFID) 27–31
Real account 154
Regional health information oragnization 6
Relative value scale 31
Retainer 30

S

Safety and health 128
Schematic drawings
Shake-down period 97
Specifications 91
Staffing 1, 14, 16
Strategy 12–13
Structure 47
Structural drawings 69

Surgical suite 110
Systems concept 110

T

Technology in healthcare 9
Telemedicine 13
Tender drawings
TQM 47
Types of layout 123

U

Ultrasound room 127

V

Value engineering 142

W

Waste management 120
Work
   measurement 140
   sampling 141
   study 137
Working drawing 91

X

X-ray room 126

Z

Zonal distribution 109